Manifestations of Aphasia Symptoms in Different Languages

MANIFESTATIONS OF APHASIA SYMPTOMS IN DIFFERENT LANGUAGES

Edited by

MICHEL PARADIS
McGill University

INTERNATIONAL ASSOCIATION OF LOGOPEDICS AND PHONIATRICS

2001

PERGAMON
An imprint of Elsevier Science
Amsterdam – London – Oxford - New York – Paris - Shannon – Tokyo

ELSEVIER SCIENCE Ltd
The Boulevard, Langford Lane
Kidlington, Oxford OX5 1GB, UK

First edition 2001

Library of Congress Cataloging in Publication Data
A catalog record from the Library of Congress has been applied for.

British Library Cataloguing in Publication Data
A catalogue record from the British Library has been applied for.

ISBN: 0 08 043662 5

∞ The paper used in this publication meets the requirements of ANSI/NISO Z39.48-1992 (Permanence of Paper).
Printed in The Netherlands.

Publisher's Preface

In recognition of the current importance of this topic, this collection was also published as Volume 14 (2-4) of the *Journal of Neurolinguistics.*

Contents

1. By way of a preface: The need for awareness of aphasia symptoms in different languages. *Michel Paradis* 1-7

2. Dialectal variants of verbs in narratives of African Americans with aphasia: Some methodological considerarions. *Hanna K. Ulatowska & Gloria Streit Olness* 9-26

3. Aphasia in Afrikaans: A preliminary analysis. *Claire Penn, Analou Venter & Dale Ogilvy* 27-48

4. Aphasia manifestations in Basque. *Itziar Laka & Lore Erriondo Korostola* 49-73

5. On manifestations of aphasia in Catalan: A case study of Broca's aphasia. *Jordi Peña-Casanova, Faustino Diéguez-Vide, Raquel Lluent & Peter Böhm* 75-93

6. Manifestation of aphasic symptoms in Czech. *Helena Lehečková* 95-124

7. Manifestations of aphasia in Persian (Farsi). *Reza Nilipour & Shahla Raghibdoust* 125-146

8. Grammatical structuring in Broca's and Wernicke's aphasia in Finnish. *Marja-Liisa Helasvuo, Anu Klippi & Minna Laakso* 147-169

9. Manifestations of aphasia in Friulian. *Franco Fabbro & Giovanni Frau* 171-196

10. Manifestations of morphological impairments in Greek aphasia: A case study. *Kyrana Tsapkini, Gonia Jarema & Eva Kehayia* 197-212

11. Aphasia in Hebrew speakers. *Mira Goral* 213-228

12. Manifestations of aphasic symptoms in Hungarian.
Andrew Kertesz & Judit Osmán-Sagi 229-235

13. A longitudinal study of agrammatism in Polish: A case study.
Hanna K. Ulatowska, Maria Sadowska & Danut Kądzielawa 237-252

14. The manifestation of aphasic symptoms in Spanish.
Alfredo Ardila 253-263

15. Agrammatic verb errors in Spanish speakers and their normal
discourse correlates. *José G. Centeno & Loraine K. Obler* 265-280

16. Grammatical features of aphasia in Swedish.
Ann-Christin Månsson & Elisabeth Ahlsén 281-296

By way of a preface: The need for awareness of aphasia symptoms in different languages

Michel Paradis

Department of Linguistics, McGill University

Abstract—The likelihood of encountering aphasic patients who speak a language other than that of the clinic in which they are assessed is rapidly increasing to the point of becoming commonplace. It is therefore more important than ever to become aware of the manifestations of aphasia in languages other than one's own. A number of factors conspire to influence the symptoms in each language, from the phonological and morphosyntactic structure of the language to the frequency of obligatory contexts, the importance of the form for the derivation of meaning, and the degree of redundancy. Therefore, the same underlying deficit may cause different surface manifestations in different languages. It is important to recognize these different manifestations as language-specific instantiations of the same underlying cause rather than symptoms of different types of aphasia.

Key words: cross-linguistic aphasia, language-specific symptoms, bilingualism, symptom manifestations

At its August 1998 meeting in Amsterdam, on the occasion of the XXIVth Congress of the International Association of Logopedics and Phoniatrics (IALP), the Aphasia Committee undertook to prepare a report on manifestations of aphasia symptoms in different languages, to be presented at the XXVth IALP congress in Montreal in August 2001.

A first draft of these investigations was discussed by the contributors at a meeting held in Santiago de Compostela, Spain, on 22 and 23 June 2000. After a thorough discussion of each contribution, each author wrote a final report which is published in the present volume. Hence, all contributions report on research conducted specifically for this publication over the past three years by members of the IALP Aphasia Committee and their collaborators.

Since Grodzinsky's (1984) article and the publication of the first sourcebook on cross-linguistic agrammatism (Menn & Obler, 1990), researchers and to some extent clinicians have become aware of the language-specificity of aphasia symptoms. The aim of this collection of papers is to provide specific indications on the characteristic manifestations of aphasia symptoms in 14 languages, in the Germanic, Finno-Ugric, Indo-Iranian, Romance, Semitic, and Slavic language families (including Czech, the most inflectional of the Slavic languages). More specifically, characteristics of African-

American English, Afrikaans, Basque, Catalan, Czech, Farsi (Persian), Finnish, Friulian, Greek, Hebrew, Hungarian, Polish, Spanish, and Swedish are described in this volume, so that researchers and clinicians may know what to look for and how to interpret the symptoms they observe, in terms not of a universal description but of specific traits linked to the language spoken by their patient. Some of these manifestations are widespread, cutting across language families, and may even be universal, whereas others are specific to a language family or even to a particular language. Such specificity may be manifested in forms of agrammatism and/or paragrammatism, and/or phonological deficits.

For the purpose of this book, it is the quality of the error which is of the greatest importance; that is, if an error is produced, the form it takes is of primary interest. The frequency of occurrence of the relevant structure in a given language is of secondary relevance, though it may have an influence on the saliency of this type of error. It is linked to some extent to the structure of the language (e.g., the extent to which it is morphology-rich or morphology-poor, from which we can predict the frequency of a particular type of error). The absolute number of errors produced by a patient is of no interest; only the percentage of errors produced relative to the number of obligatory contexts present in the sample is indicative of severity and can be meaningfully used in cross-linguistic comparisons between individuals or within polyglot individuals.

Three types of studies are provided: (1) group studies; (2) small series of single case studies; (3) experimental studies focussing on a particular salient feature of a language. Each contributor was asked to describe the relevant aspects of the language in question, give a brief review of previous findings (from the literature, if any), and give a characterization of the *types* of errors observed in their language, i.e., what the most conspicuous manifestations of agrammatism, paragrammatism, or phonological errors look like. Every author was then asked to report what is the most salient deficit in the type of aphasia under consideration in this language, based on their data, and try to infer *why* this is so, in light of the structure of the language under review.

Corollary to Murphy's Law

The manifestations of aphasia in any given language are constrained by the corollary to Murphy's Law that states that only that which can go wrong will go wrong (Paradis, 1989). In other words, the structure of the language determines what types of errors may occur. The reason why a certain type of error is salient or conspicuous in a given language may be due to one or more of several factors: (1) the incidence of obligatory contexts, (2) the importance of the form for the derivation of meaning, (3) the frequency of use of the item in a language/culture, (4) the structural complexity of the item (e.g., number of deviancies from the canonical form), (5) the presence or absence of redundancy (e.g., word order and agreement vs. either word order or agreement); (6) the presence or absence of a zero morpheme and whether nouns and verbs exist as bare roots or must necessarily be inflected; (7) whether, when inflections are omitted, the remaining form is pronounceable or not; and (8) whether the form is memorized or derivable by rule, i.e., whether it is regular or irregular. The form of the error will likely depend on the type of aphasia (e.g., omission versus substitution and/or type of substitution), but the pool of possible errors (i.e., what *can* be omitted or substituted) is restricted by the grammar of the language.

Thus, the form of the error may depend on the type of aphasia, though potential errors is constrained by the structural characteristics of each language. An agrammatic patient may substitute a default morpheme (the zero morpheme when available, but when this is not an option because it would lead to an unpronounceable form or merely to a nonword, some other, less marked, morpheme, such as the nominative case for nouns and the infinitive for verbs, again modulated by frequency of use).

Societal and geopolitical factors
In some cases (e.g., Basque, Catalan, Friulian) the inherent bilingualism of the speaking community may have to be taken into consideration and systematic interference due to the influence of the other language may be routinely observed; clinicians should therefore be reminded that certain phenomena are actually features of a local dialect in these areas rather than pathological manifestations. This influence (unidirectional or mutual) may be observed at any or all levels of linguistic structure (phonological, morphological, syntactic and lexical). Code-mixing may be common in some bilingual communities, though not in others, and may also depend on the bilingual speaker's language mode (Grosjean, 1998).

Saliency
If we assume, for example, that, clinically, agrammatism is broadly characterized as a reduction in the use of free and bound inflectional morphology, lack of grammatical agreement, reduction in the use of complex sentence structures, and use of telegraphic style (Thompson, Shapiro, & Roberts, 1993), we may expect that, given the structural characteristics of specific languages, some of these manifestations will be more or less salient. At the very least, in a language that does not contain particular items (e.g., definite articles), aphasic patients will not have the opportunity to drop them in obligatory contexts—in fact, in any context, since there are none to be dropped. Assuming that such a feature does exist but occurs only rarely, again, there will be few opportunities to show a deficit in its use. If the feature is optional, maybe patients will omit it more often than non-brain-damaged individuals, and thus show a difference in frequency of use, but the result could not be said to be ungrammatical.

Speakers of languages that are typologically different may be expected to exhibit symptoms that vary in accordance with the parametric differences of their languages. The structure of particular languages may cause them to be more vulnerable in their verb morphology (e.g., Farsi) as compared to other languages (e.g., English), as discussed in Nilipour & Paradis (1995). These differences are quantitative. Qualitative differences may also occur, as the structure of the language causes a particular deficit (e.g., a problem with tense marking) to be manifested as the substitution of one inflection for another, such as intraword substitution of vowels in Arabic and Hebrew, compared to the dropping of suffixes in English.

Yiu and Worrall (1996) showed that the fact that the Cantonese sentences of a Cantonese-English bilingual patient consisted of only simple phrases (whereas English sentences were more complex) cannot be interpreted as evidence of a better recovery of English. English may differ from Cantonese for a number of reasons; for example, there may be more elliptical sentences in Cantonese due to straightforward structural differences (i.e., fewer obligatory contexts in Cantonese), and better conservation of morphological structures in English because morphological structures convey more meaning in English and therefore are assumed to be less vulnerable to agrammatic disruption—the latter being a theoretical inference and hence only true if the inference is valid. If it is valid, however, this is another type of explanation for the role of specific language characteristics in the cross-linguistic manifestations of aphasic symptoms, not to be ignored when comparing bilingual individuals' performance in their two languages. In some languages, certain inflections may be more semantically laden while others are more structural and possibly redundant. The percentage of omissions in a language where such omissions are possible may be determined by the semantic weight attached to the form.

General principles

Cross-linguistic evidence tends to support the notion that the underlying impairment affects the patient's ability to perform certain types of implicit phonological, morphological, and syntactic procedural computations (what linguists attempt to describe as rules). It is therefore possible to predict the form of the surface manifestations of the symptoms, as long as the structure of any language is known.

By searching for the principles that, across languages, seem to underlie the various manifestations corresponding to a given deficit, a number of general principles may be observed. For example, typically, across languages, agrammatic patients tend to use short and simple sentences (i.e., avoid complexity) and favour (1) the forms most frequently used in the language (the forms themselves, of course, vary considerably in accordance with the specific structural characteristics of each language, as seen above and abundantly illustrated in the contributions to this volume); (2) the forms that are constructed from a smaller paradigmatic set (the more extensive the paradigm—i.e., the larger the number of possible choices—the more opportunities there are for selecting the wrong one). A paragrammatic patient, on the other hand, may randomly substitute one form for another, with no evidence of simplification, e.g., replacing an oblique case by another oblique case, generally from the same paradigm but occasionally even from a different one.

Patients also tend to resort to whatever devices are available in the language (e.g., stylistic possibilities of simplification) in order to avoid, or to get around, complexity. Thus, much of what is produced by some patients with agrammatism may in fact not be ungrammatical but characteristic of particular styles (Jarema, 1985). Similarly, Basque agrammatic patients produce forms that occasionally occur in child language (Laka & Erriondo Korostola, 2001).

The larger the number of choices in a paradigm, the more vulnerable the item. The more frequent, the more resistant. Whatever adds to complexity (e.g., an additional suffix) adds to vulnerability. The greater the distance from the canonical form (i.e., the number of changes from it), the more prone to errors the construction is. The derivational system is also differentially vulnerable, depending on the complexity of the system, i.e., the number of specific endings of each kind, and whether they are sensitive to gender, number, diminutive, augmentative, and/or locative.

Agrammatic patients who are insensitive to grammatical information will compensate by relying heavily on semantic information. This information will be available to the extent that it is present in the structure of each language. Also, high-frequency forms tend to be more resistent (Centeno & Obler, 2001), and order of morphemes is robust, even when the actual form of the morpheme is defective (e.g., wrong paradigm, person, number, or tense).

However, in any given language, no error type is common to all patients with agrammatism. Patients do show general patterns and tendencies but few errors (if any) are found in all patients. Moreover, a particular error type, frequent in one language, need not be observed cross-linguistically, even when the opportunity exists. For instance, while utterance-final particles are often omitted in Cantonese (Yiu & Worrall, 1996), they are generally not omitted in Japanese (Sasanuma, 1989).

Some language-specific symptoms differ from the traditional definitions. For example, in Czech there is no clear difference between the symptoms of agrammatism and paragrammatism, since, as in all languages where words do not appear as bare roots, the omission of bound morphemes is rarely an option (Lehečková, 2001). Both omission and substitution of free-standing grammatical morphemes have been reported in some agrammatic patients in Italian (Miceli et al., 1989; Fabbro, 2001). And in some languages, contrary to the general wisdom, some patients will produce nonwords by dropping affixes (Månsson & Ahlsén, 2001).

Reasons why the cross-linguistic study of symptoms is necessary

Given that different languages use different devices to mark certain features (e.g., word-order, pre/postpositions, affixes, or a combination of these), the same underlying deficit may cause different surface manifestations in different languages (Paradis, 1988). Therefore, it is essential for clinicians and researchers to be aware of cross-linguistic symptoms, for at least three basic reasons: (1) in the countries of the world where English is not a national language, patients ought not to be diagnosed on the basis of data derived from English; (2) immigration patterns around the world have created large numbers of speakers of languages other than English now living in traditionally English-speaking countries (e.g., in the United States alone, there are currently over 7.2 million persons born in Mexico, 1.1 million Filipinos, 1.1 million Chinese, 763,000 former nationals of the Soviet Union, over 600,000 Koreans, 600,000 Indians and 600,000 Vietnamese, as estimated by the Census Bureau); (3) in order to determine whether one of the languages of a bilingual or polyglot patient is recovered to a greater or lesser extent than the other language(s), once one becomes aware that the same underlying deficit may cause different surface manifestations in different languages, one must be able to interpret the patients' behavioural pattern in terms of its significance for each language.

"If therapy is to be principled, then a knowledge of the rationale behind what one is doing is an obvious prerequisite. It is important for speech-language pathologists to be familiar with the theoretical foundations of their work, i.e., why they do what they do, so that they may adapt appropriately to diverse circumstances, as well as what to expect, how to interpret findings." (Paradis, 1995, p. xxi). This is another reason why it is important for one to be aware of the particular manifestations of aphasic symptoms in a given language or family of languages, namely, to avoid misdiagnosis. As long as agrammatism was defined as the omission of grammatical morphemes in obligatory contexts and paragrammatism as their substitution, there was a risk of diagnosing agrammatism in English (or Spanish or Hungarian) but paragrammatism in Hebrew, in an English- (or Spanish- or Hungarian-) Hebrew bilingual patient who was actually agrammatic in both languages (cf. Albert & Obler, 1978, Silverberg & Gordon, 1979). The clinician and researcher should therefore be aware that what is generally true in their own language may not be in the language of the patient under assessment.

Conclusions

Possible aphasic symptoms are determined by the phonological and morphosyntactic structure of each type of language, the number of obligatory (as opposed to optional) contexts, the frequency of occurrence of items in the language and their semantic weight. The grammar (implicit linguistic competence) provides constraints (possible choices).

Pragmatics selects among these available grammatical choices (languages, registers, indirect speech acts, figurative speech, syntactic constructions). Pathology limits the available choices, either in grammar (subsequent to a left-hemisphere lesion) or in pragmatics (subsequent to right-hemisphere damage). Therefore, the same underlying deficit may cause different surface manifestations in different languages. External societal and geopolitical factors may have a specific impact: bilingual populations may give rise to local dialects, diglossia and/or code-mixing. Awareness of the characteristic symptoms in different languages is essential for clinicians and researchers in countries where English is not the national language, in countries with large numbers of immigrants, and in countries where bilingualism is inherent.

By comparing symptoms of different languages, we should eventually be able to ascertain whether some deficits are caused by what is encoded (e.g., causality, negation, etc.) or by its linguistic means of implementation (e.g., lexical vs. inflectional causation).

Acknowledgments

Thanks are due to Jennifer Mortimer for her careful formatting of the text and the production of the camera-ready copy. Dr. Zofia Laubitz revised many of the texts contributed by non-native speakers of English.

Address correspondence to: Michel Paradis, Department of Linguistics, McGill University, 1085 Dr. Penfield Avenue, Montreal H3A 1A7, Canada.. E-mail: mparad@po-box.mcgill.ca

References

Albert, M., & Obler, L.K. (1978). *The bilingual brain.* New York: Academic Press.

Centeno, J.G., & Obler, L.K. (2001). Agrammatic verb errors in Spanish speakers and their normal discourse correlates. *Journal of Neurolinguistics, 14,* 349-367.

Fabbro, F. (2001). Manifestations of aphasia in Friulian. *Journal of Neurolinguistics, 14,* 255-280.

Grodzinsky, Y. (1984). The syntactic characterization of agrammatism. *Cognition, 16,* 99-120.

Grosjean, F. (1998). Studying bilinguals: Methodological and conceptual issues. *Bilingualism: Language and Cognition, 1,* 131-149.

Jarema, G. (1985). Is "agrammatic speech" agrammatical? *Papers in Linguistics, 18,* 223-238.

Lehečková, H. (2001). Manifestations of aphasic symptoms in Czech. *Journal of Neurolinguistics, 14,* 179-208

Laka, I., & Erriondo Korostela, L. (2001). Aphasia manifestations in Basque. *Journal of Neurolinguistics, 14,* 133-157

Månsson, A.-C., & Ahlsén, E. (2001). Grammatical features of aphasia in Swedish. *Journal of Neurolinguistics, 14,* 369-384

Menn, L. & Obler, L.K. (1990). *Agrammatic aphasia. A cross-language narrative sourcebook.* Amsterdam: John Benjamins.

Miceli, G., Silveri, M.C., Romani, C., & Caramazza, A. (1989). Variation in the pattern of omissions and substitutions of grammatical morphemes in the spontaneous speech of so-called agrammatic patients. *Brain and Language, 36,* 447-492.

Nilipour, R., & Paradis, M. (1995) Breakdown of functional categories in three Farsi-English bilingual aphasic patients. In M. Paradis (Ed.), *Aspects of bilingual aphasia* (pp. 123-138). Oxford: Pergamon Press.

Paradis, M. (1988). Recent developments in the study of agrammatism: Their import for the assessment of bilingual aphasia. *Journal of Neurolinguistics, 3,* 127-160.

Paradis, M. (1989). Linguistic parameters in the diagnosis of dyslexia in Japanese and Chinese. In P.G. Aaron and R. Malatesha Joshi (Eds.), *Reading and writing disorders in different languages* (pp. 231-266). Dordrecht: Kluwer.

Paradis, M. (1995). Foreword to L. Menn, M. O'Connor, L.K. Obler, and A. Holland, *Non-fluent aphasia in a multilingual world.* Amsterdam: John Benjamins.

Sasanuma, S. (1989). Universal and language-specific symptomatology and treatment of aphasia. *Folia Phoniatrica, 38,* 121-175.

Silverberg, R., & Gordon, H.W. (1979). Differential aphasia in two bilinguals. *Neurology,* 29, 51-55.

Thompson, C.K., Shapiro, L.P., & Roberts, M.M. (1993). Treatment of sentence production deficit in aphasia: a linguistic-specific approach to wh-interrrogative training and generalization. *Aphasiology, 7,* 111-113.

Yiu, E. & Worrall, E. (1996). Sentence production ability of a bilingual Cantonese/ English agrammatic speaker. *Aphasiology, 10,* 505-522.

Dialectal variants of verbs in narratives of African Americans with aphasia: Some methodological considerations

Hanna K. Ulatowska and Gloria Streit Olness

University of Texas at Dallas

Abstract—A focus on African American Vernacular English (AAVE) verb use in narratives is advantageous for examining the effects of dialect in aphasia. The inherent variability in speakers' use of dialect features is discussed. Verb morpho-syntax is examined in speakers of AAVE who have aphasia, and compared to that of African American normal controls. Dialect features were preserved despite the presence of aphasia, although there was variability in performance that could not readily be attributed to code-switching. While individuals with less mild aphasia used fewer AAVE verb forms in this sample, they also produced shorter narratives. The challenges of research in this area are discussed, and strategies are suggested for future efforts.

Key words: African Americans, dialect, aphasia, verb system, narratives

Introduction

The current article proposes certain key methodological issues for the study of dialectal manifestations among African Americans with aphasia. Points for consideration are drawn from dialectal and clinical studies, in combination with qualitative analysis of an extensive data set of personal narratives produced by African Americans with aphasia, and African-American normal controls.

To our knowledge, there have been no systematic studies of dialectal features in the discourse of African-American adults with aphasia. Early work in this area (e.g., Anderson & Ulatowska, 1975) was performed within a traditional clinical framework of repetition, reading, and writing tasks, for purposes of differential diagnosis. Consideration of dialect in discourse would offer the opportunity to explore the robustness of ethnic dialect features among African Americans who have aphasia, in their very context of use. Not only would this offer insights on the relative complexity of the various features of African American Vernacular English (AAVE) in natural discourse contexts, but also on the clinical issues important in working with individuals with aphasia who speak an AAVE dialect. A logical first step in any such endeavor would be to plan methodological approaches and anticipate potential complications or pitfalls in such an undertaking through the use of previous clinical and dialectal research, in tandem with pilot data.

Past studies of dialect(s) used by African Americans have been heterogeneous in their goals and approaches. This very heterogeneity, however, provides insights into the mosaic of factors which impinge on the form and functions of given dialectal variants among African Americans. An impetus for much of this research has been to provide evidence that AAVE in its many dialectal variants, is a language in its own right, at all levels of structure, and not a flawed version of some sociologically determined standard. To this end, many have explored the historical roots of AAVE (e.g., Johnson, 2000). The earlier sociolinguistic studies of AAVE (e.g., Labov, 1972), while largely restricted to descriptions of the language of young urban males, explored the broad complexity of AAVE dialect as a language in its own right. In more recent years, the groups of AAVE speakers under consideration have expanded, while the language aspects being considered have narrowed and become more specific as our understanding of AAVE deepens. For instance, Green (1994; 1998a; 1998b) looks at use of AAVE dialect among African Americans in general, although her focus is largely on the complexities of the AAVE verb system. Likewise, Rickford and Rafal (1996) focus on highly specific aspects of verb-use-in-discourse among certain groups of AAVE speakers.

Discourse has often been the chosen context in which to elicit language from African American speakers. Some individuals have chosen to describe the nuances of the discourse strategies used by African Americans (e.g., Smitherman, 1977). Other waves of studies have been even more ethnographic in their approach, exploring language as an expression of cultural identity (Strevy & Aldridge, 1994; Leslie, 1998). Much of the clinical research on children's use of vernacular dialect has used discourse as the framework for study and as a means of elicitation (Seymour, Bland-Stewart, & Green, 1998). This parallels research on the origins of certain dialect forms among ex-slaves, again elicited naturally in the form of narratives (Schneider, 1989). Thus, there has been an inherent understanding that AAVE as a dialect has communicative utility in the context of use, which has been reflected methodologically in the use of discourse as a means of elicitation of dialectal, ethnic, and cultural forms.

From a sociolinguistic standpoint, AAVE cannot be viewed as a unitary dialect. As noted by Johnson (2000), AAVE "exits in a context of cultural and linguistic contact" (p. 141). Although AAVE dialects are by definition ethnic dialects, certain dialects of AAVE overlap with regional dialects (e.g., Southern dialects), and the elaborateness of their forms also depends inherently on the degree of stratification and overlap between social groups, i.e., social dialectal variants (Johnson, 2000). Thus, any consideration of AAVE dialect must minimally include a description of the regional and social origins of the speakers. Estimates of the proportion of African Americans who use at least some features of AAVE range from 60% (Spears, 1987), to 80% (Dillard, 1972).

Designing a Means of Elicitation

Traditional approaches

With regard to the study of the effects of aphasia on dialectal use among African Americans, a key consideration is how best to elicit language for such a purpose. Traditionally, studies of the structural changes associated with aphasia, or more specifically, morphological changes, have elicited language in sentential contexts which constrain the speaker to produce a given morpheme of interest. Other researchers ask speakers to retell culturally familiar stories, or describe standardized pictures, and again isolate obligatory contexts in which a given morpheme is not produced (Menn & Obler, 1990). Lack of production of the morpheme in such obligatory contexts is taken as evidence of the effect of aphasia on the ability to produce the morpheme. However, such "acontextual" elicitation procedures are also very artificial from a socio-pragmatic perspective, which poses a distinct disadvantage when one is interested in uncovering the interplay between aphasia and non-standard dialect forms. The reason is that dialects other than the standard dialect are typically reserved for more informal settings, personal topics, and familiar interlocutors.

Specific means of elicitation

Thus, if one is interested in the manifestations of the effects of aphasia in non-standard dialectal forms, one first needs to elicit the language in a context which invites the use of the vernacular in the cultural group of interest. At the same time, the language elicitation method should also be designed to have high probability of eliciting the morphological forms that maximally distinguish the dialect of interest from other dialects.

There is evidence to indicate that personal narratives may be a productive means of eliciting language for purposes of examining dialectal features of AAVE. As noted by Labov (1972), the most effective of the techniques used in the study of vernacular language are "narratives of personal experience, in which the speaker becomes deeply involved in rehearsing or even reliving events of his past" (p. 354). For instance, personal narratives of a frightening experience, especially when elicited by another speaker of AAVE, are likely to invite use of an AAVE dialect. The likelihood of using AAVE dialect in personal narratives may be largely an outcome of the central role played by highly personalized narratives in the African-American community. As noted by Smitherman (1977):

> The story element is so strong in black communicative dynamics that it pervades general everyday conversation. An ordinary inquiry is likely to elicit an extended narrative response where the abstract point or general message will be couched in concrete story form. The reporting of events is never simply objectively reported, but dramatically acted out and narrated. The Black English speaker thus simultaneously conveys the facts and his or her personal socio-psychological perspective on the facts (p. 161).

Given an interest in the grammatical features of the AAVE dialect in speakers with aphasia, one then needs to ask whether elicitation of personal narratives is also likely to elicit a broad range of morphological forms that maximally characterize the dialect. One highly productive set of morphological features are those which mark tense and aspect on verbs. Indeed, one characteristic of AAVE which distinguishes is from other dialects of English is its rich aspectual system (Labov, 1998; Martin & Wolfram, 1998; Green, 1998a). Johnson (2000) comments that "(v)arious features of the verb system provide especially compelling evidence for the continuities and distinctiveness in the linguistic expression of culture" among speakers of AAVE (p. 143). Likewise, Wolfram and Fasold (1974) and Green (1998a) comment that in the ethnic and regional dialect used by many African Americans, the verb system is one of the more complex and pivotal of the grammatical systems of those dialects. These forms can be well elicited with narratives. The temporal axis is the backbone along which the events in the narratives are organized

(Longacre, 1983), and the verb is a primary carrier of this temporal and aspectual information.

Even though narratives typically relate past events, it is not exclusively the past tense that can be elicited with narratives. A wide variety of forms, including the future tense, can be found. This is largely a function of the prominent use of direct speech within the narratives of African Americans. Speakers in the oral tradition often use direct speech to draw the listener into the narrative by acting out the events in the story line. These instances of direct speech often contain tenses such as the future and present, or aspect markers such as perfective DONE, which would not otherwise be found in reports of actions on the main event line.

In summary, for researchers interested in interactions between AAVE dialect and aphasia, methodological approach is critical. With respect to African American speakers, language is probably best elicited in non-formal contexts (e.g., with personal narratives), which at the same time offer maximal potential for elicitation of morphology which is rich and highly characteristic of the dialect (e.g., verb morphology).

On Certain Methodological and Interpretive Complexities

As discussed in the preceding section, the complexity of the verb system in AAVE is ideally suited to allow researchers in aphasia to look at particular vulnerabilities (or lack thereof) of the morphological tense and aspect markers carried in that system. Theoretically, the more complex a system, the more vulnerable it may be to the effects of aphasia. Beyond the distinctiveness and richness of the verb system in AAVE, however, there are several factors that remind us that our understanding of these complexities is in its infancy.

First, Green (1994) comments that "although there have been great strides in research in African American English (AAVE), we do not yet have a descriptively adequate grammar of the dialect" (p. 65). In addition, although in this article we discuss AAVE as a single dialect, one needs to be aware that there is no single or unitary AAVE dialect, but rather multiple dialects produced by African American speakers. Finally, numerous sources of variability in performance exist. We now consider this latter element in more detail.

Sources of variability

There are several sources of variability which contribute to between- and within-speaker differences that one may find. As noted by Seymour et al. (1998), "knowledge of patterns of variability for particular linguistic structures has important diagnostic implications" (p. 97) and "without a complete description of the rule constraints governing variable usage of AAVE features, it remains difficult to discern whether the absence of morphemes and morphemic inflections is due to dialect or disorder" (p. 97). This is an issue of the diagnostic saliency of features.

One source of variability may be the overlap that many ethnic dialects of AAVE have with regional and social dialects (e.g., Schneider, 1989). Many of the speakers in our database are African Americans who were raised in the South, and whose dialects may have been influenced by Southern regional dialects. On the other hand, the overlap between features of the ethnic dialect of AAVE and the regional dialect of Southern American English has been well documented (Baily, 1993; Labov, 1998), even among

Northern speakers of AAVE, as a result of the African-American diaspora. In other words, regional and ethnic dialect features can be expected in the speech of any given speaker of AAVE. For this reason, some researchers choose to study AAVE features without making any claims for their uniqueness (e.g., Martin & Wolfram, 1998).

As another potential source of variability, Whatley (1981) comments that African American speakers generally have a broader range of styles of speaking, in their verbal repertoire, than Caucasians (p. 103). Use of non-standard dialects is largely conditioned by the overall interactive and discourse content, the ethnic and regional origins of the conversational partner, and the nature of the relationship between the speaker and the interlocutor. It is often difficult to know the socio-pragmatic rules and individual choices that govern this code-switching.

In addition, certain individuals may code-switch more readily across contexts than other individuals; others may code-switch from standard to non-standard dialect even within a given interaction. This variability both within and across individuals makes comparisons difficult. For example, females may code-switch less readily than males (Fordham, 1993; Houston Stanback, 1985). Additionally, one's social class influences use of grammatical forms. As noted by Wolfram (1969), grammatical morphemes often reveal sharp rather than gradient stratification between the different social groups, while phonological variables more often reveal gradient stratification between the social groups (p. 204). Yet as commented upon by Whatley (1981, p. 103), variability of forms in the speech of the African-American community tends to be greater than in other varieties of American English.

Finally, multiple levels of language converge to govern the application of morphological rules that constitute a given dialect, making naïve any attempt to treat the morphological rules of this dialect simplistically. Awareness of the morphological rules of a dialect, as well as the linguistic contexts that condition them, is imperative. For instance, in the description of AAVE to come later in this article, one notices how linguistic context at several levels influences application of the structural rules of the language. For instance, at the phonological (segmental) level, consonant cluster reduction may condition presence or absence of the –ed morpheme in certain dialects of AAVE (Wolfram & Fasold, 1974). At the phonological (suprasegmental) level, auxiliaries may be seen in contexts of emphatic stress, but not in unstressed environments (Green, 1994); likewise stressed and unstressed *been* function very differently in AAVE (Rickford, 1983). At the morphological level, *-z* can attach itself to any person in present tense in some AAVE speakers. This morphological pattern may sometimes be hypercorrected to appear even on non-finite forms (Wolfram & Fasold, 1974). At the syntactic level, verb sequencing sometimes precludes the use of tense marking. Dillard (1972) notes that "whereas in Standard English every verb in a sequence (in a sentence or in a related series of sentences) must be marked as either present or past, in Black English only one of the verbs needs to be marked—although more than one may be so marked" (p. 42). As another example, both the syntactic and discourse levels condition alternations between the historical present and the preterite. Historical present may be used by AAVE speakers in contrast with surrounding use of the past tense in narratives, in order to highlight the vividness of the action with the historical present. However, these shifts may only occur across sentences, and not within sentences. As an example of lexical conditioning of morphological variants in AAVE, some irregular past tense formations of verbs may be expressed in the present tense by some AAVE speakers, although such regularization may occur only on certain irregular verbs (e.g., *come*, *say*) and not others (Poplack & Tagliamonte, 1994). Finally, discourse level considerations may affect use of dialectal features at the morphological level. Rickford and Rafal (1996) comment that while the past perfective (e.g., *She had died*) indeed marks past tense and perfective aspect in AAVE, its use as a discourse means of highlighting information may be on the increase across speakers of certain dialects. Specifically, this form, especially when preceded by the simple past and when it occurs at the climax of a story, may also function to highlight a given event within the on-going series of events in the narrative.

An Overview of the AAVE Verb System

With the preceding variability issues in mind, a general overview of the AAVE verb system is provided. Wolfram (1991) comments that dialect speakers who are learning Standard American English (SAE) should "focus on systematic differences between the standard and nonstandard English forms" (p. 220). It would follow that if one speaks SAE, one should systematically compare it to AAVE if one wants to learn AAVE. Thus, in the following description, we recognize the full linguistic status of AAVE, while describing it relative to SAE for those readers not familiar with AAVE. The description here is gleaned from a variety of sources, thus reflecting AAVE characteristics potentially found across a variety of African-American speakers, rather than features of a unitary dialect.

Of the verb features described below, certain can be thought of as relatively unique to AAVE. These include the dual function of the past perfect; the variable non-expression of '-ed' and third person singular '-s'; the auxiliary 'come'; the aspectual markers 'been', 'be' and their combination with perfective 'done'; and the use of 'be' to mark future tense.

Dual function of past perfect

The form of the past perfect or pluperfect *HAD + past participle / HAD + preterite* (e.g., *I had seen it*) is similar in AAVE dialects to that used in SAE. However, its frequency of use, meaning, and function, may be different in the two dialect groups. Wolfram and Fasold (1974) comment that "the use of the past-perfect tense ... is a striking feature of Vernacular Black English narrative style. The construction is used liberally in stories about events in the past" (p. 152). Beyond its frequency of use, there is emerging evidence to suggest that this form may increasingly be used in some AAVE dialects to fill an additional discourse function, namely to highlight an event within the complicating action of a story, when other surrounding verbs are expressed in the simple past tense (Rickford & Rafal, 1996; Cukor-Avila 1995). This function, alternatively viewed, may be used by the narrator at the climax to evaluate or indicate the point of the narrative. This essentially represents a spread of this form from the orienting clauses of a narrative to the complicating action. (See other sections on past participle vs. preterite.)

The '–ed' suffix as marker of past tense and past participle

The suffix *–ed* is part of the grammar of both AAVE and SAE, although speakers in of certain AAVE dialects may not always pronounce it. Its expression in some AAVE dialects appears to be largely phonologically conditioned (Wolfram & Fasold, 1974), e.g., through rules of consonant cluster reduction and deletion of syllable-final *d*. Not only may this be conditioned phonologically, but it may also be conditioned by surrounding context; when the surrounding context indicates past tense, the past tense morpheme may not be used (Johnson, 2000).

Lack of distinction between preterite and past participle

Among some speakers of non-standard dialects, the distinction between preterite and past participle may not be made for irregular verbs (Wolfram & Fasold, 1974). At times, the past-participle form serves both functions (*He taken it*; *He has taken it*), although more often the preterite is used in both contexts (*He came*; *He has came*). Some speakers may generalize the one, and other speakers may generalize the other. This fluidity of form use sometimes leads to use of hypercorrection, e.g., creating a novel past participle, such as *cutten*.

Use of present tense form as a marker of past tense

While the use of present tense forms in a past context appears to be relatively rare in AAVE, there are certain irregular past tense formations of verbs in SAE that may be expressed with the present tense form in some dialects of AAVE. For instance, *say* may be used for SAE *said* (Wolfram & Fasold, 1974). Notably, this is a pattern that is manifested not only in AAVE dialect, but also in other non-standard dialects.

Regularization of irregular past tense

Some speakers of non-standard dialects, including dialects of AAVE and Southern English (Baily, 1997) will occasionally replace irregular past tense forms with regular *–ed* past tense forms, for example *knowed* for *knew*. Wolfram and Fasold (1974) note that even though such usage may be relatively rare, it may be more noticeable than other dialect differences when it does occur.

'Done' as perfective aspect

Some non-standard dialects, including ethnic dialects of AAVE, as well as certain regional dialects of the Southern United States (Baily, 1997; Labov, 1998), may use *done* as an auxiliary with the past tense or past-participial form, as another means of expressing perfective aspect (e.g., *He's done went home; You done aced the test*). (Wolfram & Fasold, 1974; Green, 1994; Labov, 1998; Green, 1998a; Johnson, 2000). It is used to emphasize the completeness of the action, and is not found in SAE. Aspectual *done* can also be combined with other aspectual particles, such as in *be done* or *been done*, to achieve even more complex aspectual meaning in AAVE (Labov, 1998; Green, 1998a), although this will not be considered here in detail.

'Come' as auxiliary

When *come* precedes a verb + *ing* construction, its role is similar to that of an auxiliary verb, and its meaning implies indignation, e.g., *She come going in my room—didn't knock or nothing* ('She had the nerve to go in my room') (Johnson, 2000; Martin & Wolfram, 1998).

'Been' as marker of remote time aspect

Been has been used in AAVE as an auxiliary to emphasize the remoteness of an action from the current interests of the speaker (Wolfram & Fasold, 1974). For example, the *been* in *You won't get your dues that you been paid* does not involve a passive construction. Rather *been* indicates that the payment occurred in the remote past. Johnson (2000) comments that it may not only be used to indicate that something started a long time ago, but also that it is not news, or that it occurred in the past. Green (1994, 1998a) and Labov (1998) indicate that this form, when used as an aspect marker, receives emphatic stress. More recent analyses of its semantics across various contexts (Green, 1998b; Martin & Wolfram, 1998) indicates that *been* situates the initiation of a state in the remote past, and the state continues up until the moment of utterance.

Invariant 'be'

In AAVE, uninflected *be* can be used as the main verb, with any subject (*I be here this afternoon; Sometime he be busy*). In some instances, this may be a result of non-use of the contracted forms of the auxiliaries *will* (*'ll*) (*He be here pretty soon*), or *would* (*'d*) (*If you gave him a present, he be happy*). It is notable that this also happens in other non-standard dialects, and occasionally in SAE (Wolfram & Fasold, 1974).

An additional source of the invariant *be* in AAVE is to use *be* as marker of habitual aspect, marking action that occurred in the past but continues, is ongoing or recurs (*Sometime he be here and sometime he don't; They be telling us*...) (Johnson, 2000; Labov, 1998). This use of invariant *be* is exclusive to AAVE (Wolfram & Fasold, 1974). It is quite irregular and is heavily favored by certain speakers, and not by others. This habitual be may also take the form of *bees* in the third person, or when preceding a vowel-initial word (Berstein, 1988).

Absence of concord with forms of 'be'

According to Wolfram & Fasold (1974), some speakers of AAVE may use present-tense *is* and past-tense *was* for all persons (I/You/He/We You/They is/was), although hypercorrected present-tense forms from SAE may infrequently be seen (*There she are* or *You am a teacher*).

Auxiliary/copula deletion

It is common in AAVE to delete auxiliary forms (e.g., *I gone there three times* (no *have); He go there tomorrow* (no *will*); *He gonna go* (no *is*)). Notably, many speakers of regional Southern dialects may also delete auxiliaries, especially auxiliaries with *gonna* (e.g., *He gonna go*) (Wolfram & Fasold, 1974). Likewise, copulas may not be used in AAVE (*He good*; *They over there all the time*). Johnson (2000) comments that non-use of the copula and auxiliary is common with *be*. Notably, however, these auxiliaries and copulas are not completely absent from the AAVE system. As noted by Green (1994), the auxiliaries *be*, *do*, and *have* are retained when they are stressed, when marked for negation, and in yes/no questions. Labov (1972) also comments on the syntax-dependent presence or absence of the copula in AAVE.

Use of non-past third person singular –s

In SAE, the *–s* suffix is placed on the third-person singular forms of verbs, e.g., *he walks*, although no suffix is used to mark present tense with other persons (Johnson, 2000). Some speakers of AAVE dialects will regularize the paradigm, by eliminating any use of the *–s* morpheme (Wolfram & Fasold, 1974), although use of the regularized paradigm is not necessarily consistent, even within speakers who sometimes display its use. In AAVE, *don't* as in *He don't walk* may demonstrate this pattern more than other verbs.

At other times, speakers of AAVE may hypercorrect in violation of the grammatical rules in their dialect, by adding the *–s* to verbs in the non-past tense which are not in the third-person singular (e.g., *I/You/We/They walks*). According to Wolfram & Fasold (1974), this may extend even to non-finite verbs among certain speakers of the dialect, as in *He want to goes*.

Future tense

In AAVE, *be* is sometimes used to mark future tense (e.g., *She be there later*) (Smitherman, 1994).

Double modals

The use of double modals in AAVE (e.g., *I might could go*) overlaps with use of double modals in Southern English.

Zero passive voice

Jordan (1985) asserts that "there is no passive voice construction possible in Black English" (p. 129) because the cultural importance of asserting human presence, survival, and truth are paramount among African Americans.

Multiple negation

Certain speakers of AAVE may use double or multiple negatives (e.g., *Nobody doesn't like it; He doesn't know nothing*; *We ain't had not trouble about none of us pulling out no knife*), although this may also occur in other non-standard dialects (Wolfram & Fasold, 1974; Johnson, 2000). Notably, such negative concord was quite common historically prior to the 18th century, when grammarians imposed the rule that negatives should be marked only once (Labov, 1972).

Description of Group

Data was taken from transcripts of personal narratives of a frightening experience, produced by two different groups of African-Americans: one group of 36 individuals with mild and moderate levels of aphasia, and a second group of 38 neurologically normal controls. Time post onset for the group with aphasia ranged from 3 to 252 months, with an average of 46 months. Each group included comparable proportions of males and females. Ages across groups ranged from approximately thirty-six to seventy-one years. Mean educational level was twelve to thirteen years. Participants were primarily semi-skilled or unskilled employees. All but 3 of the normal control subjects and all but 4 of the subjects with aphasia were raised in the South. Two-thirds of the participants were interviewed by an African-American clinician, and one-third were interviewed by one of two Caucasian clinicians. Notably, the African-American interviewer used multiple features of AAVE during the interviews, and one of the Caucasian interviewers, a Southerner, reported code-switching into Southern American English during the interviews.

Description of Data

The narrative data used as the corpus for this study were derived from a larger study of discourse in African Americans. In addition to the request for a personal narrative of a frightening experience, individuals were also asked to retell a story (an Aesop's fable), and to describe a story depicted in pictorial form. Notably, the speakers used their ethnic dialect in neither the story retell task nor the picture description task. The retell was produced by all but one of the speakers in SAE, similar in dialect to the form in which they heard it. Only one person used ethnic dialect in completing this task. The picture description task was also inappropriate for the examination of ethnic features of dialect as they interact with aphasia. Many of the normal-control speakers use abbreviated sentential forms, similar to a telegraphic style, in addition to using the standard dialect.

In contrast to the other two tasks, most of the personal narratives of frightening experiences were produced in non-standard dialect. The topic of frightening experience, because it is emotionally laden and salient to the speakers, invited free use of code-switching to the most natural style of the speaker. Notably, the fact that the speakers used SAE in the retell and picture description tasks, and AAVE in personal narratives, suggests the ability of these speakers to code-switch. All but seven of the individuals with aphasia used at least one verb form associated with AAVE in their personal narratives, and all but three of the normal control subjects used at least one verb form associated with AAVE in their personal narratives. Thus, it would appear that the presence of aphasia did not affect overall use or non-use of AAVE features. There was a slight tendency for individuals with more severe aphasia to use none, or fewer, of the features, especially those associated exclusively with AAVE, as compared to individuals with less severe aphasia. However, these individuals also had shorter narratives, so the effects of sample length and aphasia severity are confounded in these data. Those individuals with more severe aphasia who did use relatively more AAVE verb features were also those who produced longer narratives.

In addition, the use of forms exclusively found in AAVE, and not in Southern American English, was also examined because ethnic AAVE features often overlap with other non-standard regional dialects such as Southern American English, and also because the majority of subjects were from the South. Approximately one-half of the normal control subjects, and slightly less than one-half of the subjects with aphasia used at least one AAVE verb feature associated exclusively with AAVE. However, the language sample for this task consisted of a single narrative per subject, some of these narratives were relatively short, and most AAVE-exclusive features occur in less-frequently-expressed and context-specific forms associated with the AAVE aspectual system. The key point here is that the large majority of subjects used features associated with AAVE in their personal narratives, whether subjects were using features exclusively found in AAVE, or only AAVE features that overlap with regional dialects.

The relative use of AAVE verb features in the narratives of the subjects did not shift by race of interviewer. Comparable proportions of users and non-users of AAVE were found in the interviews by an African-American clinician and a Caucasian clinician, and relative frequency of subjects' use of AAVE-exclusive features was also unaffected by race of interviewer.

The narratives were on a variety of topics, many of them describing events from adolescence and childhood. Because of the "frightening experience" theme being elicited, many were quite dramatic in topic, similar to the narratives of near-death experiences in adolescence described by Labov (1972). In addition, many of the narratives were quite long, ranging from 4 propositions to 161 propositions for the individuals with aphasia, and from 5 to 119 propositions for the non-neurologically impaired individuals, with a mean of 22 and 29 propositions for each of the groups respectively. Each of these features taken together provided a context in which a wide range of verb forms could be elicited.

AAVE Verb Use in Context

The narratives of both groups (African Americans with aphasia and African-American normal controls) are similar with respect to the frequent occurrence of non-standard dialectal features. When the two groups are compared, it is their overall similarity in use of the non-standard dialect, rather than differences due to presence or absence of language pathology, which are the most striking. The overall similarity between the groups is probably largely associated with the fact that most of the individuals with aphasia had a relatively mild aphasia. For this reason, and also because the data used in this study were not originally designed to elicit agrammatic features *per se*, the data presented here will not be dealt with comprehensively for group contrasts. However, these data are significant for the fact that dialect features are preserved despite the presence of aphasia, and projections of the effects of aphasia on use of non-standard dialect can be discussed.

The narratives were carefully examined for presence of dialect features in the overall lexicon, functor words, the nominal system (e.g., noun pluralization and reflexive pronouns) and the verb system. However, the dialect features in the narratives were concentrated, in frequency, variety and range, in the verb system. While certain verb forms such as the past tense were more frequent, the future and the present tenses were also found in instances of direct speech, yielding a full range of tenses and aspects.

The most conspicuous features of the verb system of AAVE are evident in both normal controls and individuals with aphasia. In the following section are examples of the use of these verb forms. A special emphasis is placed on certain features specific to the individuals with aphasia, such as variability in use of a form, which may be instances of either code-switching or compensatory self-corrections. We do not claim to give a comprehensive view of verb use in this group, but rather a focused highlight of those forms which feature prominently in the narratives of this group. The examples are accompanied by comments on the nature of the forms and their use.

One prominent morphological form is the past perfect, which is the most varied in terms of form and function. With regard to form, the speakers often displayed a lack of distinction between preterite and irregular past participle forms. The use of the preterite form was more frequent. Functionally, most were used in discourse setting. For example:

(Normal control) *I remember once when I was real small and I had, um, went into my mother's bedroom.*

(Normal control) *She thought I had went down the hall, and when she came out of the bathroom she said, "I thought you was down the hall, and I said, "No, I wasn't."*

(Individual with moderate aphasia) *I had a dream. I was very scared. Thought someone had died.*

(Individual with moderate aphasia) *Oh, yeah, a long time ago. Because uh, what had happened, a lady had died that time. Me and some more people, some children come and scared people about the lady, the lady done died you know. So the lady died, when they come back, and they say...*

In other instances, the past perfect is used to emphasize a key event in the narrative, often at the climax. In such instances, the past perfect is preceded and followed by the use of the past. For example,

(Normal control) *But by the time it was getting dark, nobody had showed up. I was sitting on the porch.*

This discourse highlighting function of the past perfect is also evidenced among the individuals with aphasia.

(Individual with moderate aphasia) *So my father said, "Don't, don't be playing with those guns." And I was looking at it to see if I was going to shoot, and uh, I said "Naw" but, but I then, I had pulled the trigger on the r-r-rifle. Just just a little bit and uh and uh one of our friends uh you know a guy who was about the same age as I was, he said....*

Among the individuals with aphasia, there are two points of note. One is the variability in the use of the past perfect form, which is not necessarily associated with systematic code-switching. The other is repetition of the accompanying auxiliary. For instance, the following individual uses both the preterite and the past participle with the auxiliary.

(Individual with moderate aphasia) *I was so scared that I had, I had broken my hip or somethin'. And so that was when I was really scared that I had broke a hip bone.*

The auxiliary *had* is repeated twice by this speaker, which may indicate difficulty in accessing the main verb. Thus, the variation between the preterite and the past participle in this individual may be code-switching, or may be the result of aphasic difficulties.

Similar variability of form among the individuals with aphasia is seen with the variable absence or presence of concord with *be.*

(Individual with mild aphasia) *We was chopping cotton ah my mother said XXX* (unintelligible). *We went across the ah, get some water and while we were gone, going the wind started blowing.*

(Individual with mild aphasia) *But I remember we were afraid to get up. We was scared to get up.*

Although in the current data set such variability of use was seen primarily among the individuals with aphasia, one still does not know whether it is also evidenced among individuals who do not have aphasia. Thus, one cannot be sure whether this is a function of code-switching or compensatory code-mixing secondary to the aphasia. For instance, one normal control variably uses the auxiliary:

And he said, "We looking for him." And I said, "What is you talking about" because I was already married to him by then.

In other more obvious instances of aphasic interference, an individual may be unable to access the main verb when attempting formation of the past perfect, despite repeated attempts, as indicated through repetition of the auxiliary, seen below. Note that this same individual also demonstrates variability in use of the plural forms of *child* and *card*, further indicating aphasic difficulties.

(Individual with moderate aphasia) *My childrens was playing card...My children was playing cards, and somebody had, somebody had up to my door, not front, the back door. And they had, had trying to, I don't know to, it wasn't cut.*

Across all individuals, the past perfect was not evidenced in direct speech. Whether in setting or climax, it was used in description of the main event line. In certain instances, the remoteness of the action indicated by the past perfect was redundantly encoded in accompanying adverbial phrases, e.g., *...when I was real small.* Use of such adverbial phrases can be used to reinforce interpretations of remote time in contexts which might be otherwise ambiguous, e.g., when aphasic errors are present.

The individuals with aphasia show a surprising command of a variety of forms beyond the complexities of the past perfect. Consider, for example, the following individual with aphasia.

(Individual with moderate aphasia) *Oh, yeah, a long time ago. Because uh, what had happened, a lady had died that time. Me and some more people, some children come and scared people about the lady, the lady done died you know. So the lady died, when they come back, and they say...*

In this citation, setting information is first expressed with the past perfect. The narrative then moves into the preterite, using present tense form "come" as the dialectal variant for expression of past tense. This is followed by use of perfective marker "done" in "done died." In the following sentence, simple past is again displayed, with "come" and "say" in the past tense forms commonly used in AAVE (i.e., what would be the present tense form of SAE).

Many forms are seen primarily in direct speech, because direct speech simulates the natural speech of members of the speakers' dialectal community. For instance, the future tense, which would not be otherwise seen in a narrative of a past event, is seen in direct quotes.

(Normal control) *"Girl, you sure got you a nice husband, he'll buy you anything you want." Girl, I tell you that was terrifying XXX* (unintelligible), *but you know the women are killing the men and they have, probably have, a good reason.*

(Normal control) *And they said, "Maxine, girl, they gon get you tonight. They gon get you."*

(Individual with mild aphasia) *One day I decided, "I'm gon walk to the store without this cane, and if I just fall, I fall." I tried it ...*

Notice the AAVE dialectal form *gon*, which is a morpho-phonemically reduced form similar to *going to* or *gonna* in SAE.

Likewise, the present tense is found, not only in direct quotes, but also to highlight information for the listener within the main event line:

(Normal control) *Just looked like a person, you know. And he is watching me and he's saying, "She is there by herself." But by the time it was getting dark, nobody had showed up. I was sitting on the porch.*

Notice how this use of the present tense is surrounded by use of past tense in the narrative.

Not only is direct speech likely to provide instances of the future and past tense forms, but it is more likely to include dialectal forms. A very good example to illustrate this point is a quote from one of the individuals with aphasia:

(Individual with moderate aphasia) *So my father said, "Don't, don't be playing with those guns." . . . . But then I had pulled the trigger on the rifle.*

Here, the father, as a member of the older generation, is advising the son using a dialectal form. In other words, the relative age of the speaker who is being quoted, his relationship to the narrator, and the speech act being performed through the direct quote (directive), all contribute to the likelihood of AAVE dialect use in this instance of a direct quote.

Throughout the narratives, one sees multiple additional features of AAVE, both among the normal controls and the individuals with aphasia. Many of these features also occur in non-standard regional dialect. Thus one cannot necessarily discriminate between the ethnic and regional dialect use among the speakers in this sample. Again, these forms appear even among the individuals with aphasia. These include a) variable deletion of AUX copula:

(Normal control) *And he said, "We looking for him." And I said, "What is you talking about" because I was already married to him by then.*

(Normal control) *Once my ex-husband abusive and he use to throw things at me and I was in the kitchen peeling potatoes and he was having one of his spells, I call it.*

b) regularization of irregular past tense, as well as double negative:

(Individual with mild aphasia) *The lady had some sheets hanging on the line and the wind blowed the sheets and they made noise, made noise like whup whup (E: Right) And we thought sho the cows was coming at us and ran and throwed down the water. We didn't have no water.*

c) *been* as remote time aspect:

(Normal control) *Oh, girl, don't say that I been scared a lot of time.*

(Normal control) *But of course these were high school students cause they went to high school with my brother and we couldn't been more than sixth grade.*

(Normal control) *And it was a tornado coming. That's the only time I been real scared.*

and d) non-use of third person singular *–s*, and *done* as completive aspect:

(Individual with mild aphasia) *And then my pastor, and he came down there and he said, "It kinda look like she done had a stroke."*

Concluding Remarks

As seen in these data, individuals with mild and moderate aphasia do use features of AAVE dialect, albeit intermingled with aphasia-associated difficulties. Overall, AAVE features in the verb appear to be preserved, despite the presence of aphasia. The question still remains how robust the dialectal features would be among individuals with more severe aphasia. Although individuals with moderate aphasia in these data tended to use fewer types of AAVE features than individuals with mild aphasia, the difference by aphasia severity level was not an absolute. Furthermore, individuals with more severe aphasia also produced shorter narratives; this restriction in sample length may have precluded attempts at contexts necessary to elicit a variety of AAVE verb forms. Considering the complexity of the verb system in AAVE, though, one might imagine special vulnerability of AAVE verbs when a more severe aphasia is present. One might conjecture that, in more severe forms of aphasia, primarily the phonological characteristics of the dialect (both segmental and suprasegmental) would survive.

The key question in any attempt to look at the interaction between dialect and aphasia is discerning which differences are attributable to the dialect, and which are attributable to pathological processes. This takes not only a thorough understanding of the ethnic dialect (cum regional and social dialects) which an individual might be expected to use, but also the degree to which one can expect that individual to use a non-standard dialect in the context in which language is being elicited. As highlighted in earlier portions of this article, a thorough understanding of AAVE is still in its infancy, and use or non-use of AAVE by any given individual may not always be predictable.

When one is not fully familiar with the ethnic dialect of a particular speaker, there is an additional confound. Namely, there is the possibility that the processes used by individuals with aphasia to compensate for their language impairment may also be very natural processes cross-linguistically (and across dialects) among non-neurologically impaired speakers (Kolk & Heeschen, 1990). The issue here is one of discerning natural processes from pathological processes when one is not familiar with the dialect (Seymour et al., 1998). For instance, there are several linguistically natural features of AAVE which parallel deletions and substitutions which one might anticipate among SAE speakers with aphasia. These include the following: deletion of past-tense endings, deletion of auxiliaries (especially in their contracted forms), deletion of the copula BE, regularization of irregular past-tense forms, and use of the preterite instead of the past participle in the present and past perfect forms (e.g., *I have wrote*). Thus, minimally, one cannot necessarily assume that an AAVE speaker with aphasia is using such forms because of the aphasia. These are natural features of the AAVE dialect as a linguistic system.

Operationally, then, interactions between dialect and aphasia are extremely difficult to study. Given a limited understanding of AAVE in its various manifestations, however, there are certain strategies that can be used to make progress in such an endeavor. One strategy is to begin work in connected language, as exemplified in the current article, and only then move into elicitation through specific contexts which have been built on a thorough understanding of how the AAVE dialect works in discourse. As noted earlier in this article, it is most useful to focus on aspects of the dialect which are relatively complex and also maximally differentiate the dialect of interest from other dialects (as seen in the verb system of AAVE). Assumed in this approach is to select individuals for study who are ethnographically as similar as possible, to control as much as possible for inter-individual variation related not only to ethnic dialect, but also regional and social dialects.

Another promising avenue is to explore relative variability in use of dialect forms between individuals with aphasia and normal controls. As seen in the data discussed in this article, variability in use of dialectal forms within a given speaker may indicate either code-switching (a rule-governed process) or code-mixing (a result of pathology or aphasic compensation). A careful comparison of variability of dialect use between ethnographically similar speakers with and without aphasia may provide insights on whether this variability is rule-governed or not among the individuals with aphasia.

Seymour et al. (1998) suggest an entirely different strategy for studying the relationship between dialect and language pathology. They note that shared features (non-contrastive) between AAVE and SAE may be more diagnostically salient than features not shared (contrastive) when identifying children of AAVE language backgrounds with language disorders. This may be an optimal approach with regard to the issue of differentiating difference from deficit, at least until more information is known regarding the deficit/difference distinction for AAVE features alone. Their recommendation is to "direct diagnostic objectives to detecting productions that cannot be explained by dialect divergence" (p. 107), a strategy which can be applied to differentiating dialect from aphasia, as well.

Finally, there are certain characteristics of AAVE that can help us to discern language use related to AAVE dialect from that related to aphasia. Specifically, repetition as a narrative device for information emphasis and evaluation appears to be a salient characteristic in AAVE; this can be systematically contrasted to repetition as a means of language formulation or lexical search, as seen in aphasia (Ulatowska, Olness, Hill, Roberts, & Keebler, 2000). The *nature* of repetitions which contain morpho-syntactic features of the AAVE dialect, as well as the nature of the repetitions which precede and follow use of AAVE features, can be used to evaluate the degree to which the productions of a given speaker are driven by aphasic compensations or not.

Acknowledgments

This research was supported in part by a grant, C888-2RA, from the Department of Veterans Affairs Rehabilitation Research and Development Program. The authors also gratefully acknowledge the contributions of LaKena Cowley and Jennifer Thompson in preparation of this article.

Address correspondence to: Hanna K. Ulatowska, Ph.D., University of Texas at Dallas, Callier Center for Communication Disorders, 1966 Inwood Rd., Dallas, Texas 75235, U.S.A.
E-mail: hanna@utdallas.edu

References

Anderson, E. T., & Ulatowska, H. K (1975). A problem of diagnosis: Black English or aphasia? In R. Brookshire (Ed.), *Clinical Aphasiology Conference Proceedings* (pp. 104-109). Minneapolis: BRK Publishers.

Baily, G. (1993). A perspective on African-American English. In D. R. Preston (Ed.), *American dialect research* (pp. 287-318). Amsterdam: John Benjamins.

Bailey, G. (1997). When did Southern American English begin? In E. W. Schnieder (Ed.), *Englishes around the World,* vol. 1, (pp. 255-276). Amsterdam: John Benjamins Publishing Company.

Berstein, C. (1988). A variant of the "invariant" *be. American Speech, 63,* 119-124.

Cukor-Avila, P. (1995). *The evolution of AAVE in a rural Texas community: An ethnolinguistic study.* Dissertation, University of Michigan.

Dillard, J. L. (1972). *Black English: Its history and usage in the United States.* New York: Vintage Books.

Fordham, S. (1993). "Those loud black girls": Black women, silence, and gender "passing" in the academy. *Anthropology and Education Quarterly, 24,* 3-32.

Green, L. (1994). Study of verb classes in African-American English. *Linguistics and Education, 7,* 65-81.

Green, L. (1998a). Aspect and predicate phrases in African-American Vernacular English. In S. S. Mufwene, J. R. Rickford, G. Baily, & J. Baugh (Eds.), *African-American English: Structure, history, and use* (pp. 37-68). London: Routledge.

Green, L. (1998b). Remote past and states in African-American English. *American Speech, 73*(2), 115-138.

Houston Stanback, M. (1985). Language and black woman's place: Evidence from the black middle class. In P. A. Triechler, C. Kramarae, & B. Stafford (Eds.), *For alma mater: Theory and practice in feminist scholarship* (pp. 177-193). Urbana, IL: University of Illinois Press.

Johnson, F. L. (2000). *Speaking culturally: Language diversity in the United States*. Thousand Oaks, CA: Sage.

Jordan, J. (1985). *On call: Policital essays*. Boston: South End Press.

Kolk, H. & Heeschen, C. (1990). Adaptation and impairment symptoms in Broca's aphasia. *Aphasiology, 4,* 221-231.

Labov, W. (1972). *Language in the inner city: Studies in the Black English Vernacular*. Philadelphia: University of Pennsylvania Press.

Labov, W. (1998). Co-existent systems in African-American Vernacular English. In S. S. Mufwene, J. R. Rickford, G. Baily, & J. Baugh (Eds.), *African-American English: Structure, history, and use* (pp. 110-153). London: Routledge.

Leslie, A.R. (1998). What African American mothers perceive they socialize their children to value when telling them Brer Rabbit stories. *Journal of Comparative Family Studies, 29*(1), pp.173-185.

Longacre, R. (1983). *The grammar of discourse*. New York: Plenum Press.

Martin, S., & Wolfram, W. (1998). The sentence in African-American Vernacular English. In S. S. Mufwene, J. R. Rickford, G. Baily, & J. Baugh (Eds.), *African-American English: Structure, history and use* (pp. 11-36). London: Routledge.

Menn, L., & Obler, L. K. (Eds.) (1990). *Agrammatic aphasia: A cross-language narrative sourcebook*. Amsterdam/Philadelphia: John Benjamins.

Poplack, S. & Tagliamonte, S. (1994). '-s' or nothing: Marking the plural in the African-American diaspora. *American Speech, 69*(3). 227-233.

Rickford, J. R. (1983). Carrying the new wave into syntax: The case of Black English BIN. In R. W. Fasold (Ed.), *Variation in the form and use of language: A sociolinguistics reader* (pp. 98-119). Washington, DC: Georgetown University Press.

Rickford, J. R., & Rafal, C. T. (1996). Preterite-Had + V-ed in the narratives of African-American pre-adolescents. *American Speech, 71*(3), 227-254.

Schneider, E. W. (1989). *American earlier Black English: Morphological and syntactic variables*. Tuscaloosa, AL: University of Alabama Press

Seymour, H. N., Bland-Stewart, L., & Green, L. J. (1998). Difference versus deficit in child African-American English. *Language, Speech, and Hearing Services in Schools, 29,* 96-108.

Smitherman, G. (1977). *Talkin and testifyin: The language of Black America*. Detroit, MI: Wayne State University Press.

Smitherman, G. (1994). *Black talk. Words and phrases from the hood to the Amen corner*. Boston: Houghton Mifflin.

Spears, A. K. (1987). Are black and white vernaculars diverging (Papers from the NWAVE XIV Panel proceedings). *American Speech, 62,* 48-55, 71-72.

Strevy, D. & Aldridge, J. 1994. Personal narratives themes of African-American mothers. *Perceptual and Motor Skills, 78,* 1143-1146.

Ulatowska, H. K., Olness, G. S., Hill, C. L., Roberts, J. A., & Keebler, M. W. (2000). Repetition in narratives of African Americans: The effects of aphasia. *Discourse Processes, 30*, 265-283.

Whatley, E. (1981). Language among Black Americans. In C. A. Ferguson, & S. B. Heath (Eds.), *Language in the U.S.A.* (pp. 92-107). Cambridge: Cambridge University Press.

Wolfram, W. A. (1969). *A sociolinguistic description of Detroit negro speech*. Washington, DC: Center for Applied Linguistics.

Wolfram, W. (1991). *Dialects and American English*. Washington, DC: Center for Applied Linguistics.

Wolfram, W. & Fasold, R. W. (1974). *The study of social dialects in American English*. Englewood Cliffs, NJ: Prentice-Hall.

Aphasia in Afrikaans: A preliminary analysis

Claire Penn*, Analou Venter°, Dale Ogilvy°

**University of the Witwatersrand °University of Cape Town*

Abstract—The language of a group of mildly impaired aphasic subjects speaking Cape Afrikaans in South Africa was compared with a group of matched controls. A narrative task was used to elicit samples and analysis methods included productivity, syntax and coherence measures, as well as ethnic, stylistic and pragmatic variables. The strongly bilingual tradition of this group became apparent in the results. Syntactic and productivity measures differentiated the groups to some extent, particularly in relation to the mechanism of verb movement. More marked differences were noted in aspects of coherence. Features such as code-switching, word order changes and stylistic intensification are interpreted as providing a robust compensatory and scaffolding structure for some of the primary aphasic deficits in this sample.

Key words: Aphasia, Afrikaans, Narrative, Bilingual, Verb, Coherence.

South Africa is a country with a wide diversity of cultures and languages, earning its epithet of "the rainbow nation." Most of its inhabitants speak at least two languages, if not several. Eleven of these languages have been afforded official status but many more exist. Further, there is wide dialectal and regional variation.

One of the languages unique to South Africa which has a relatively short history, yet ironically is one of the most comprehensively documented, is Afrikaans. It has existed much in today's form from about 1850, and was given legal recognition in 1925 when it became the language of the church and government. It is a language that is diverse in terms of region, dialect and social class, originating from not only the Dutch used by the 17th century settlers in South Africa, but also having features of Malay, Portuguese, Khoekhoe, French and German as well as English (Combrink, 1978; Roberge, 1995).

This language is the home language of a large number of people in South Africa (seven million) and until very recently was the medium of education for a number of non first language speakers (Kroes, 1978). Viewed as the "language of the oppressor" for many years, it has been the topic of extensive debate among politicians and educationalists and in the formulation of the language policy of the new South African government (Herbert, 1992; Alexander, 1996).

Structure of Afrikaans

The structure of Afrikaans has been described in detail by authors such as Combrink (1978), Donaldson (1993), Raidt (1994) and Oosthuizen (1996). Because of a relative paucity of early documentation, there remain debates about the issues such as its exact genesis and its status as a partially creolized language. However, among points of note for the aphasiologist are the following:

- Afrikaans has been classified both as an SVO and an SOV language because both patterns are seen (McCormick, 1995). However, like Dutch, it is probably best described as an SVOV language, meaning that the base generated position of the verb is after the object and that the auxiliary is in the verb second position.
- It lacks verb inflections in the present indicative and has no inflectional endings for number or person, attributed by Combrink (1978) to early contact situations between Germanic dialects.
- It has a regular orthography.
- There is reduplication (hypothesized to be of Malay origin) of all major categories such adjectives, adverbs, nouns, verbs and numbers – intensifying the meaning of the message e.g. Hy het staan-staan die koffie gedrink and toe gery.
  He drank the coffee while standing (standing-standing), and then he rode away. (Combrink, 1978)
- There is a reduplication of the negative marker. If the VP of a sentence consists of a single verb, the negative *nie* is placed directly after the verb. If the VP is more complex two *nies* are used, one after the verb and one at the end. Complicators include Object NPs, additional verbs, adverbials, adjectives or subordination. This double *nie* was inherited from 17th century Dutch though it has been noted that the second *nie* is dropped in modern forms of Afrikaans (Oosthuizen, 2000).
- There is a high proportion of compound words.
- There is a marked use of loan words primarily from English, present particularly in colloquial speech and somewhat frowned upon by the early purists (Donaldson, 1995).
- The preposition *vir* (for) is frequently used before a human indirect object (hypothesized to be of Portuguese origin) e.g. gee dit vir hom *give it to him* (Donaldson,1995:343)
- There is a retention of some Dutch forms, some of which are present in older, less mobile users of the language e.g. *gaat/gaan* (go), *slaat/slaan* (hit).

Cape Afrikaans

One group, for whom a distinctive dialectal version of Afrikaans has developed, is a group of mixed racial heritage, the so-called 'Coloured' group, largely resident in the Cape Province. This community developed through events of Dutch colonization in the seventeenth century and the interaction between the settlers and the indigenous people of the Cape. There are estimated to be more than 3 million users of Cape Afrikaans, which differs from the language of standard Afrikaans speakers in a number of different ways. These have been highlighted by van Rensburg (1997), McCormick (1989;1995), Kotze (1993), van der Reede (1983) and others, and include differences in phonology, lexicon, syntax and stylistic variables. Code-switching and code-mixing is another aspect which has been documented extensively in this dialect and which reflects important socio-cultural factors. The strong oral tradition of this group as well as its unique dynamic position in society account for some of these aspects including "intensive linguistic exchange" (McCormick, 1995:204) and language contact factors with a very strong effect of English, often spoken to children in the home and at school by second language speakers.

Cape Afrikaans lexicon draws heavily on English loanwords which are mostly nouns, followed by verbs, adjectives and adverbs and conjunctions (mainly *but* and *because*) (McCormick, 1995). Nouns retain English number marking but verbs adopt Afrikaans morphology. Syntactic convergence is also noted. According to McCormick (1995), the most striking aspect is violation of verb placement rules, or optional use of such rules, allowing the verb to precede the object as in English. This change from SOV is often triggered by a specific type of main clause verb (I know, I think, I see) and by the use of the copula in the subordinate clause following the verb complementizer *wat* (what) which in standard Afrikaans will require the verb to be in clause final position. Other features documented include:

- reduplication of articles, adjectives, prepositions and auxiliaries
- reduplication of conjunctions, especially *toe* (then)
- possession with the personal pronoun
- the use of the article *die* (the) before a proper noun
- a change of word function such that the demonstrative adjective *daai* (this) serves a subject or object noun

Aphasia in Afrikaans

There has to date been relatively little work undertaken on aphasic manifestations in Afrikaans and nothing, as far as we know, on Cape Afrikaans aphasia. Several studies have explored the translation and adaptation of English aphasia tests into standard Afrikaans (e.g. Rautenbach, 1973). Among these was the study by Jones (1989) who developed an Afrikaans version of the *Bilingual Aphasia Test* (Paradis, 1987) and Millar (1998) who developed an Afrikaans version of the PALPA and used a psycholinguistic framework to explore the reading and writing skills of a bilingual aphasic patient.

Kemp's work on verb movement in standard Afrikaans is ongoing. Schoeman (1997) examined verb movement in topicalised sentences in five Afrikaans-speaking agrammatic patients and used specific triggers (adverbial phrase) to elicit second sentence position for the verb. This was compared to a Dutch study which used the same methodology (Cahana-Amitay, 1997) and was analysed in relation to Chomsky's Minimalist Program.

This framework was also used as the basis for a study on the use of the negative in two Afrikaans agrammatic subjects (Millar, 1998) whose performance on an anagram task data was incorporated into a larger study on the negative in Dutch and French aphasia by Rispens (1997).

Some preliminary evidence from these studies and from clinical experience suggests that in Afrikaans, areas particularly susceptible to aphasic breakdown, *for agrammatic patients at least,* are the verb or any operations surrounding verb movement. Extrapolating from the extensive and explicit work of Kolk et al (1990) and Bastiaanse and colleagues on Dutch aphasia (e.g. Vermeuelen, Bastiaanse and van Wageningen, 1989; Bastiaanse and van Zonneveld, 1998; Bastiaanse and Jonkers, 1998; Edwards and Bastiaanse, 1998) verb movement and retrieval difficulties as well as problems with prepositions and articles, and sentence embedding would be anticipated.

Given some of the characteristics of Afrikaans, specifically Cape Afrikaans, in addition to these potential trouble spots in this language for the person with aphasia, various predictions can be made. We suggest that a number of the stylistic and syntactic aspects we are seeing in Cape Afrikaans discourse reflect the compensatory efforts of a group whose sociolinguistic status (specifically great diversity, lexical borrowing, code-switching and diverse daily interface/contact) provides well practiced shift strategies. Those individuals with aphasia therefore have a particularly well-stocked armamentarium of strategies for deployment during conversational interchange and that this feature is thus well worth exploring.

Rationale for studying discourse

It should be noted that the focus of much of the syntactic work in aphasia has been conducted with agrammatic aphasic patients and using tasks which are sentence or clause based, including picture and sentence matching, sentence completion and anagrams. Certainly the cross-linguistic material available to date focuses primarily on structural and syntactic aspects. The impact of task has been commented on as affecting the accuracy and nature of the language obtained (Hofstede and Kolk, 1994) and there remains a scarcity of studies on discourse level, identifying grammatical and narrative features of more fluent patients. This is a particularly fruitful field of study in a group such as the Cape Afrikaans group where literacy is limited (especially in older members of society) and for whom the oral narrative is a strong tradition.

STUDY

As part of a larger ongoing collaborative comparative study on discourse skills across cultures (Ulatowska, 1998), a group of seven subjects with fluent aphasia and seven matched controls were examined. These subjects came from the Western Cape Afrikaans community (hereafter CA) and as such can be viewed as having a strong bilingual tradition.

All aphasic subjects were right handed subjects who developed aphasia as a result of a single cerebrovascular accident. Subjects had to be at least three months post onset of stroke and were rated as having mild to moderate aphasia on the WAB (Kertesz, 1983). An adapted Afrikaans version of the WAB was used and as is the case with any aphasia measures developed in North America, the results of this testing should be viewed with extreme caution, bearing in mind the significant cultural, linguistic, educational and literacy differences between the standardized sample and the subjects under study. Subjects with severe aphasia were excluded from the study as the task involved connected language. Subjects were required to be under the age of 69 years and to be from the Cape Coloured Afrikaans-speaking community. The subjects were sourced from a local stroke club. Unfortunately, because of an underdeveloped health care system in the community from which the subjects were drawn, detailed medical records were difficult to obtain in most cases.

Control subjects who had no history of neurological or psychiatric problems were matched for age, gender, language, cultural group, education and occupation.

An adapted version of Paradis' bilingualism questionnaire was administered to each subject (Paradis, 1987) to ensure first language status of this group and to document patterns of language exposure. All subjects presented with Afrikaans as their first language. As is typically the case in the Cape, all subjects were exposed to English (L2) from an early age in the home. They were further exposed to English at school, socially or in the workplace. The nature of exposure varied and is documented below. Many of these subjects thus can be characterized as being bilingual, reinforcing the impression that this group as a whole has high contact patterns. Table 1 presents relevant subject details.

Table 1: Relevant case history variables for subjects with aphasia

Subject	Age (years)	Gender	Years of formal education	Premorbid vocation	WAB AQ	Severity of aphasia	Time post onset	Primary Exposure to English	Secondary Exposure to English (L2)
S1	63	M	9	Machinist	56.6	Mild	3.4 years	L2 of parents	English instruction at school School friends
S2	63	M	10	General assistant	55.9	Mild	3 years	L2 of parents	English instruction at school Work environment
S3	64	M	7	Maintenance	54	Moderate	4 months	L1 of father	English instruction at school
S4	30	F	8	Seamstress	50.6	Moderate	2.6 years	L2 of parents	English instruction at school Work environment
S5	66	F	8	Housewife	54.5	Mild	2 years	L1 of mother	English instruction at school School friends
S6	57	F	10	Typist	53.8	Mild	4 years	L1 of mother	English instruction at school School friends
S7	69	M	12	General assistant	49.6	Moderate	7 years	L1 of mother	English instruction at school Work environment

METHOD

An Afrikaans-speaking examiner elicited the narratives from all the subjects. Tasks included picture description, fable tasks, proverb tasks and narrative of personal experience. The most frightening experience was chosen for the purposes of this analysis as it yielded very rich data and consistently longer and richer samples than the other tasks both in this and a prior study (Sinoff, 1993). These samples were videotaped and later transcribed to allow for the coding of critical non-verbal information such as gesture which became important in the analysis of evaluation.

Analysis method

The transcripts were analysed along the following dimensions: productivity, lexical and syntactic aspects, quality/macrostructure, ethnic markers and stylistic and pragmatic aspects with an emphasis on evaluative elements. It became clear however that particularly in the genre of narrative, such headings are somewhat artificial and that there was considerable overlap between categories.

1. Productivity measures

Narrative length, proposition (defined as an informational unit that contains a verb and an argument (Ulatowska, 1998)) analysis, T Units (main clause and any subordinate clause), words per T Unit and correctness/error analysis were examined.

2. Lexical and Syntactic aspects

A number of specific syntactic features of aphasia were examined which appeared to be prominent in the data base and which have been identified by others as being important areas of concern/characterization:

2.1. The verb

We chose to focus on verbs in the analysis as they are very important in consideration of agrammatism (Saffran et al, 1980; Thompson et al, 1997; Bastiaanse and Jonkers, 1998), and they contribute substantially to coherence, providing a window onto the structure of narrative (Sinoff 1998). Verbs are generally well documented and several successful treatment frameworks for the verb have been identified. There is however, relatively little research on the verb in more fluent types of aphasia. Further an analysis of the verb enables comparison with the work on the verb and aphasia by Bastiaanse and colleagues in the Dutch language in both agrammatic and fluent Dutch aphasic subjects. A comparison between Dutch and Afrikaans aphasia has potentially fascinating parallels, given their strong historical link.

Measures of verb in this study included productivity as well as complexity and variety measures. A number of verb measures were examined (after Sinoff, 1993). Measures obtained were: total verbs (each separate verb, including Aux and Cop was tallied with the exception of the infinitive form which was counted as one verb), mean verbs per T Unit, mean auxiliaries per T Unit, mean copulas pr T Unit, verb types and tokens (using the same method as Edwards and Bastiaanse, 1998) and number of subordinations. In addition, tense shifting in relation to the use of the historical present tense and instances of direct speech were examined separately as part of the verb analysis.

2.2. Negatives
Negatives were examined with regard to placement and application of reduplication rules.

2.3. Conjunctions
Conjunctions were analyzed as they are important structures for between-sentence cohesion and are linked to verb movement in Afrikaans. Specifically the conjunction *toe* (then) was examined as it has been identified as triggering historical present tense which was found to be a prominent feature of the narratives analyzed.

2.4. Prepositions
As reduplication of prepositions is considered to be an important feature of Cape Afrikaans, this aspect was examined together with the incidence of *vir* (for).

3. Quality
A rating scale for quality of narrative was applied. This was based on the work of Labov (1972) and included the categories suggested by Ulatowska (1998) as well as the dimensions of Relevance, Character, Supporting Description and Ending (Sinoff 1993). The ratings were conducted by a culturally matched speech pathologist from the Cape Afrikaans community as well as the researchers. Three raters reached acceptable agreement on these measures

4. Ethnic markers
Lexical and syntactic convergence were examined as well as other features singled out by authors to be characteristic to the Cape Afrikaans dialect.

5. Stylistic and pragmatic aspects
There are a number of devices which have been used in discourse of aphasic patients which have been documented to reflect compensatory attempts on the part of the speaker (Penn, 1999; Schnitzer, 1974 and Kolk and Heeschen, 1990). Aspects such as ellipsis, topicalization and the use of comment clauses which have been identified in previous research were analyzed in the samples. In addition, evaluation, as a construct, was analyzed according to the method of Labov (1972). Evaluative devices are used to express the narrator's feelings about characters and events. Labov identified intensifiers, comparators, correlators and explications as the 4 major categories of evaluation. The category of intensifier was focused on as Ulatowska (1998) has indicated that her aphasic subjects used intensifying elements more than other types of evaluative elements. Aspects examined were: gesture, phonology, quantifiers, lexical items, repetitions, ritual and WH exclamations. Evaluative elements have been identified by Menn et al (1998) as being empathic aspects well retained in Japanese and English aphasia. In the following section these results will be illustrated with reference to some individual transcripts.

Table 2: Group Data for Productivity Measures (means)

Variable	Subjects (n=7)	Controls (n=7)
Number of words*	167 SD = 122.31	316.57 SD = 111.98
Number of propositions*	28 SD = 14.81	38.26 SD = 12.57
Words per T Unit	9.16	10.23
Number of T Units*	25.3 SD = 11.7	31.7 SD = 11.6
Verbs per T Unit	2.0 SD= 0.37	2.24 SD= 0.28
Auxiliaries per T Unit	0.52 SD= 0.27	0.47 SD= 0.27
Tense shift per T-Unit	0.44 SD= 0.17	0.4 SD= 0.14
Copulas per T-Unit	0.3 SD= 0.11	0.2 SD= 0.11
Tokens*	27.5 SD= 10.58	50.86 SD= 21.42
Types*	16.7 SD= 5.82	26.6 SD= 8.66
TTR	0.53 SD= 0.22	0.54 SD= 0.13
Tokens/T Unit	0.86 SD= 0.23	0.88 SD= 0.19
Subordinates/T Unit*	0.12 SD= 0.076	0.18 SD= 0.09
Verbs – verb tokens	24.71 SD= 37.69	18.57 SD= 6.425
Number of verbs*	38.33 SD= 17.9295	69.42 SD= 25.178

Note: - *indicates significance without outlier

RESULTS

1. Productivity measures

The productivity measures for the aphasic subjects and the controls are summarised in Table 2. These results reflect group means but exclude where relevant S2 whose very lengthy sample (1288 words) rendered him an outlier.

In general the control subjects produced longer narratives with a greater number of T Units. The mean length of the narrative for the aphasic sample was 167 words (range 83-285), indicating generally a shorter and more diverse sample size for the aphasic group than for the controls, whose range was 226-512 words. This difference was found to be statistically significant (Mann Whitney U test, U=5.0, p=0.22).

The number of T Units and propositions were comparable when the sample of S2 was included in the tally of the means, but significantly fewer for aphasic subjects when S2's sample was excluded. This is similar to the findings of Ulatowska et al (in press) who found a lower number of propositions in her aphasic African American group.

Because of the wide variation in sample size, direct comparisons of other productivity measures were possible only through ratios expressed in relation to the T Unit. The mean length of the T Units was 9.16 words for the aphasic subjects (range 7.5-12) and 10.23 for the control subjects (range 8.3-14). This was not statistically significant.

The mean number of verbs per T Unit was also found not to differentiate groups, however, the total number of verbs, the number of verb types and tokens and the number of subordinations per T Unit were significantly higher in the control sample and will be discussed in more detail in the following section.

2. Syntax

In general, more errors, incomplete and minor utterances and paraphasias were noted in the samples of the aphasic subjects. Not unexpectedly, however, with aphasic subjects at the mild end of the severity continuum, few frank errors were noted.

Their samples suggested slightly reduced syntactic complexity with fewer complex or non canonical sentences. For example the total number of subordinate sentences in the aphasic data was 19 whereas the control subjects used 37 subordinate sentences. This is reflected in a significant difference between subordinates per T Unit (p=O.25). There were some instances of incomplete subordination attempts in the aphasic subjects suggesting false starts induced by syntactic complexity.

Verbs

Some interesting differences emerged between the aphasic and control groups when the verb was analyzed using complexity and variety measures. The mean number of verb words was higher for the controls than for the aphasic subjects but there appeared to be no difference between number of verbs and the number of auxiliaries per T Unit. No significant difference emerged between groups for copula verbs.

This is slightly at variance with the findings of Vermeulen and Bastiaanse (1984) and Edwards and Bastiaanse (1998) who found that their anomic patients produced not only more copulas but also more auxiliaries and modals than normal controls, but Bastiaanse and Jonkers (1998) found a normal number of modals and copulas in their subjects. These differences can probably be explained in terms of task differences.

The finding regarding reduced verb complexity in the aphasic group was strengthened by examining the mean difference between the number of verbs (actual verb words) and the number of verb tokens (verbs in their simple or expanded form) for each group. The difference is smaller in the control group (18.57) when compared to the aphasic group (24.71) suggesting more elaboration (via tense markers and auxiliaries) of the verb for the control group.

With regard to verb variety, like previous studies (Edwards and Bastiaanse, 1998) a significantly lower diversity of verbs (p= 0.06) was found, reflected in the mean number of 16.7 verb types (range = 9-23) for the aphasic group versus 26.6 (range = 16-39) for the control group. The verb TTR mystifyingly did not prove significant (0.53 versus 0.54). Again S2 was an outlier and was not included in this analysis.

Auxiliary Analysis

Auxiliary doubling was found, as in the following instance:

Maar ek het nog altyd gebid het
But still I always prayed

It is suggested that the second *het* is spelling out a trace which is usually omitted and lends support for the SOV nature of Afrikaans (Oosthuizen, 2000).

That we found fewer, rather than disrupted auxiliaries, was somewhat unexpected given the findings of Kolk et al (1990) but the sample of S4 is interesting. She demonstrated a moderate (rather than mild aphasia) and produced a more restricted sample with more syntactic problems than others. Interestingly, her difficulties with the auxiliary are manifested in each attempt at use. She produced 12 T Units, 9 of which were complete and 3 of which were inaccurate or abandoned attempts. All these false starts related to management of the past tense auxiliary:

Auxiliary omission: Ek ge- gedink hy gaat my klap (omission of het)
I thought he would hit me

Incomplete auxiliary: Ek het ged gedink (incomplete)…. Ek was baie bang
I thought…I was very scared

(arguably changed from auxiliary to copula form)

Abandoned auxiliary: Ek het die man wat vir my geslaat het so ----
I (past tense Aux) the man who hit me so---

(abandoned, presumably because of processing demands induced by syntactic complexity/embedding)

The rest of her verb use consists of copulas and the use of historical present tense.

The samples were also examined for the presence of English word order. This change (SOV) is often triggered by a specific type of main clause verb (e.g. I know, I think, I see) and by the use of the copula in the subordinate clause. In Cape Afrikaans an optional rule allows the verb to precede the object.

Some evidence was found for such optional word order changes

e.g. S2: "En ek sien hier staan 'n ry trokke"
And I see here stands a row (of) trucks

Dink ek iets is darem nie reg hier nie
I think something is really not right here

versus
ek dink ek gaan darem nie so na aan hom draai nie
I think I will really not turn so close to him (with verb final position kept)

Ek het gedink ek gaan nou nooit weer uit die hospitaal uit kom nie
I thought I would never again get out of the hospital.

(Note in this example retained verb position and duplication of the preposition *uit* (out)).

Negatives

In Afrikaans, as for the fourteen languages studied in the cross-language aphasia study (Menn and Obler, 1989), negatives seemed well retained in these data, probably because, as Menn (1989) suggests, despite syntactic complexity, they bear a heavy semantic load. Most instances suggest adequate management of the negative rules despite syntactic complexity:

E.g. As 'n mens nie notisie vat nie, dan gebeur daar ook baie dinge
If one does not take notice then many things also happen

Of the 45 instances of negative which appeared in the expressive samples of the aphasic and control subjects, there were several examples from both groups in which the second negative marker *nie* was not expressed at the end of the utterance. Variation occurred both between and within subjects. Oosthuizen (2000) suggests such data are evidence that a theory of tree pruning in which functional (versus substantive) categories (Chomsky's theory of minimalism) are pruned, does not necessarily hold true (personal communication).

Ek kan nie onthou
I can't remember

Ek weet nie want nie want hulle sê
I don't know why because they say

The following pairs (from the same control subject) are particularly interesting suggesting within-subject variation, clearly not accounted for by pathological mechanisms.

Ons het nie soos vandag se kinders gewees nie.
We were not like today's children
(Note in this example the regularisation of the past tense verb *het gewees* in place of *was gewees*, to be discussed in a following section)
and
Ons wil nie huis toe gaan.
We did not want to go home

Ek was nie bewus
I was not aware,
and
ek het nie geweet daar's twee OKs.
I did not know there were two OKs

Other aspects of syntax examined, namely preposition and conjunctions will be discussed under Ethnic Markers.

3. Quality

A coherence rating was undertaken for all the transcripts using Sinoff's (1993) five point rating scale for Temporal Organization, Relevance, Character, Supporting description and Ending. These results are presented in Figure 1.

The mean for aphasic coherence was 19 (out of 25), and for controls 24.5 which was statistically significant ($t = 4.894$; $p = 0.05$). When an analysis of each of the constructs of coherence was undertaken, these differences were all statistically significant. This finding suggests that there are elements of the aphasic narrative that are lacking in relation to the control narrative and has several implications.

Firstly, the obvious differences between the aphasic and control subjects in the coherence of the narratives is markedly in contrast to many of the productivity and complexity measures utilised, in which no significant differences could be found. This finding has important implications both for assessment and therapy and seems to reflect the sensitivity of narrative and discourse features not solely to linguistic factors but to cognitive and social aspects as well.

Following from this, it suggests that for patients with mild aphasia, a focus on macrostructure or quality aspects may prove to be more relevant than on syntactic or productivity aspects, though obviously there is a strong correlation between structural aspects (such as verb management) and coherence (as Sinoff's (1993) findings suggest).

The differences found between aphasic and control subjects for the categories of Character, Relevance and Temporal organization suggest that, for this type of narrative at least, a more fine tuned analysis may yield more data than the Ulatowska rating scale which is a three point scale and which collapses certain categories of setting, complication action, resolution and coda into a single global structure.

4. Ethnic markers

Several ethnic markers were examined in the samples, many of which failed to differentiate aphasic and control groups. These will be discussed at a lexical and syntactic level.

As predicted by the literature, a change in the standard Afrikaans word forms was noticed in both groups of subjects (1) the contracted form *daai* (of demonstrative adjective *daardie* (that)) was frequently used as a pronoun in subject or object position indicating an extended grammatical function, (2) a change of standard Afrikaans word forms was also noted in production of *gaat*/gaan (go) which seems to be equivalent to the "light verbs" discussed by Bastiaanse and Jonkers (1998), *slaat*/slaan (hit) (S4) and some lexical items considered to be "old Afrikaans" e.g. *kooi*/bed (bed), (3) the possessive form after the pronoun was also seen: Ons *se*.

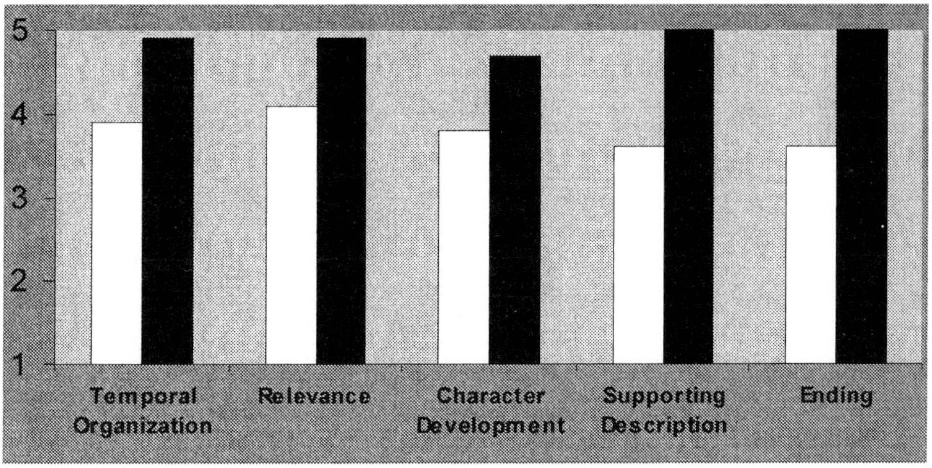

Figure 1. Coherence ratings for aphasic subjects and controls

The most common feature of the samples were the plentiful examples of code-switching and code-mixing in the transcripts. McCormick (1995) has pointed out that Cape Afrikaans is a mixed code in itself and mixing and switching cannot therefore be clearly differentiated. As Romaine (1995: 51) and McCormick (1995: 194) have suggested, such behaviours are common practice of bilingual speech communities. No evidence of pathological code-mixing as defined by Fabbro et al. (2000) was observed.

Lexical convergence

There are many examples of loan words in the samples, mostly from English, reflecting the high contact patterns between languages in the Western Cape. Examples of loan words were found in most word classes as illustrated:

Nouns
Examples include:
Predicament (C7)
Pavement (S2)

C6: Hy't sommer daai wreede *look* soos 'n mal mens
He had that wild look like a mad person.

En die kêrels, ons is groot *pals*.
And the fellows, we are big pals
(Note: the noun characteristically has retained the English number marking)

S2: hy het 'n overall aan van daai met die *strappy* het
He had an overall on, of that (kind) with the strap

Conjunctions
Examples include:
because why? (S1)
because (S7;S8)
But (S8)

Adjectives
Examples include:
C6: Maar dit was *terrible*
C7: Die *one way* strate
29 *thousand odd* rand

Verbs
Examples include:
Ek het nie ge*panic* nie (S5)
I did not panic
(Note how the loan verb adopts Afrikaans morphology with the past tense marked with *ge-*)

C6: Met daai gedagte jy *doze* af
With those thoughts, you doze off
(Note in this example that the verb particle remains in Afrikaans)

Adverbials
oraait (allright) (S2 and S6)
Anyway (C6)

With regard to lexical convergence, one would predict, given that aphasia influences lexical access, that this may precipitate more frequent use of loan words, particularly in more strongly bilingual subjects. There is sparse quantitative evidence in the sample to confirm this, but 6 out of 7 aphasic subjects used loan words (as opposed to 4 out of 7 controls). No differential level of bilingualism could be used to account for differences between subjects.

Syntactic convergence

Features found by Venter (2000) include:

Regularizing irregular past tense form
The past tense form of the verb 'to be' (*om te wees*) is *was* in standard Afrikaans e.g. *het gewees* (instead of *was gewees)*. Cape Afrikaans speakers often make use of the auxiliary *het* instead of *was* as in the following examples:

e.g. S3 "Ek het nou gewees in die Wetton".
I was in Wetton
(Note also the use of die (the) plus Proper noun which is a typical feature of CA)
Ons het nie gewees soos vandag se kinders nie
We were not like today's children.

Word order
English word order XV was observed replacing VX in the samples:
e.g. S2 " Ek dink toe en ek wil gaat na haar toe met 'n bos blomme"
I then thought and wanted to go to her with a bunch of flowers.

S6: Miskien my spraak gaan weg
Perhaps my speech would go away.

Explanations for verb movement have varied from diachronic ones to those based on trace theory (see for example Rispens, 1997). A pragmatic explanation for verb movement however is compelling, specifically in relation to the aphasic data. With limited processing capacity as well as lexical difficulties, earlier rather than later, realisation of the verb slot will presumably affix and consolidate the argument of the utterance. Such an explanation is compatible with explanations about the nature of the aphasic deficit as a processing limitation and can obviously also account for control examples (Kolk, 1990 and Schnitzer, 1974). This has interesting therapeutic implications, suggesting that SVO therapy may be more effective than SOV with such cases.

Prepositions
Some examples of reduplication were noted in the transcripts of preposition reduplication for the words *uit* (out), *in* (in) and *af* (off).

Toe sukkel ek om uit te kom die dam uit.
Then I struggled to come out of the dam

S8: 'n jaar gevat voor daai afgegaan het van my af
(It)took a year before that left me.

C6: So in 'n sak in
As in a sack

C1: "een dag het ek uitgeskiet ,gestap in die veld in"
One day I shot out, walked in the veld

(Note this example of a loan word from Afrikaans which has been adopted into English, of which there are many fascinating examples in international use (Bramford and Claughton, 1995)

e.g. " ek het gedink ek gaan nou nooit weer uit die hospitaal uit kom nie"
I thought I would never again come out of the hospital

The preposition vir (for) preceding a person object was also evident:

e.g. S2: Ek vra vir hom
I ask him

Conjunctions
Reduplication of conjunctions was common, particularly in the context of historical present tense and the conjunction *toe* (then). The preterite is avoided when relating past events where it is obvious from the context that the action occurred in the past. In Afrikaans colloquial narrative, it is common to insert an adverbial *toe* (then) in the main clause while starting the subordinate clauses with a conjunctional *toe* (Donaldson, 1993), obviating the necessity for past tense.

C5: Toe die aand, toe kry hulle die vrou beet.
Then (in) the evening, then they beat up the woman

There are numerous examples of this in the narratives, particularly in those of the aphasic subjects who use of *toe* both in the main clause and subordinate clauses. Of the 44 uses of this conjunction in the aphasia samples, 34 are followed by the present tense, while 53 of the 73 uses of this conjunction in the control samples were followed by the present tense.

Specific samples illustrate this well. S6 for example used a total of 33 verbs, only 3 of which were in the past tense. C6's sample was also exceptional in this regard. She used no fewer than 31 instances of *toe* over a sample of 433 words, with multiple examples of reduplication.

Toe kom sy toe gaat sy mos nou huis toe.
Then she comes then she just goes home.

S2 used *dan* (then) in the same way:
En dan wat maak hulle? Dan't my pa gevat, dan sit hy 'n doek om hom
And then what did they do? Then my father took, then he put a cloth around him.

It could be argued that use of these conjunctional forms together with the historical present is a simplification strategy, enabling an avoidance of syntactic complexity through past tense marking and verb movement.

Tense Shifts
The number of tense shifts per T Unit was compared in the two groups as it was hypothesized that there would be fewer tense shifts in the aphasic group. The difference between the groups was not, however, significant (see table 3).

Direct speech
Direct speech provides another well documented mechanism to avoid tense shift, exploited fairly frequently in the samples of the aphasic subjects. There were 31

instances of direct speech in the samples of the aphasic group and 15 in the control samples.

S3: "Die water is; Oe Vader jy moet my nou help"
The water is--- "Oh Father, you must help me now"

S1: Maar die doktor ...se die Doktor "Nee man"
But the doctor ----the doctor says "No man".

In both the above instances, arguably the speakers stopped midstream and chose direct speech as an alternative to more complex forms.

Code-switching
As the discussion on lexical and syntactic convergence above demonstrates, code-switching was a marked feature of the samples. It is defined here as the alternation of elements longer than one word. There may be conversational code-switching, which has a range of pragmatic and stylistic functions, or situational code switching due to the influence of the interlocutor (McCormick, 1995, p.202). This may also act as a verbal strategy to compensate for word finding problems in the first language (see also Paradis, 1998).

The most delightful example of both of these types is supplied by S2 who demonstrates at the same time code switching, code mixing and interestingly direct speech and comparative evaluation:

En ek se vir hom "Ek wil Kaap toe gaan." Hy se "Yes but you've just missed the train" ah uh" Hy se vir my "But you are not alone" Maar ek is alone. Ek se vir hom "Of course I'm alone. Daar's niemand by my nie. I'm not alone!"

5. Stylistic and pragmatic factors

Certain stylistic features have been identified as enhancing the properties of narrative. Some of these are syntactic, others relate to aspects such as reduplication. Ideally, non verbal aspects should always be considered in such an analysis.

Grammatical aspects such as ellipsis have been identified by Kolk and Heeschen (1990) as "positive" and preventative strategies used by aphasic patients. There are stylistic aspects which can be seen in the same light (see also Penn, 1988; 1999). Menn et al (1998) have indicated that pragmatic factors are well retained in the narratives of English and Japanese aphasic patients. They identify markers of empathic focus (evaluation, topicalization, attribution of mental state).

Evaluation conveys the narrator's feelings about characters and events (Labov, 1972) and Ulatowska (1983) and Sinoff (1995) have found that the narrative of personal experience produced a high number of evaluative elements. This was the case in this study.

The narrative task is a particularly fruitful one for the examination of intensifier. Venter (2000) has undertaken a detailed analysis of the intensifier elements in the samples of the present subjects. She found that a mean of 7.7% of the aphasic samples and 10.2% of the control subjects' samples were intensifier elements. The breakdown of type of intensifiers were as follows: Ritual (74 instances), Phonological (29 instances), Repetition (18 instances), Lexical (17 instances), Gesture (10 instances), Quantity (3 instances) and WH (3 instances)

Ritual utterances included tag question markers such as *nê*, *okay* and *oraait* (Anglicisms), empathic markers such as *natuurlik*, *mos*, *ja* (yes) and *nee* (no) (like Dutch).

Phonological intensifiers included lengthening of a word for emphasis.

Lexical items included *darem* and *regtig.*

Repetition was apparent in the following examples:

C7: En ons wag en ons wag en ons wag.
And we wait and we wait and we wait

S4: Maar ek sal nooit vergeet nie. Ek is nou ... Ek sal dit nooit vergeet nie
But I shall never forget it. I am now—I shall never forget it.

McCormick (1995) has commented on repetition as a strategy to create emphasis in CA.

Repetition has been identified by Ulatowska et al. (in press) as an ethnic stylistic feature but also as an aphasic strategy (Oelschager and Damico, 1998, Penn, 1988). This is particularly interesting because of the strong oral narrative tradition in our country and the observation that repetition as the core component of the traditional narrative is relatively well preserved.

Comparators such as comment clauses were also noted.

S2: U sal seker nie weet van n tiekie nie
You probably won't know about a tickie.
Dis nou n ware storie, nê?
This is now a true story. OK?
Snaaks genoeg
Funnily enough

Ellipsis and topicalization were felt to have a stylistic function in the samples but can also be explained as compensatory devices which facilitate the production in aphasia (Schnitzer, 1974; Kolk and Heeschen, 1990; Menn et al., 1998).

e.g. Maar ongelukking is ek daai dag.
But unlucky was I that day

Hoe het ek deur die drade gaan, weet ek nie
How I got through the wires, I don't know

When the individual results of the subjects are examined, it is possible to account for some of the pragmatic and stylistic features observed in terms of case history variables. For example S3 whose aphasia was of only four months standing, is apparently using more gestural intensification than the other aphasic subjects possibly as the more available compensatory strategy in the absence of more verbal skills. Similarly, different exposures and levels of English proficiency may well account for some of the features seen, specifically code switching. Further testing (in the second language of these subjects) may well yield intriguing data in this regard. The fact that the interlocutor, though Afrikaans-speaking, was not culturally matched may also account for some of the situational code switching observed.

CONCLUSIONS

In the small sample of fluent Cape Afrikaans aphasic subjects studied, we found a range of linguistic and stylistic features in their narratives, reflecting unique aspects of Afrikaans and its regional Cape form, and also aspects which can be hypothesized to be aphasic in origin. It is argued that the "default mode" of Cape Afrikaans with its strong bilingual tradition, includes patterns of code switching, flexible word order and stylistic intensification and that this provides a robust compensatory and scaffolding structure for some of the primary aphasic deficits. Further, it can be concluded that the genre of narrative provides a strong basis for such pragmatic strengths to emerge.

While certain productivity and syntactic measures clearly differentiated the two groups, these differences were not always easy to separate from stylistic and ethnic aspects. It is possible that this arises from both severity and task factors. The subjects were at the mild end of the continuum and the narrative task may camouflage such differences. The study certainly suggests however that verb movement, management of the auxiliary and word order aspects tax the compromised system. What does seem to be important with this group is that measures beyond the sentence level such as the coherence analysis have a stronger differentiating role and this has important clinical implications.

Many areas of future research present themselves and ongoing research includes (1) correlation of specific symptomatology with neurological and cognitive information; (2) comparing the present data with that from standard Afrikaans aphasic subjects; (3) careful consideration of bilingual informants and their performance in English and other South African languages on similar tasks; (4) comparison of the narrative of personal experience with performance on other tasks, including specifically constructed tasks which also tap comprehension and probe some of the hypotheses proposed. Menn et al (1998) correctly suggest that "Clinical experiments make clear the extent of these losses; naturalistic elicitations bring out the ability to compensate for them". A replication and expansion of this study's methods to include an agrammatic group will enable closer comparison with studies in other languages and allow further insight into the syntactic features highlighted here.

Clearly international collaborative efforts will yield and reinforce such efforts, and the unique socio-cultural context of language use in South Africa provides no shortage of opportunity to those interested in such challenges.

Acknowledgements

I would like to acknowledge the following persons who greatly assisted in the production of this chapter: Lisa Kalmek for her able and patient research assistance, Nicki Millar for her insights, Dr Johan Oosthuizen, Department of African Studies at the University of Cape Town, Heila Jordaan, Department of Speech Pathology and Audiology, University of the Witwatersrand for her support and Dr Hanna Ulatowska for her encouragement and vision in matters cultural.

Address correspondence to: Prof. Claire Penn, Department of Speech Pathology and Audiology, University of the Witwatersrand, Private Bag 3, Wits 2050, South Africa.
E–mail: 053penn@muse.wits.ac.za

References

Alexander, N. (1996). *Towards a national language plan for South Africa.* Department of Arts, Culture, Science and Technology. Pretoria: Government Printer.

Bastiaanse, R., & van Zonneveld, R. (1998). On the relation between verb inflection and verb position in Dutch agrammatic Aphasics. *Brain and Language, 64,* 165-181.

Bastiaanse, R., & Jonkers, R. (1998). Verb retrieval in action naming and spontaneous speech in agrammatic and anomic aphasia. *Aphasiology, 12,* 951-969.

Branford, W., & Claughton, J.S. (1995). Mutual lexical borrowings among some languages of Southern African: Xhosa, Afrikaans and English. In R. Mesthrie (Ed.), *Language and social history.* Cape Town: David Philip.

Combrink, J.G.H. (1978). Afrikaans: Its origins and development. In L.W. Lanham and K. P. Prinsloo (Eds.), *Language and communication studies in South Africa* (pp. 69-95). Cape Town: Oxford University Press.

Donaldson, B.C. (1993). *A grammar of Afrikaans*. Berlin: Mouton de Gruyter.

Edwards, S., & Bastiaanse, R. (1998). Diversity in the lexical and syntactic abilities of fluent aphasic speakers. *Aphasiology, 12,* 99-117.

Fabbro, F., Skrap, M., & Aglioti, S. (2000). Pathological switching between languages after frontal lesions in a bilingual patient. *Journal of Neurology, Neurosurgery and Psychiatry, 68,* 650-652.

Herbert, R.K. (1992). *Language and society in Africa.* Johannesburg: Witwatersrand University Press.

Hofmeyr, I. (1987). Building a nation from words: Afrikaans language, literacy and ethnic identity 1902-1924. In S. Marks and S. Trapido (Eds.), *The politics of race, class and nationalism in the twentieth century.* London: Longman.

Hofstede, B.T.M., & Kolk, H.H.J. (1994). The effects of task variation on the production of grammatical morphology in Broca's Aphasia: A multiple case study. *Brain and Language, 46,* 278-328.

Jones, D. (1989). The assessment of English/Afrikaans bilingual aphasic patients using the Bilingual Aphasia Test. Unpublished research report, University of the Witwatersrand.

Kemp, M.A. Dept of Linguistics, University of Stellenbosch. PhD in progress.

Kolk, H., & Heeschen, C. (1990). Adaptation and impairment symptoms in Broca's aphasia. *Aphasiology, 4,* 221-231.

Kolk, H., Heling, G., & Keyser, A. (1990). Agrammatism in Dutch. In L. Menn and L.K. Obler (Eds.), *Agrammatic aphasia: A cross-language narrative source book.* New York: John Benjamins

Kertesz, A. (1982). *Western aphasia battery.* The Psychological Corporation Harcourt Brace Jovanovich, Inc. USA

Kotzè, E.F. (1993). Variasie patrone in Maleier-Afrikaans. Unpublished PhD Thesis. University of the Witwatersrand: Johannesburg.

Kroes, H. (1978). Afrikaans in Education. In L.W. Lanham and K.P. Prinsloo (Eds.), *Language and communication studies in South Africa.* Oxford University Press: Cape Town.

Labov, W. (1972). *Language in the inner city: Studies in the black English vernacular.* Philadelphia: University of Pennsylvania Press.

McCormick, K. (1989). *A sociolinguistic study of English and Afrikaans in District 6.* Unpublished PhD Thesis. University of Cape Town.

McCormick, K. (1995). Code-switching, code-mixing and convergence in Cape Town. In R. Mesthrie (Ed.), *Language and social history.* Cape Town: David Philips.

Menn, L. and Obler, L.K. (1990). *Agrammatic aphasia: A cross-language narrative source book.* New York: John Benjamins.

Menn, L., Reilly, K.F., Hayashi, M., Kamio, A, Fujita, I., & Sasanuma, S. (1998). The interaction of preserved pragmatics and impaired syntax in Japanese and English aphasic speech. *Brain and Language, 61,* 183-225.

Menn, L. (1989). Comparing approaches to comparative aphasiology. *Aphasiology, 3*(2), 143-154.

Mesthrie, R. (1995). *Language and social history.* Cape Town: David Philip.

Millar, N. (1998). Unpublished research, University of the Witwatersrand.

Oelschager, M.L., & Damico, J.S. (1998). Spontaneous verbal repetition: a social strategy in aphasic conversation. *Aphasiology, 12*(11), 971-988.

Oosthuizen, J. (1996). Minimalisme en woordordevariasie in Afrikaanse Vraagsinne. In R.P. Botha et al (Eds.), *SPIL plus linguistics for the language professions.* University of Stellenbosch.

Oosthuizen, J. (2000). Department of African Languages, University of Cape Town. Personal communication.

Paradis, M. (1987). *The assessment of bilingual aphasia.* Hillsdale: Lawrence Erlbaum Associates.

Paradis, M. (Ed.) (1998). *Pragmatics in neurogenic communication disorders.* Oxford: Pergamon Press.

Penn, C. (1988). The profiling of syntax and pragmatics in aphasia. *Clinical Linguistics and Phonetics, 2,* 170-207.

Penn, C. (1999). Pragmatic assessment and therapy for persons with brain damage: What have clinicians gleaned in two decades? *Brain and Language, 68,* 535-552.

Raidt, E.H. (1994). *Histories Taalkunde: Studies oor die geskiedenis van Afrikaans*: Johannesburg: Wits University Press.

Rautenbach, S.H. (1973). 'n Vertaalde Afrikaans afasie toets. Unpublished research report. University of Pretoria.

Rispens, J. (1997). Negation of agrammatic aphasia: A cross-linguistic comparison. Unpublished PhD Thesis: Rijksuniversiteit.

Roberge, P.T. (1995). The formation of Afrikaans. In R. Mesthrie (Ed.), *Language and social History.* Cape Town: David Philip.

Romaine, S. (1995). *Bilingualism.* Oxford: Blackwell Publishers.

Saffran, E.M. (1980). The word order problem in agrammatism. *Brain and Language, 10,* 163-280.

Schnitzer, M.L. (1974). Aphasiological evidence for five linguistic hypotheses. *Language, 50,* 300-315.

Schoeman, M. (1997). Werkwoordverskuiwing in getopikaliseerde sinne geproduseer deur vyf Afrikaanssprekende Broca Afasie. Unpublished Research Report. University of Stellenbosch.

Sinoff, A. (1993). Coherence and the verb in the narratives of Hearing Impaired Children. PhD Thesis, University of the Witwatersrand.

Thompson, C. K., Lange, K.L., Schneider, S.L.., & Shapiro, L.P. (1997). Agrammatic and non-brain-injured subjects' verb and verb argument structure production. *Aphasiology, 11*(4), 473-490

Ulatowska, H.K., Freedman-Stern, R., Weiss Doyle, A., & Macaluso-Hayes, S. (1983). Production of narrative discourse in aphasia. *Brain and Language, 19,* 317 – 334.

Ulatowska, H.K. (1998). *Narrative discourse battery.* Callier Communication Centre: University of Texas.

Ulatowska, H., Streit Olness, G., Hill, C.L., Roberts, J., & Keebler, M. W. (in press). Repetition in narratives of African Americans: The effects of aphasia. *Discourse processes*

Valkhoff, M.F. (1972). *New light on Afrikaans and "Malayo-Portugues"*. Louvain: Peeters.

Van der Reede, I. (1983). 'n Sosiolinguistiese ondersoek na taalgebruik in Bellville-Suid. MA Thesis. University of the Western Cape: Bellville.

Van Rensburg, C. (1997). *Afrikaans in Afrika.* J.L. van Schaik: Pretoria.

Venter, A. (2000). Narrative discourse of Afrikaans speaking coloured aphasics in the Western Cape. Ongoing Masters research report, University of Cape Town.

Vermeulen, J., Bastiaanse, R., & Van Wageningen, B. (1989). Spontaneous speech in aphasia: Correlational study. *Brain and Language, 36,* 252-274.

Aphasia manifestations in Basque

Itziar Laka, Lore Erriondo Korostola

Linguistics Dept.& Psycology Dept. Euskal Herriko Unibertsitatea-University of the Basque Country, Paseo de la Universidad 5, Apdo 2111, E- 01006 Vitoria-Gasteiz

Abstract—This paper presents a description of the main symptoms of agrammatism found in a corpus of spontaneous speech production of 59 Basque-speaking aphasic patients. The main symptoms relate to deficits in the production of inflectional morphology. From the standpoint of grammatical structure, the deficits involve the production of the syntactic category Infl, that heads the sentence (IP). Basque has a morphologically complex Inflection, containing up to three agreement markers, plus tense and modality specifications. The most outstanding symptom of agrammatism is the absence of inflected verbs, or its extremely low frequency, correlated with a high frequency of uninflected participial forms. The study of the inflected forms produced in aphasic speech reveals a significant number of errors in the selection of appropriate morphemes, particularly number and dative agreement markers, and a considerable number of newly coined impossible forms, resulting form the combination of morphemes from conflicting paradigms. However, the relative order of the morphemes in the auxiliary is correct, which could indicate that the basic structure of Inflection is not affected, at least in the case of patients that produce inflected forms. Errors in case-marking also appear, mostly involving ergative and absolutive markers.

Key words: Aphasia, Basque, Agrammatism, Inflectional morphology, Inflection, Case-marking.

1. Introduction: the corpus

This paper presents and discusses data from a corpus of Basque speaking aphasic subjects, focussing on *agrammatism*. The only work done up to now on manifestations of aphasia in Basque speaking subjects is Erriondo Korostola (1995); the corpus examined in this paper is taken from this seminal work. We have studied records of spontaneous speech of 59 subjects with cerebral damage that caused aphasia. The spontaneous speech of these subjects varies widely: some are rather fluent, with few errors, and others are almost incapable of producing syntactically connected sequences.

The subjects studied in this corpus had been patients in various hospitals of the Basque country, during 1986 and 1989, and had some form of cerebral damage; most of them were originally not diagnosed with aphasia.. 25 subjects were diagnosed with aphasia; eight of them were diagnosed as Broca, and nine of them as Wernicke. Nine subjects were diagnosed as having global aphasia, three as having symptoms of anomia, and one as having transcortical aphasia. In 46 cases were aphasia was originally not diagnosed, the clinical history of the patients contains information concerning the cerebral hemisphere that was damaged; out of these 46 patients, 39 had damage in the left hemisphere, one had right hemisphere damage and six of them had lesions in both hemispheres.

The age distribution of the subjects is as follows: three subjects belong in the 0-19 age group, two male and a female. Two subjects belong in the 30-39 age group, male and female. In the 40-49 age group there is one male subject. There are thirteen subjects in the 50-59 age group, ten male and three female. "3 subjects belong in the 60-69 age group, seventeen male and six female. Twelve subjects belong in the 70-79 age group, nine male and three female. Finally, there are five subjects in the 80-89 age group, two male and three female.

All subjects in this corpus are bilingual; 55 of them have Basque as their native language, and Spanish as their second language. The remaining four have Spanish as their native language and Basque as their second language.

The subjects were interviewed at different times since their original lesion, ranging from a day, a month and eleven months from the time of the lesion. 13,5% of the subjects were interviewed around two years after the lesion; 10,1% of the subjects were interviewed seven months after the lesion; 8,5% five moths after, 6,8% within a month after the lesion. There are three subjects (5,1%) who were interviewed fifteen months after the lesion, and two subjects (3,4%) who were interviewed after a month.

Given the fact that the paper concentrates on symptoms of agrammatism, we have ignored deficits that are clearly phonological. Whenever a piece of data could be interpreted as mispronunciation rather than an effect of agrammatism, it has been discarded for the purpose of this discussion.

2. A brief description of Basque grammar

Since our discussion on the data from aphasic patients will concentrate on agrammatism, our description will focus on aspects of Basque grammar directly related to the phenomena under discussion. Laka (1996), a document available at <http://www. ehu.es/grammar>, contains an general overview of the language, in a broader and more accessible format. Whenever relevant, the interested reader is referred to particular points of that hypertext document for details.

Basque (or Euskara, as it is known to its speakers) is an isolate language; it does not pertain to any known language family. Typologically, Basque is an SOV language, of the agglutinative type. It has overt case markers and rich inflectional morphology, including up to three agreement markers on the inflected verb (subject, object and dative agreement). Euskara is a free-word order language, with a preverbal position for the focus of the sentence. Basque is an ergative language; that is, subjects of intransitive clauses and objects of transitive clauses are morphologically identical, while subjects of transitive clauses are morphologically distinct, bearing ergative case (Levin (1983), Ortiz de Urbina (1989)).

2.1 Basic elements of the sentence.

A declarative sentence in Euskara contains: a main verb and its arguments, an aspect marker attached to the main verb, and an auxiliary verb, which contains agreement morphemes, tense and modality markers and an attached complementizer in the case of embedded sentences. It can also contain other phrases, such as adverbials or postpositional phrases. Examples are provided in (1):

(1) a. ume-a kale-an eror-i da
child-the street-in fall-asp is
'the child fell in the street'

b. emakume-a-k gizon-a ikus-i du
woman-the-erg man-the see-asp has-him
'the woman has seen the man'

c. gizon-a-k ume-a-ri liburu-a ema-n dio
man-the-erg child-the-dat book-the given has-it-tohim
'the man has given the book to the child'

(For the purposes of this initial description, the gloss is notional rather than grammatical. As the discussion proceeds, they will be substituted by the grammatical gloss; thus, for instance, the inflected verb glossed as "is" in (1), will eventually appear glossed as "3rd-be", or the determiner *-a*, glossed here as "the", will eventually be glossed as "det".)

In (1a), the sentence is constructed with the intransitive verb *erori* 'to fall'. The verb is marked for perfective aspect with the morpheme *i*; it denotes a completed event. The auxiliary verb is *da*, a form of *izan* 'to be', which is inflected for present tense, third person singular. The subject *umea* 'the child' is marked with absolutive case, which bears a zero morpheme, that is, no manifest ending for the case. There is also a locative postpositional phrase *kalean* 'in the street'. The word order in (1a) is said to be neutral, that is, the sentence in (1a) is a natural answer to a question such as *zer gertatu da?* 'what happened?'. In other words, the entire sentence is informationally relevant.

In (1b), the sentence is constructed with a transitive verb, *ikusi* 'to see', which has the perfective aspectual morpheme *i* attached. The auxiliary verb is a form of *ukan* 'have', inflected for present tense, third person subject, and third person object. The subject *emakumea* 'the woman' is marked for ergative case (morpheme *k*), and the object *gizona* 'the man' is case marked absolutive (morpheme zero). The word order in (1b) is neutral.

In (1c), the sentence contains a ditransitive verb, *eman* 'give', which has a variant of the perfective aspectual morpheme, namely, the final *-n* on the verb. The auxiliary verb carries the Inflection, which in this case is specified for present tense, third person object, third person dative and third person subject. The subject *gizona* is marked for ergative case (morpheme *k*), the dative phrase is marked for dative case (morpheme *i*) and the object is marked for absolutive case (morpheme zero). The word order in (1c) is neutral. The neutral order of phrases in the sentence is schematized in (2):

(2) [Ergative Noun Phrase] [Dative NP] [Absolutive NP] [verb + auxiliary]

That is, given the language typology proposed by Greenberg (1963), (1978), Euskara is a Subject-Object-Verb (SOV) type language (de Rijk (1969)). Within the Government & Binding Theory (henceforth GB), Basque is a Head-final grammar: the syntactic head of phrases appears at the end of the phrase (Ortiz de Urbina (1989)). Regarding constituents that do not agree with verbal inflection, such as adverbs and postpositional phrases, it is not as clear what the neutral word order is. For instance, the EGLU grammar provides example (3) as neutral word order, where the locative phrase *San Martin kalean* 'in San Martin street', follows the verb. :

(3) duela bi ordu sekulako istripua izan da San Martin kale-an
ago two hours huge accident been is Saint Martin street-in
'there has been a huge accident in Saint Martin street two hours ago'

Euskara is a 'free word order' language; this means that the order of phrases (not really the words) in the sentence can vary. Some of these variations yield different informational patterns. Consider sentence (1a) above. The variations on the order of phrases of (1a) shown in (4) are all possible:

(4) a. kalean umea erori da
street-in child-the fallen is
"The child fell on the street"

b. umea erori da kalean
c. kalean erori da umea

Sentences with initial verb and auxiliary are also possible, as shown in (5a, b).

(5) a. erori da umea kalean
fallen is child-the street-in

b. erori da kalean umea

where the order of the phrases following the [verb+auxiliary] complex allows for variation as well, as shown in (5b). Leaving aside neutral word orders like the ones shown in (1), the phrase immediately preceding the main verb is interpreted as the focus of the sentence, the informationally relevant phrase. That is, Basque has a preverbal focus position.

The Noun Phrases (henceforth NPs) that agree with the verb need not be overtly manifest in the sentence: Ergative, dative and absolutive NPs can be absent and understood. In terms of Government and Binding theory, Basque is a *pro*-drop language, like Spanish or Italian. In (6a), we repeat example (1c), a sentence with ergative, dative and absolutive NPs, in order to illustrate the absence of verbal arguments:

(6) a. gizonak umeari liburua eman dio
man-the-E child-the-D book-the given has
'the man has given the book to the child'

b. umeari liburua eman dio
child-the-D book-the given has
'(someone) gave a book to the child'

c. gizonak liburua eman dio
man-the-E book-the given has
'the man gave a book (to someone)'

d. gizonak umeari eman dio
man-the-E man-the-D given has
'the man gave (something) to the child'

e. eman dio
given has
'(someone) gave (something) (to someone)'

In example (6b), the ergative NP has been omitted. It is understood that someone gave a book to the child. In (6c), the dative NP is omitted. It is understood that the man gave a book to someone. In (6d), the absolutive NP is omitted. It is understood that the man gave something to the child. More than one of these arguments can be omitted simultaneously, as shown in (6e), where all three are absent, and understood.

It should be kept in mind that the possibility of *pro*-dropping all three verbal arguments is often used in actual speech; in fact, it is usually the case that only informationally relevant NPs are expressed overtly if they belong to the agreeing group. This fact makes the frequency of overt subjects, objects or dative arguments much lower than in languages such as English which do not have this possibility. The relative low frequency of overt NP arguments must be kept in mind when considering the relative low frequency of deficits in nominal case morphology found in the corpus.

2.2. Case Morphology

There are three grammatical cases in Euskara: Ergative, dative and absolutive. NPs bears absolutive case under two conditions: (a) if it is the subject of an intransitive verb, as shown in (7a); (b) if it is the object of a transitive verb, as shown in (7b).

(7) a. **otso-a** etorri da
wolf-the-A arrived is
'The wolf has arrived'

b. ehiztari-a-k **otso-a** harrapatu du
hunter-the-E wolf-the-A caught has-it
'the hunter has caught the wolf'

Absolutive case is morphologically null, that is, there is no overt morpheme for this case. Absolutive case is glossed A in these examples.

NPs bear ergative case if they are subjects of transitive verbs, as shown in (8):

(8) **zazpi gizon-ek** piano-a ekarri dute
seven man-E piano-the-A brought have-it
'seven men have brought the piano'

There is a small set of verbs that require ergative subjects, despite the fact that they do not appear to be transitives. Most of them are agentive predicates. Sentence (9) illustrates one example, the verb *iraun* 'to remain', which does not fall clearly in the agentive category:

(9) gure etxeak zutik irauten du
our house-det-E standing remain-impf has
'our house remains standing'

Dative case is assigned to indirect objects (benefactives, goals):

(10) etxe-ko **txakurr-a-ri** hezur bat eman diozu
house-of dog-det-D bone one given have-it-to him-you
'You have given a bone to the dog of the house'

Some diadic verbs require that one argument be marked with dative case. An example is shown in (11), with the verb ekin 'to start on, to engage on' :

(11) lanari ekin behar diogu
work-det-D engage must have-it-we
'we must engage in work'

Although Basque is often described as having declensions, much like Latin, it is by now agreed that the concept of declension is rather misleading in order to describe the language (Eguzkitza (1977)). Euskara's morphology works rather like a child's construction game: constituents are constructed by attaching elements, typically at the end of the previous phrase. This way of constructing phrases by attaching morphemes is known as *agglutination.* Euskara is therefore an agglutinative language. This agglutinative strategy is used to mark NPs with case, as shown above, and this strategy is maintained when building postpositional phrases. Let us consider a couple of examples:

(12) a. [Bilboko kale bat]ean
[Bilbo-of street one]in
'in one street of Bilbao'

b. [zazpi leiho]tatik
[seven window]from
'from seven windows'

In (12a), the locative postposition has been attached to the last word of the Noun Phrase in brackets, the numeral *bat* 'one', but it is the entire NP that the postposition takes as its complements, as the bracketed structure indicates. Similarly, in (12b), the postposition is attached to the last word of its complement NP, in this case the noun *leiho* 'window'.

2.3. Verbal Inflection.

Inflection, the category that manifests itself as the auxiliary verb in Basque, is comparatively complex. This might help understand why the vast majority of symptoms of agrammatism in this language involve the inflected auxiliary. Inflectional morphology in Basque contains: (a) Agreement with ergative, dative and absolutive Noun Phrases; (b) Tense: present past or irrealis; (c) Modality: potentials and conditionals; (d) Complementizer: whether the auxiliary belongs to an embedded sentence, and what type; (e) In some varieties and registers, Inflection includes an agreement marker for the person addressed in the speech (addressee agreement).

The morphological combinations of these four or five categories yield a wide array of auxiliary forms. For a detailed account of the structure of verbal inflection in Basque, see *<http://www.ehu.es/grammar>*, in particular chapter 5, which is entirely devoted to the structure of Inflection, and to showing step by step how the auxiliary system works. Schematically, the order of morphemes in the auxiliary verb is as shown in (13):

(13) absolutive+auxiliary root+dative +modal+ergative+tense+complementizer

There is an additional marker for the plurality of the object, which surfaces in different positions depending on the type of auxiliary or the variety of the language. Given the array in (13), the plural marker for the object can appear either before the root or immediately after, or immediately preceding the tense morpheme in some varieties. As it will be shown in section 3.2., one salient deficit found in aphasic speech involves the absence of this plural marker when required.

Basque displays auxiliary selection: In general terms, the root of the auxiliary ukan 'to have' is used when there is ergative agreement in the auxiliary form. Otherwise, the root of the verb *izan* 'to be' is used. We illustrate this contrast in (14):

(14) a. igela agertu da
frog-the appeared is
'the frog has appeared'

b. Josebak igela ikusi du
Joseba-E frog-the seen has
'Joseba has seen the frog'

As the pair illustrates, an intransitive sentence with no ergative phrase like (14a) selects a form of the auxiliary *izan* 'to be', in this case a present tense third person singular form. However, a sentence with an ergative phrase, such as (14b) selects a form of the auxiliary *ukan* 'to have', in this case a present tense third person singular subject and third person singular object.

3. Symptoms of agrammatism in Basque

Most symptoms of agrammatism manifested in this corpus of spontaneous production of aphasic subjects in Basque, are related to deficits in morphology, and more specifically, in inflectional morphology (mainly auxiliary verbs, and less frequently case endings). From the standpoint of grammatical structure, and given the data available in this corpus, it can be claimed that the most outstanding symptom of agrammatism in Basque involves a deficit in the production of the syntactic category Infl, which contains tense and agreement morphology. In terms of GB Theory (Chomsky (1981), Infl is the head of IP (Inflectional Phrase), which is in turn the syntactic projection of the sentence. Thus, the main symptom of agrammatism in Basque involves deficits in the production of the syntactic head of the sentence. We have not detected clear deficits in word order, a fact that is not surprising given the free-word order nature of this language. This does not necessarily mean that those errors do not surface, but rather, that they are extremely hard to detect in a free word order language simply by observation of spontaneous speech production.

Before entering our discussion of the data, a few considerations are in order, about the way in which the data are presented. Spoken Basque presents a wide variety of different linguistic varieties; the standard language currently used for education and writing was created in the second half of the XXth century, and most speakers do not use it in everyday speech. Hence, our corpus contains examples from many different spoken varieties. In order to make the significant aspects of the data more readily available, irrelevant variations have been omitted, and we have adapted the oral record to the standard version, whenever it did not interfere with the exposition of the deficit under discussion.

3.1. Deficits in the production of Inflection: missing auxiliaries.

One of the most salient symptoms found in the corpus is the low frequency of auxiliary verbs in spontaneous speech of aphasics. Some of the subjects present spontaneous speech completely lacking inflected verbal forms; such is the case of subjects 5, 50 and 57 for instance. These subjects present a form of speech which is relatively fluent, but where the verbs are always uninflected participial forms, or nominalizations of the lexical verb. Sometimes, lack of inflected verbs yields ungrammatical outputs, as in example (15) below, but sometimes the output is not clearly ungrammatical, as in example (16), because it resembles a process of auxiliary deletion that is available in the language. However, even when the output cannot be categorized as clearly ungrammatical if taken sentence by sentence, the high frequency of participial forms lacking inflected auxiliaries renders the speech anomalous, as in (16). The examples in (15) and (16) illustrate this type of symptom: the words highlighted in the utterances from aphasic speech are verbal participles or nominalizations of verbs, all of which lack inflectional morphology.

(15) ba ni zapata hone-kin nen-go-en etxe-an
well I shoe these-with 3rd/pst-be-pst home-loc
"well, I was home with these shoes"

ba ni zabata honeki ba **egon** etxe-an
well I shoe these-with well been home-loc (subject 50)

Throughout the paper, the examples present first the target sentence, that is, the sentence presumably intended by the subject in its grammatical form, with glosses and translation, followed underneath by the actual utterance produced by the subject.

In (15), the verbal perfective participle produced is *egon* 'to stay'; the target sentence contains an inflected form of this verb, *nengoen*, although it would also be possible to create a grammatical sentence by combining the perfective participle with an auxiliary verb, denoting a different aspectual relation (as it has been described in the previous section). In any instance, the aphasic utterance in (15) is ungrammatical because it lacks inflectional morphology completely. From the standpoint of linguistic theory, the sentence is ungrammatical because it lacks any sort of overt specification for the category Infl, the head of the syntactic phrase corresponding to a full sentence.

Consider now the example in (16), which is not clearly ungrammatical, although it pushes to its limits a phenomenon available in Basque grammar. The example displays a series of verbal participles in a chain. The patient is answering a question about what it is he does in the morning:

(16) pix-a egi-te-a lenengoa, arpegia garbitu ta komunera joan da gero gosaldu
pee-det do-nom-det first face-det wash-prf and bathroom-to go-prf and then have-breakfast
"First to pee, yes then wash (my) face and go to the bathroom and then to have breakfast"

pixa **egitea** lehenengoa, bai arpegia **garbitu** ta komunera **joan** da gero **gosaldu**
pee do-to first-the, yes face-the wash and bathroom-to go and later have-breakfast (subject 5)

In (16), the first form, *egitea,* is a nominalization of the ver *egin* 'to do'. The subsequent verb forms are all perfective participles: *garbitu* "to wash", *joan* "to go", *gosaldu* "to have breakfast". The utterance in (16) is not sharply ungrammatical, because Basque has a phenomenon of auxiliary deletion (Amundarain (1997)), illustrated in (17):

(17) etxera **etorri**, mahaian **jezarri**, eta **afaldu** zuen
home arrived, table-at sat, and dined 3rd-root-pst
"She arrived home, sat at the table, and dined"

This phenomenon of auxiliary deletion is legitimate when the auxiliaries corresponding to each participle are similar enough. In the case in (17), for instance, they share all relevant morphological features: person, number, and tense. The difference between (16) and (17) is that (16) lacks inflected auxiliaries completely, thus rendering the utterances anomalous, even though it is possible to rescue the complete meaning, given the fact that the question to which the subject replies did contain an inflected auxiliary.

Thus, in many cases, aphasic speech yields sequences that are not strictly ungrammatical, but it must be pointed out that the frequency of perfective participles relative to the frequency of inflected auxiliaries is much higher than in colloquial speech, where constructions like (17) are common. Examples of this high frequency of uninflected participles are found throughout in the corpus, even in subjects with relatively fluent speech, such as subject 5, from example (16).

3.2. *Deficits in the production of Inflection: ungrammatical auxiliary forms.*
Within the general symptom of deficits in the production of inflectional morphology, spontaneous speech of Basque aphasics presents auxiliary forms that are not grammatical in the sentences where they appear, although the forms themselves are well-formed. The ungrammaticality of the forms produced results from a mismatch of person and/or number features: either because they do not contain plural markers in cases where the object of the sentence is plural, or because the agreement markers do not match the features corresponding to the Noun Phrase they should agree with. We have not found examples where the ungrammaticality of the form was due to a mismatch in tense specifications.

(a) Number agreement deficits. Example (18), from subject 42, illustrates this symptom. The auxiliary forms are well formed, but not grammatical for the sentence where they appear, because they lack plural markers for the object:

(18) a. hitz-ak nahas-i egi-ten d-it-u-t
word-det$_{pl}$ mix-perf do-impf 3rd-pl-root-1st
"I mix the words"

hitz-ak nahas-i egi-ten **d-u-t**
word-det$_{pl}$ mix-perf do-impf 3rd-root-1st (subject 42)

b. bakarrikan euskera-z d-aki-zki-t abesti-ak
only Basque-ins 3rd-know-pl-1st song-det$_{pl}$
"I only know the songs in Basque"

bakarrikan euskera-z **d-aki-t** abesti-ak
only Basque-inst 3rd-know-1st song-det$_{pl}$ (subject 4)

In (18a), the inflected form that appears in the aphasic speech is *d-u-t*, which would be grammatical for a sentence with a singular object. A sentence containing a plural object like the one exemplified in (18a) requires the auxiliary form *d-it-u-t* "I have them", where the plural marker *it* is inserted after the object agreement marker and before the root of the auxiliary verb *ukan* "to have". In (18b), the inflected form produced is *d-aki-t* "I know it", and the grammatical form for the target sentence should have been *d-aki-zki-t* "I know them". Again, the plural marker for the object, in this case the morpheme *zki*, has been ommited.

Another instance of this symptom is found in example (19):

(19) ema-ten d-i-zki-zu beste lau karamelo
give-impf 3rd-root-pl-2nd other four sweet
"they give you four more sweets"

ema-ten **d-i-zu** beste lau karamelo
give-impf 3rd-root-2nd other four sweet (subject 22)

This example contains the imperfective participle *ematen* "giving", and a tripersonal auxiliary form *dizu* "it-have-you-someone" highlighted in bold, which is not grammatical for this sentence, given the plural nature of the object. In (19), as in the previous example (18b), the auxiliary should contain the plural morpheme, *zki*, shown in the target sentence.

All errors involving number agreement involve forms lacking the plural morpheme for third person object. There are no instances in the corpus where the subjects produce forms with plural morphemes that are not required (with the only possible exception of example (26), which contains an extra plural marker even though there is not third person involved). Although the number of errors involving missing plural markers is not very large in absolute terms, it is nevertheless one of the most frequent type of error involving ungrammatical auxiliary forms.

From the perspective of the grammatical structure of Basque, the morphemes involved in this type of error, that is, the plural markers for the object, are rather peculiar in their behavior within the structure of Inflection: (a) they are the only morphemes that display different positions in different varieties of the language; (b) there are varieties of the language that do not have them at all (which is not the case of the variety spoken by subjects 42 and 22); (c) they behave as separate from the person agreement paradigm, and are thus not affected by morphological phenomena that apply to third person agreement markers. From the standpoint of the morphological structure of Inflection in Basque, plural markers of the type illustrated in (18) and (19) are autonomous from person agreement, and behave as if they were less central to the structure of Inflection than person and tense morphemes (Laka (1993), (1996)). It has been argued (Laka (1993)) that these morphemes are in fact adjuncts in the structure of the inflected forms in Basque; that is, structurally they would have the same status as non-subcategorized adverbial phrases have in the structure of the sentence, as opposed to the status of subcategorized arguments.

(b) Dative Agreement: third person instead of first person. These type of deficit surfaces in a variety of auxiliary forms involving dative markers. The subjects produce third person dative agreement markers, instead of the required first person singular dative agreement morpheme. Let us consider some instances of this symptom:

(20) a. mareoa bezela egin z-i-da-n
dizziness like do-prf 3rd/pst-root-1st-pst
"It sort of made me dizzy"

mareoa bezela egin **z-i-e-n**
dizziness like do-prf 3rd/pst-root-3pl-pst (subject 9)

b. hau dena hilda bezela geratu z-i-tzai-da-n
this all dead like stay-prf 3rd-root-1st-pst
"All this went like dead on me"

hau dena hilda bezela geratu **z-i-e-n**
this all dead like stay-prf 3rd-root-3pl-past (subject 9)

In (20a), the target auxiliary is a tripersonal form, containing a 3rd person singular object/absolutive marker, a first person singular dative marker, and a third person singular subject/ergative marker. The form produced by the subject contains what looks like a third person dative morpheme, *-e-*, instead of the first person marker. It is clear in the discourse that the intended form is *z-i-da-n*, with a first person singular dative agreement marker *da* "to me" which refers to the patient, who is describing the symptoms of his illness.

There is however one caveat we must make regarding example (20a): it has been pointed out to us (Ezeizabarrena p.c.) that in the general area this subject comes from, there is a variety were the standard from *zidan* can be phonologically reduced to *zien* or *zin*. Even if the subject were producing a grammatical form in (20a) given his native variety, the second example from his spontaneous speech, (20b) displays a clear deficit, and this is the ultimate reason that leads us to consider (20a) as an error.

In (20b), the same auxiliary form appears, constructed with third person agreement markers only. In this example, the target form is an intransitive form, containing a first person dative agreement marker. The produced form is transitive, as the different roots illustrate, and the dative marker is a third person plural morpheme *-e-*.

Consider more examples of more inflectional deficits, also involving dative agreement markers:

(21) a. ni-ri gaixo-ak gusta-tzen j-a-t-az-an
I-dat patient-det$_{pl}$ like-impf 3rd-root-1st-pl-pst
"I liked patients"

ni-ri gaixo-ak gusta-tzen **j-a-ko-n**
I-dat patient-det$_{pl}$ like-impf 3rd-root-3rd-pst (subject 20)

b. esan eu-st-e-n aste betera joa-teko
say-prf 3rd-root/1st-pl-pst week full-in go-to
"they told me to go in a week's time"

esa-u-tze-n ea, aste betera joateko
said-3rd-root/3rd-pl-past eh, week full-in go-to (subject 20)

In these utterances, as in the previous examples, the subject produces inflected forms with a third person dative agreement marker, instead of a first person dative, even though they refer to themselves in the discourse. It is clear that the target form is a first person singular dative in this case, given the context in which this form appears; the patient is talking about her illness. In fact, in the discourse of this subject, the examples selected above in (21) appear next to forms with the correct first person dative agreement markers, one of which, immediately preceding example (21b), is displayed in italics in example (22):

(22) ordun baja emon *z-i-da-te-n-* eta ...
then leave give-prf 3rd/pst-root-1st-3rdpl-pst
"then they gave me a sick leave and ..." (subject 20)

This deficit in the production of agreement markers appears to fit with a well known claim in Linguistic Theory: third person agreement markers have widely been argued to constitute the unmarked forms or "zero forms" in verb-paradigms of many human languages. Specifically for the case of Basque, it has been argued that there are no actual forms for third person agreement, and that the markers glossed as third person are in fact null in their initial representations (Laka 1993). Thus, it seems that the deficit involves the production of the empty form in the paradigm, instead of a form with content, in this case the first person marker. The fact that we do not have examples of second person markers missing is probably not significant: in this corpus, the subjects are mostly talking about themselves, their experiences and feelings. They are not addressing the hearer, and thus there are hardly any forms containing second person agreement markers.

Regarding the nature of dative agreement morphology, and if we were to speculate as for the motives why it is that all examples of errors in agreement markers found in the corpus involve exclusively dative makers, it is tempting to bring into the discussion two observations: The first one is typological, and the second one concerns the history of the dative agreement paradigm of Basque. Typologically, it is well known that grammars with dative agreement markers incorporated onto verbal inflection are very rare among human languages. One of the implicational universals proposed by Greenberg (1963), (1978), sets dative agreement at the top of a hierarchy: if a language has dative agreement, then it has object agreement as well. Moreover, if a language has object agreement, then it has subject agreement as well. Although it is not clear whether this typological implication has any bearing on the internal organization of a given grammar, such as the grammar of Basque, it appears to fit with the findings from this corpus, since it is only dative agreement that appears affected with a high frequency.

From the standpoint of the historical evolution of the verbal paradigm of Basque, it has been claimed (de Rijk (1981)) that the dative paradigm is the latest addition to the structure of Inflection in this language. This claim is based on the morphological peculiarities of the dative agreement paradigm, and its similarities with the demonstrative system of the Noun Phrase. Finally, it is also suggestive to consider that there are eastern varieties of Basque (not spoken by the subjects whose speech we have illustrated here), where dative agreement can be optionally absent under certain conditions, but there are no varieties of the language where object or subject agreement can be absent. In a sense that can only be impressionistic at the moment, it appears that the high frequency of this deficit is somehow linked to the relative "markedness" of dative agreement in the inflectional system.

(c) Transitive auxiliaries instead of intransitive auxiliaries: The data in the corpus show instances of transitive auxiliary forms (*have* auxiliaries) attached to verbs that require intransitive auxiliaries (*be* auxiliaries). We have found no instances where intransitive auxiliaries surface instead of transitive auxiliaries. Consider the following two examples:

(23) hare-kin joa-ten gara
that-with go-impf 1stpl/be
"we go with that one"

hare-kin joa-ten **d-u-gu**
that-with go-impf 3rd-have-1stpl (subject 1)

In (23), the subject uses a transitive "have" auxiliary for the intransitive verb *joan* "to go", which selects a "be" type auxiliary, as shown in the target sentence. In errors like this, it is difficult to ascertain whether the error concerns strictly the selection of the auxiliary, or whether it also implies an error in the assignation of case to the arguments of the sentence, a type of error we discuss in section 3.2. The reason why this is hard to asses is because NPs need not be overt in Basque; thus, for instance, in (23), we fail to see any overt NP corresponding to the subject of the sentence, and we cannot see whether it is marked with ergative case, as we do in the examples in section 3.2. We can only assert that the auxiliary form is transitive instead of intransitive.

Example (24) illustrates another instance of this type of error:

(24) ta gero jausi egiten dira lurrera
and then fall-prf do-impf 3rdpl/be ground-to
"and then they fall on the ground"

ta gero jausi egiten **dabe** lurrera
and then fall-prf do-impf 3rd-root-3rdpl ground-to (subject 58)

In (24), once again we find a transitive auxiliary form *dabe* (from the Biscayan variety) "they have it", instead of the intransitive "be" form, *dira* "they are" shown in the target sentence. The verb is the unaccusative predicate *jausi* "to fall", which selects intransitive auxiliaries. The imperfective form of the verb *egin* "to do" is used here as an emphatic device, and does not change the valence of the sentence. As in the previous example, it cannot be said whether this error is also an instance of mistaken case marking, since there are no overt NPs whose case can be determined, but it is plausible that the subject is turning the entire sentence into a transitive format, and not only the auxiliary form. If this were the case, this deficit could be merged with errors in case marking like the ones illustrated in section 2.3.

Finally, consider (25), where there is a failure to produce an intransitive form in the progressive aspect:

(25) idaz-ten n-u-en hitz-eta-n pentsa-tzen ari n-intz-en hitz-ak
write-impf 1st/pst-root-pst word-pl-loc think-impf prog 1st-be/pst-pst/comp word-det_{pl}
"I wrote in words the words that I was thinking"

idaz-ten n-u-en hitz-eta-n pentsa-tzen ari **n-it-u-en** hitz-ak
write-impf 1st/pst-root-pst word-pl-loc think-impf progr 1st-pl-have-pst/comp word-det_{pl} (subject 18)

In (25), the subject produces a transitive form, *nituen* "I had them", which is not grammatical in the progressive construction. This type of progressive, marked by the element *ari*, requires an intransitive auxiliary, regardless of the type of lexical verb heading the sentence. In this example, for instance, the verb *pentsatu* "to think" requires a transitive auxiliary, but the presence of the progressive marker *ari* turns the sentence into an intransitive format. The subject appears to have failed to satisfy the requirements of the progressive. Interestingly, this last type of error does occur, occasionally, in child-language, during the acquisition of the progressive form, and there are certain varieties of Basque were this type of progressive allows transitive forms (Ezeizabarrena p.c.).

3.1.3. Inflectional deficits: neologisms in auxiliary forms.

A third main type of symptom that appears frequently in aphasic speech in Basque, also involving Inflection, is the creation of impossible auxiliaries, or neologisms in the class of inflected verbs. These newly coined forms often result from combining morphemes from conflicting paradigms, but the order of morphemes in the forms tends to be correct. Consider the following examples:

(26) a. zelatan nen-go-en?
how 1st/pst-be-pst
"How was I?"

zelatan **nen-go-ez-en**?
how 1st/pst-be-pl-pst (subject 57)

b. nik zazpi seme-alaba dauzkat, horrenbeste urte dauzkate
I-erg seven son-daughter 3rd-root-pl-1st that-many year 3rd-pl-root-3rdpl
"I have seven children, they have so many years"

ba nik se zazpi seme-alaba dauzkat....**dauza**...urte
well I se seven son-daughter 3rd-root-pl-1st.....3rd-root-pl...year (subject 53)

In (26a), the auxiliary form combines an agreement morpheme from the singular paradigm (*nen-* is a first person singular absolutive agreement marker for the past tense paradigm) with a plural marker *ez*, which results in an impossible form, although the morphemes are recognizable. The possible and grammatical form, *nen-go-en* "I was", excludes the plural marker, which is not required for the first person singular.

In (26b), the first inflected form is correct, *dauzkat* "I have them", but the second one, highlighted in bold, is not. It combines the object marker *da-* and a plural marker for the object, *-z-*, which is appropriate since the subject is talking about her children, but the root of the verb is ill formed; it should contain *ka*, for the verb *eduki* "to have" that means possession. Finally, either the form is missing the agreement marker for the ergative subject, which should presumably be a third person plural (she is talking about her children's' age, which is conveyed as possessing a given number of years), or it surfaces as a third person singular, a zero morpheme.

More examples of impossible auxiliaries are found in subject 52:

(27) a. erraminta trankila ge-unka-n
tool quiet-det 1stpl-root-pst
"we had quiet tools"

erraminta trankila **ge-u-n**
tool quiet 1stpl-root-pst

b. eta gero graziak etorri gin-e-la
and later thank-pl come-prf 1stpl-be-pst/comp
"and then thank (God) we arrived"

eta gero graziak etorri **gin-e-n-la**
and later thank-pl come 1stpl-be-pst-comp

c. eta medikuak denak ze-ude-n han
and doctor-pl all-pl 3rd-root/pl-pst there
"and the doctors were all there"

eta mediku-ak den-ak **ne-ude-n** han
and doctors-pl all-pl 1st-root/pl-past there

d. eta ikus-i z-u-an dena mekauen Don Isidro-k
and see-prf 3rd-root-pst all shit Mr. Isidro-erg
"and Mr. Isidro, shit, saw everything"

èta ikusi **u-an** dana mekauen Don Isidro-k
and see-prf root-pst all shit Mr. Isidro-erg

The array of examples in (27), are all impossible auxiliaries. The first form, in (27a), contains a first person plural subject marker, and a past tense morpheme, but the root of the verb is not appropriate in this paradigm. Given the western variety spoken by this subject, the correct form is either *gendun* "we had it" or *geunkan* "we possessed it". Notice that the only affected part of the auxiliary is the choice of root, while the agreement and tense markers are appropriate. Example (27d) is morphologically identical in this sense: the form is wrong in the choice of verbal root, but it contains a third person singular agreement marker (zero morpheme) and a past tense that are identifiable and well-placed.

Example (27b) is particularly interesting from a linguistic point of view, because the impossible form that surfaces, *ginenla*, is the underlying form of the correct auxiliary, *ginela* "that we were", before the application of a phonological rule that turns the sequence */nl/* into */l/*. The past tense form of the first person plural of the copula is indeed *ginen*, and the addition of the complementizer *la* "that" yields the underlying form *ginenla*, to which the deletion rule applies. It would appear that the subject has ommited the application of this phonological rule.

Finally, example (27c) shows an impossible auxiliary that combines an agreement marker from the singular paradigm, *ne*, a first person singular morpheme, with a root from the plural paradigm *ude*, much like the previous example in (26a), where first person singular was also combined with a plural marker. However, in this case, the intended meaning is "they were", and thus the error lies in the choice of agreement marker, and not of the plural root. The target form is *ze-ude-n* "they were".

All impossible auxiliaries found in the corpus present a well-formed order of morphemes. That is, there are no cases of impossible auxiliaries were the output presents morphemes in an order different from the canonical one. This is particularly noteworthy in the some past tense forms involving ergative agreement markers, where the canonical order given in (13) is altered, and the ergative agreement appears at the beginning of the auxiliary and not at the end (this phenomenon is known as *ergative displacement;* for a description, see chapter 5 of the Internet grammar, section 1.3.1., "Past tense and ergative agreement", or see Laka (1993)). Acquisition data show that children often produce forms where the displacement of the ergative has not taken place (Ezeizabarrena (1996)), but we have not found forms in the corpus where subjects failed to locate the ergative agreement marker at the beginning of the form, whenever this had to be done. Thus, for instance, the impossible form in (27a) correctly displays an initial agreement marker corresponding to the ergative subject of the sentence.

Similarly, in (28a), we find an ill-formed auxiliary involving past tense and ergative marking. Once again, the subject has not failed to locate the ergative agreement at the beginning of the auxiliary (which is not the canonical location, except for these type of transitive and past tense forms), but the auxiliary is impossible because the choice of root is not correct:

(28) a. Franko-ri egin gen-izk-i-o-n egun bat-ean bigote-ak
Franco-dat do/prf 3rdpl/pst-pl-root-3rd-pst day one-loc moustache-det$_{pl}$
"One day we did (painted) a moustache on Franco"

Franko-ri egin **gin-tza-n** egun bat-ean bigote-ak
Franco-dat do/prf 3rdpl/pst-root-pst day one-loc moustache-det$_{pl}$ (subject 1)

b. zergatik ni-re ama-k esa-ten z-i-da-n den-etik ikas-i behar zela
because I-gen mother-erg say-impf 3rd-root-1st-pst all-from learn-prf must
"because my mother told me that one must learn from everything"

zergatik nire ama-k esa-ten **na-u-n** ba denetik ikasi behar zela
because I-gen mother-rg say-impf 1st-root-pst well all-from learn-prf must
(subject 20)

The utterance in (28b) contains a form composed of: first person absolutive of the present tense paradigm, *na*, followed by the root of the transitive verb *ukan*, *-u-*, and followed by the past tense morpheme *-n*. The target form, as shown above is one with third person subject and first person dative, combined with the auxiliary root for tripersonal forms, *-i-*. In the inflected form produced by the patient, the dative marker does not surface, and instead, first person agreement surfaces in the absolutive. It appears that the subject is producing a form with *ergative displacement* (that is, a form where the agreement corresponding to the transitive subject appears in the first position within the auxiliary), but where the fronting of the agreement marker has affected the first person dative marker.

However, there is another possible account of (28b): the form *naun* could also be a present tense transitive form *nau* "(s/he) has me" to which the past tense marker *-n* has been attached. This type of forms, containing present tense morphology (in the agreement markers and choice of root), and a past tense marker attached appear rather frequently in acquisition data (Barreña (1993), Ezeizabarrena (1996)).

Consider now the utterance in (29). In the example, we provide a first line of context from the subject's discourse, from which it can be seen that he is talking about himself and his illness. In the next line we provide some context for the actual utterance that contains the newly coined auxiliary form:

(29) eta gero behin joan nintzen eta arnas estua neukan
and later once go-impf 1st/pst-be-pst and breath short-det 1st/pst-root-pst
"and then once I went and I had short breath

eta esa-n z-i-da-te-n ez egi-teko lan-ik eta orduan baja ema-n z-i-da-te-n
and say-prf 3rd/pst-root-1st-3rdpl-pst not do-to work-prt and then leave give-prf 3rd/pst-root-1st-3rdpl-pst
and they told me not to work and they gave me sick-leave"

eta esan **n-itx-en** ez egite-ko lan-ik eta orduan baja eman z-i-te-n
and say-prf 1st-root-pst not do-to work-prt and then leave give-perf 3rd/pst-root 3rdpl-pst (subject 20)

In (29), the subject is narrating the events around his illness, and in this narration the highlighted impossible form surfaces, *nitxen*, where a first person agreement marker *n* can be identified, perhaps intended as a dative marker, but placed in a position where it can only correspond to a subject or an object first person. Following the agreement morpheme, there is the element *-itx-*, which could be intended as a tripersonal root *-i-*, or as the past tense root of the intransitive auxiliary, *-intz-*. In any case, the form is an impossible one.

Finally, from the same subject, we have the following example:

(30) orain ere bai zergatik esan z-i-da-n kardiologu-k ezin n-eza-ke-ela lan-ik egin
now also yes because say-prf 3rd/pst-root-1st-pst cardiologist-erg cannot 1st/pst-root-mod-comp work-prt do
"now also because the cardiologist told me I could not work"

orain ere bai zergatik esa-n z-i-da-n kardiologu-k **ezin-e-ke-la** lanik egin.
now also yes because say-prf 3rd/pst-root-1st-pst cardiologist-erg cannot-root-mod-comp work-prt do (subject 20)

The highlighted form appears to contain the negative modal verb *ezin* "cannot", which is a main verb, uninflected, a modal marker *ke* and a complementizer *la*. It does not display a first person agreement marker for the subject.

To conclude, the category Inflection, which manifests itself in Basque in the auxiliary verb, is one of the most evidently damaged piece of grammar in the production of aphasic speech. Thus, auxiliaries are far less frequent in aphasic speech than in normal language; in severe cases, auxiliaries are missing completely. Mistaken forms of auxiliaries are also found, where number agreement of the object is missing, or where third person agreement substitutes first person agreement. Finally, impossible auxiliaries, or neologisms involving auxiliary forms are frequently found. In general, with the only possible exception of (30), the correct order of morphemes has not been altered: even in the case of newly coined forms, these are structurally/linearly well-formed, and their ill-formedness derives from the combination of morphemes of different paradigms, or the combination of conflicting, non-matching features (such as singular and plural, for example).

3.2. Inflectional morphology on Noun Phrases: Case, determiners and postpositions.
We will now review symptoms related to case morphology, the determiner system, and postpositions. We will begin with case morphology.

3.2.1. Case morphology.
Given the possibility of omitting agreeing NPs in Basque, there are a large number of cases where no overt NPs are found in the utterances, and thus deficits in case morphology are probably not as easily detected as they are in the auxiliary system, where auxiliaries are obligatory. However, some instances are found in the corpus where such errors do occur. The frequency of these errors appears not to be as high as in the case of auxiliary verbs.

The errors in the production of case-endings found in the corpus involve ergative case and absolutive case. We have found no instances of errors involving dative case. There are instances where NPs have been marked with Ergative case instead of Absolutive case:

(31) a. ba ni joa-ten naz lane-ra egun guzti-eta-n
well I go-impf 1st-be work-to day every-pl-loc
"well, I go to work everyday"

ba, **nik** joa-ten naz lan-era egun guzti-eta-n
well, I-erg go-impf 1st-be work-to day every-pl-loc

b. hanka apurtu da
leg/det break-prf 3rd/be
"the leg is broken"

hanka-k apurtu da
leg/det-erg break-prf 3rd/be (subject 58)

These examples illustrate an error in the assignation of case to the subject of the sentence. In (31a), an intransitive subject of an unaccusative predicate, *joan* “to go”, has been marked with ergative case, when it should be absolutive, the unmarked case. That is, the pronominal form *nik* should not bear the ergative morpheme *k*. The correct pronominal in this case is *ni*, the absolutive form of the first person singular pronoun. Notice that the case ending of the pronoun in the utterance in (31a) does not match with the agreement marker on the auxiliary, which is also absolutive; that is, the error involves only case-marking, and not the inflected form chosen.

In (31b), the subject of the intransitive verb *apurtu* "to break" should be marked with absolutive case, but it surfaces with the ergative case ending, *hanka-k* "leg-erg". In the case of subject 58, some of whose utterances are shown in (31), this deficit is particularly manifest: out of a total of ten sentences, six of which contain overt subject NPs, we find four instances of this type of deficit.

More examples of mistaken assignation of ergative case are found in the following utterances:

(32) a. baña seminario-n, oso gutxi egi-ten zan, eta gu has-i giñan
but seminary-loc very few do-impf 3rd/be/pst and we start-prf 1stpl/be/pst
"but in the seminary very little was done, and we started"

baña seminario-n, oso gutxi egi-ten zan, eta **gu gu-k** hasi giñan
but seminary-in, very little do-impf 3rd/be/pst, and we we-erg start-prf 1st/be/pst (subject 18)

b. beste-a zen fabrikan
other-det 3rd/be/pst factory-loc
"the other one was at the factory"

beste-a-k e .... zen e fabrike-an
other-det-erg e ...3rd/be/pst e factory-loc (subject 53)

Both examples involve ergative case-marked NPs in intransitive sentences, containing intransitive auxiliaries with absolutive agreement markers. In (32a) the subject repeats the pronoun *gu* "we", first without an overt case ending, which would correspond to the absolutive form, and then with the ergative case-ending *k*. In the second example, the subject does pause between the ergative marked NP and the intransitive auxiliary, which might indicate they belong to two different, unfinished sentences, in which case the ergative-marked subject might not correspond to the auxiliary.

We have found only two instances of a subject NP that should have been marked with ergative and was not:

(33) a. barku-a-k joan egin behar d-au
ship-det-erg go-prf do-prf must 3rd-root
"The ship must go"

barku-a joan egin behar d-au
ship-det go-prf do-prf must 3rd-root (subject 52)

b. neskatila-k esaten da-u
girl/det-erg say-impf 3rd-root
"The girl says"

neskatila esaten dau
girl/det say-impf 3rd-root (subject 58)

In (33), the subject NP bears no ergative case-marking, even though the presence of the modal verb *behar* "must" requires ergative case on the subject and a transitive auxiliary with ergative agreement for the subject. Note that the auxiliary is the correct transitive form. Since absolutive is the unmarked case, bearing a zero morpheme, it is not possible to now whether the subject NP is case marked absolutive, or whether it simply fails to bear case altogether.

The frequency of errors in case endings is low, relative to the frequency of errors in inflected auxiliaries. Moreover, it does not favor the morphologically unmarked form, the Absolutive, since there are more examples of overgeneration of Ergative-marked forms, rather than Absolutive-marked forms.

3.2.2. Determiners.
There is only one type of symptom found in the corpus, related to the determiner system of the language. This symptom involves the determiner *a*, which can be considered the unmarked determiner, in the sense that it appears in the widest contexts. From a linguistic point of view, the semantic and syntactic nature of this determiner is still unclear, and data from acquisition show that children take a relatively long time to acquire it fully (Barreña (1993), Ezeizabarrena (1996)) . Most instances of errors involve sentences where this determiner is missing, yielding determinerless forms, that are ungrammatical:

(34) a. seme-a esan-go d-e-t maestro-a da
son-det say-fut 3rd-root-1st teacher-det 3rd/be
"the son, will I say it, is a teacher"

seme e esan-go d-e-t e, **maestro** da
son say-fut 3rd-root-1st teacher 3rd/be (subject 53)

b. beste-a hor ego-ten da
other-det there be-impf 3rd/be
"The other one is usually there"

beste hor egoten da
other there be-impf 3rd/be (subject 53)

c. lema bapore-a-ri apurtu eta etxera giñ-oa-z-ela
helm/det boat-det-dat break-prf and home-to 1st/pst-go-pl-comp
"The boat's helm having broken and as we went home"

lema **bapore**-ri apurtu eta etxe-ra giñ-oa-z-ela
helm/det boat-dat break-prf and home-to 1st/pst-go-pl-comp (subject 52)

In all these three examples, the highlighted nouns do not carry the determiner *a*, lack of which renders the utterances ungrammatical. Only in one instance in the corpus do we find the opposite symptom: a determiner *a* appears attached to a noun that should be bare:

(35) ezin d-u-t hitz egin euskera-z
cannot 3rd-root-1st word do-prf Basque-inst
"I cannot speak in Basque"

ezin d-u-t **hitz-a** egin euskera-z
cannot 3rd-root-1st word-det do Basque-inst (subject 42)

In (35), the noun *hitz* "word" belongs to the complex predicate *hitz egin* "to speak". Insertion of the determiner is not allowed in the noun of these complex predicates; the sentence produced by the subject would however be grammatical if the intended meaning were "I cannot make the word in Basque", which is presumably not the meaning intended by the subject, who is describing her symptoms.

Finally, and related to the presence of the determiner *a*, it should be noted that the repetitions of Nouns and Noun Phrases produced by the subjects are distinctive and different from the kinds of repetitions that might be found in normal speech. Let us consider the following examples:

(36) a. pinta-tzea eta arotza-n **lan lan-a**
paint-to-det and carpenter-gen work work-det
"Painting and carpenter's work" (subject 4)

b. ari nitzen e txabol bat **artzai artzai-a-ri** egi-ten
progr 1st/be/pst hut one sheperd sheperd-det-dat do-impf
"I was making a hut for the sheperd" (subject 4)

c. **alanbre, alanbre-k, alanbre-ak** sartu ta **amabi amabi-ak** ego-ndu giñan itsaso-a-n
wire, wire-pl, wire-det$_{pl}$ put and twelve twelve-det$_{pl}$ stay-prf 1stpl/be/pst sea-det-loc
"we put in wire, wires, the wires, and twelve, the twelve (of us) stayed at sea"

(subject 52)

Example (36a) illustrates the type of repetition frequently found in this corpus of aphasic subjects, where the bare noun, in this case *lan* "work" is produced before the correctly determined form *lana.* It must be pointed out that the semantic value of this particular determiner *a* is not always definite, as the translation of example shows. The abnormality of this kind of repetition has to do with the absence of the determiner in the first instance of the name. The determiner *a* is obligatory in citation of nouns in Basque. That is, in order to answer the question "how do you say "work" in Basque?", any speaker will reply with the determined noun *lana*, and not with the bare form **lan*. In (36b), we find the same type of repetition, with the noun *artzai* "sheperd", which is produced bare in the first instance, and fully inflected in the second one, with the determiner and the dative case marker. In (36c), the repetition occurs three times, first as a bare form, *alanbre* "wire", then as in impossible form **alanbre-k*, which appears to be an attempt to construct a Noun with a plural marker and no determiner. Such a form is not possible because plurality is marked directly on the determiner. Finally, the third form contains the correct form, consisting of the noun plus the plural determiner, *alanbre-ak*.

In some cases, the repetitions display nouns completely lacking determiners:

(37) txoria habi-a-n da-go-ela
bird-det nest-det-loc 3rd-be-comp
"tha the bird is in the nest"

txori txori habia dagoela
bird bird nest-det 3rd-be-comp (subject 58)

In (37), the subject repeats a bare noun *txori* "bird", without any determiner, which renders the utterance ungrammatical. The second noun in the sentence, *habi* "nest", carries the determiner *-a*, however. This second Noun Phrase does not display the locative postposition *-n*. In this sense, (37) also illustrates the symptom we discuss next: deficits in the postpositional system of the language.

3.2.3. Postpositions.

We have found very few instances of errors in the production of postpositions in the corpus. The two instances encountered involve the production of the participial morpheme *-ik* instead of the locative postposition *-n*.

(38) a. Beste-a, etxe-an da-go-n-a, soltero da-go
other-det home-loc 3rd-be-comp-det, unmarried 3rd-be
"The other one, the one who is at home, is unmarried"

Beste-a, **etxe-ik** da-go-n-a, soltero da-go
other-det, home-prt 3rd-be-comp-det, unmarried 3rd-b (subject 29)

b. Saturraran-en beatzi urte ta gero-z-tik ia Donosti-n hogei
Saturraran-loc nine year and then-ins-from almost Donosti-loc twenty
"Nine years in Saturraran and since then almost twenty years in Donosti"

Saturraranen beatzi urte ta geroztik ia Don **Donostik** hogei
Saturraran-loc nine year and then-ins-from almost Don Donosti-prt twenty
(subject 18)

The scarcity of errors in the distribution of postpositions other than case markers seems to indicate that these grammatical elements are not affected by the language pathology. The fact that there is a greater number of errors in the distribution of case markers and the determiner *a* can indicate that postpositions do not belong in the group of inflectional categories, but rather, that they belong in the group of lexical categories (Abney (1987)).

4. Conclusion

Agrammatism in Basque presents a number of symptoms related to categories of inflectional morphology. The most outstanding symptom is the total absence or the extremely low frequency of inflected verb forms in the speech of aphasic patients. When inflected verb forms are produced, they often present morphological errors.

The most common errors involve the absence of the plural marker for the object, and the absence of person specification in the dative agreement paradigm. It might be significant to point out that these two aspects of the morphology of inflection in Basque share certain properties: (a) for both plural marking and dative agreement marking, there exist spoken varieties of the language where these morphemes are not obligatory. (b) these morphemes are probably the latest additions into verbal morphology in the language (de Rijk (1981) (c) they belong in the group of morphological specifications that are acquired later than the core morphemes of Inflection. (Barreña (1993), Ezeizabarrena (1996)).

Within the realm of verbal inflection, another important symptom is the creation of impossible inflected forms. Examination of these forms indicates that the deficit involves the combination of morphemes from conflicting paradigms, usually keeping the canonical order of morphemes. We have found only one instance where the error could be attributed to a mistake in the ordering of morphemes in the inflected form. It has been argued (Laka (1993) that the order of morphemes in inflected verb forms in Basque stems from the internal structure of Inflection in this language. If this claim is correct, and since patients tend to keep this canonical order, it appears that the inflectional deficits in the verbal paradigm involves the capacity to retrieve the appropriate morphemes for each form, rather than the structural representation of Inflection.

We have also found some errors in the selection of intransitive forms, were subjects produced transitive instead of intransitive auxiliaries. In some cases it is difficult to determine whether this error affects only the inflected verb or the entire transitive versus intransitive format of the sentence, because there are no overt case marked NPs. In cases where the NPs are overt, we can see that they remain marked intransitively, which indicates that the error affects only the inflected form. In these cases, this type of error can be merged with the type discussed in the previous paragraph, and it could involve a failure in the retrieval of the correct morpheme for the root of the inflected form (that is, the selection of a "have" type root instead of the selection of a "be" type root).

Turning to the nominal system, there are two main types of symptoms: deficits in case-morphology and deficits in the determiner system. Regarding case morphology, the most frequent type of symptom is the production of NPs with ergative case (the case for transitive subjects) where absolutive case is required (the case for intransitive subjects). Ergative and absolutive constitute two structural cases of Basque grammar (Levin (1983), Ortiz de Urbina (1989), Fernandez (1996), Laka (2000)), equivalent to nominative and accusative in English (Chomsky (1981)). Regarding the determiner system, one type of symptom arises, affecting only one determiner of the language, the determiner *-a* (Artiagoitia (1997)). This determiner is acquired relatively late by children and its semantic content is unclear (it does not signal definiteness or indefiniteness, and it surfaces in predicative contexts). The determiner *-a* seems to be the most grammaticalized element of the determiner class in Basque; this might be a reason why it is the only determiner affected in cases of agrammatism. We have hardly found any errors in the production of postpositions, with the exception of examples (38) above.

From the standpoint of linguistic structure, all of the elements affected by agrammatism in Basque constitute functional categories. Syntactic categories have been argued to belong into two main groups (Chomsky (1981)): (a) the group of lexical categories, containing the Noun, the Verb, the Adjective and the Preposition; and (b) the group of functional categories, which includes Inflection (Infl), the head of the sentence (IP) and Determiners (D), which head the Determiner Phrase (Abney (1987)). Recently, proposals like Bittner & Hale (1996a,b) have included case morphology in this group (as a category K); this proposal has been argued to fit with the structure of Basque case marked NPs (Laka (2000). Basque is a heavily inflected, free word order language; the grammatical structure is thus largely encoded by means of inflectional morphology. The symptoms of agrammatism found in this corpus seem to involve a defective encoding of this morphological information.

Acknowledgements

The authors would like to thank Xabier Artiagoitia and Mari Jose Ezeizabarrena for their comments and suggestions. This research has been funded in part by the Basque Government's Department of Education, Universities and Research (Grant reference PI-1999-18).

Address correspondence to: Dr. Lore Erriondo, Department of Linguistics, Euskal Herriko Unibertsitatea, Paseo de la Universidad 5, Apdo 2111, E- 01006 Vitoria-Gasteiz.
E–mail: hdperkol@sf.ehu.es

References

Abney, S. (1987). The English noun phrase in its sentential aspect. PhD Dissertation, MIT, Cambridge: MA.

Amundarain, I. (1997). Juntadura eta elipsia euskaraz. PhD Dissertation, University of the Basque Country, UPV-EHU, Vitoria-Gasteiz, Spain.

Artiagoitia, X. (1997). DP predicates in Basque. In A. Taff (Ed.), *University of Washington Working Papers in Linguistics, 15,* 161-198.

Barreña, A. (1993). Haur euskaldunen hizkuntzaren jabekuntza-garapena: INFL eta KONP funtzio-kategorien erabileraz. PhD Dissertation, University of the Basque Country, UPV-EHU, Vitoria-Gasteiz.

Bittner, M., & Hale, K. (1996a). The structural determination of case and agreement. *Linguistic Inquiry, 27*(1), 1-68.

Bittner, M., & Hale, K. (1996b). Ergativity: towards a theory of a heterogeneous class. *Linguistic Inquiry, 27*(2), 531-604.

Borer, H. (1984). *Parametric syntax: Case studies in Semitic and Romance languages.* Dordrecht: Foris.

Chomsky, N. (1981). *Lectures on government and binding.* Dordrecht: Foris.

Chomsky, N. (1989). Some notes on economy of derivation and representation. In I. Laka & A. Mahajan (eds.), *Functional heads and clause structure,* MITWPL Vol. 10, Dept. of Linguistics & Philosophy, MIT, Cambridge, MA.

Erriondo Korostola, L. (1995). Afasiko elebidunen hizkuntz trebetasunen azterketa. PhD Dissertation, Universidad del País Vasco/ Euskal herriko Unibertsitatea, tesis y disertaciones académicas, Bilbao: Servicio de Publicaciones de la UPV-EHU.

Eguzkitza, A. (1977). Kasuak eta postposizioak: deklinabidea eta postposiziobidea. Hizpide, 40, 39-52.

Eguzkitza, A. (1998). Postposizioak euskal gramatikan. In I. Túrrez, A. Arejita and C. Itsaso (Eds.), *Studia philologica in honorem Alfonso Irigoien* (pp. 83-88). Bilbao: University of Deusto.

Ezeizabarrena, M.J. (1996). Adquisición de FLEX en euskera y castellano por niños bilingües. PhD Dissertation, University of Hamburg, Germany.

Greenberg, J. (1963). *Universals of language*. MIT Press, Cambridge, MA.

Greenberg, J. (1978). *Universals of human language* 4 vols., Stanford University Press: Stanford.

Jackobson, R. (1968). *Child language, aphasia and phonological universals*. Mouton: The Hague.

Laka, I. (1993). The structure of inflection: A case study in X^0 Syntax. In J. I. Hualde & J. Ortiz de Urbina (Eds.), *Generative studies in Basque linguistics. Current issues in linguistic theory 105* (pp. 21-70), Amsterdam/Philadephia: John Benjamins.

Laka, I. (1996). A brief grammar of Euskara, the Basque language, <http://www.ehu.es/grammar>

Laka, I. (2000). Thetablind case: Burzio´s Generalization and its image in the mirror. In E. Reuland (Ed.), *Arguments and case. Explaining Burzio's Generalization.* Linguistik Aktuell/ Linguistics Today, vol 34, (pp. 103-129). Amsterdam/Philadelphia: John Benjamins.

Levin, B. (1983). On the nature of ergativity. PhD Dissertation, Cambridge, MA: MIT.

Ortiz De Urbina. J. (1989). *Parameters in the grammar of basque*. Foris, Dordrecht: Foris.

de Rijk, R. (1969). Is Basque an SOV language? *Fontes Linguae Vasconum*. 319-351.

de Rijk, R. (1981) Euskal Morfologiaren Zenbait Gorabehera. Euskal Linguistika eta literatura: Bide berriak. University of Deusto, Bilbao: Deustuko Unibertsitateko Argitarazioak, 83-101.

On Manifestations of Aphasia in Catalan: A Case Study of Broca's Aphasia

Jordi Peña-Casanova*, Faustino Diéguez-Vide°, Raquel Lluent*, Peter Böhm*.

**Section of Neuropsychology, Hospital del Mar, Institut Municipal d'Assistència Sanitària (IMAS), Barcelona, Spain; °Department of Linguistics, Universitat de Barcelona, Barcelona, Spain.*

Abstract—This paper discusses a case of Broca's aphasia in light of the impact of the structure of the patient's mother tongue, Catalan, on the types of errors he makes. What seems to be most affected in the present case, in terms of Kolk's (1995) theory of "structural simplification" —proposed originally for sentence production and comprehension—are those linguistic levels that are most complex in Catalan: closed class word morphology and verb morphology as well as production and comprehension of sentences with non-canonical word order. The types of errors presented always occur in structurally obligatory contexts where the semantic or propositional content of the omitted or misused elements is rather small. Another important fact to bear in mind when studying Catalan aphasics is that, due to the bilingualism of all speakers, some of the signs and symptoms of aphasic speech have to be interpreted in light of the rival language, Spanish.

Keywords: Aphasic symptoms, Catalan, Morphology, Syntax, Broca's aphasia, Bilingualism

Introduction

Catalan, which dates back to approximately 990 AD, is a Romance language. Like many languages in the same family (such as Castilian (Spanish), Portuguese and French), it has substantially modified many of the characteristics of its parent language, Latin: amalgamation of long and short vowels, nearly total elimination of the neuter gender, substitution of case markers by prepositions, and liberalization of syntactic rules (especially word order) are only a few examples.

This paper will describe some of the semiological landmarks of Broca's aphasia in Catalan. Furthermore, we will try to place our descriptions in a larger context, whenever possible, comparing the most important findings with results for other languages, whether closely related to Catalan (e.g. Spanish), or farther removed but important for theoretical considerations (French, English).

The study is divided into three parts: First, a very brief introduction will situate Catalan among the world's languages. Second, we will briefly review some of the major linguistic features of Catalan, including only those pertinent to our discussion of aphasic symptoms. Third, we will try to provide a linguistically guided cognitive interpretation of some of the aphasic symptoms and generalize about possible mechanisms underlying these symptoms which are due to the fact that the patient speaks Catalan.

Although Catalan has various dialects (mainly distinguished at the phonetic and lexical levels), we have focused on patients who produce and understand the standard form of Catalan (*koiné*). This standard form of Catalan corresponds substantially to the dialect of Barcelona, which is propagated by the media and standardized by the Institute of Catalan Studies (*Institut d'Estudis Catalans*).

Catalan Around the World

Catalan is the mother tongue of about eight and a half million people and is spoken in several countries. Within the Iberian peninsula, it is spoken in the Principality of Catalonia (corresponding to the Spanish provinces of Barcelona, Girona, Tarragona and Lleida), the old kingdom of Valencia (at present consisting of the provinces of Valencia, Castelló and Alacant), a strip of eastern Aragon, the region of Carxe (province of Murcia) and the Balearic Islands. In France, Catalan is also spoken in what has come to be called French Catalonia: Roussillon and Cerdanya. In the Co-Principality of Andorra, Catalan has joint official status with French. Finally, Catalan is also spoken in the city of l'Alguer in Sardinia. Although Catalan extends beyond the borders of Spain, its nucleus is situated in Catalonia and Andorra, where the majority of its speakers live. Within the Spanish territories mentioned, Catalan has joint official status with Spanish. More people speak Catalan than speak Danish, Finnish or Norwegian, and the Catalan regions are greater in area than five modern European states: Denmark, Switzerland, Holland, Belgium and Albania (Yates, 1975).

One important thing to bear in mind is that Catalan, like many other minority languages, always has to be considered in the context of bilingualism. In France and Italy, its speakers use French and Italian as "major languages". In the territory of Spain and Andorra, Catalan speakers also speak Spanish due to political factors and the phenomenon of immigration. Media and linguistic policies in Catalonia are therefore bilingual.

A Brief Historical Sketch

Although Catalonia has its own government and laws, it depends politically on the government of Spain (with its seat in Madrid), and is always dependent, in the final instance, on the resolutions and laws of the Spanish government. Nevertheless, some 10 years ago, the Catalan government put in place a linguistic policy in order to standardize the Catalan language and its use on the Catalan territory. Since then, Catalan has been the mandatory language of schooling (even some schools in so-called French Catalonia have started to teach classes in Catalan), and companies started to receive subsidies for advertising and distributing their products in Catalan. The main aims of this policy, though, were to collect a corpus of the language and to develop a standard variant of Catalan.

For the second phase of this linguistic policy, the planning of a standard variant, the development of media in Catalan was another important step, quite apart from the implementation of Catalan in schools. At present there are six TV channels in the autonomous region of Catalonia: four of them broadcast in Spanish (with very short news programs in Catalan) and two are solely in Catalan. The situation for radio is similar: only 15% of the radio stations broadcast their programs in Catalan. The same is true for the press. In other words, the linguistic policy regarding the establishment of a standard variant of Catalan has been fruitful with regard to education (universities, schools, etc.), and the majority of the student population speaks Catalan. Nevertheless, for the time being it seems to have failed with respect to the media and the law.

This situation has its roots at the end of the 1930s. A military dictatorship was established in Spain at that time and remained in power until 1975, promoting a policy of centralization. One of the consequences of this policy was the prohibition of Catalan in every respect; it could not even be spoken in public. All schools and all media were in Spanish and censored. Only after the dictatorship ended could the Catalan language start to flourish once again. The *Catalan Statute of Autonomy* of 1979 and the *Linguistic Normalization Act* of 1983 were two of the necessary steps towards the re-establishment of the Catalan language.

This historical overview is necessary as history influences the current linguistic reality of Catalonia and, consequently, the effects on its aphasic population. Nearly all aphasic patients were students under the dictatorship and therefore received their education in Spanish. For this reason, in the following discussion, we practically do not take problems affecting reading and writing into account.

Relevant Linguistic Aspects of Catalan

The following paragraphs will briefly review some of the basic facts about Catalan phonetics, phonology, morphology and syntax, as they are pertinent to our discussion of aphasic symptoms. We will try to describe those areas which we believe are structurally the most vulnerable in Catalan and which will therefore be the ones impaired in pathology.

With respect to Catalan phonetics and phonology, the following facts are noteworthy: its phonotactic system is governed by the universal hierarchy of sonority (Selkirk, 1982). There are some morphophonological exceptions to this hierarchy. A consonant may have a higher index of sonority than its predecessor if and only if it follows a morphological boundary. The phonotactic system of Catalan is more complex than that of the language with which it competes on the Spanish territory, Castilian, as vowels in unstressed position are reduced in Catalan.

As mentioned above, Catalan is a Romance language, derived ultimately from Latin. With regard to its morphology, the Latin system of declensions and cases for nouns and adjectives has been replaced by a complex prepositional system. Closed class words (prepositions, articles and pronouns) have evolved in diverse directions from their Latin origins. The number of prepositions has increased substantially, the article system has preserved the number and gender information, and the pronoun system has maintained the information about number, gender, and case.

Catalan nouns carry information about number (singular/plural) and gender (masculine/feminine). Each of these grammatical functions must be expressed by a separate morpheme. The structural information may be presented as follows: [[[root] gender-morph] number-morph]. At the surface level, though, the only nouns that present a morphological distinction between masculine and feminine gender are double forms such as: *noi* – *noi**a*** (boy – girl), *mestre* – *mestr**a*** (teacher$_{male}$ – teacher$_{female}$). The other Catalan nouns do not carry the morphological marker of gender at the surface level: *la*$_{fem}$ *casa*$_{fem}$ (the house$_{fem}$), *el*$_{masc}$ *camió*$_{masc}$ (the truck$_{masc}$).

Catalan verbs specify, at the morphological level, information about tense, mood, and person, all expressed at the surface level by a single morpheme. The language has one morphological marker for the present tense, four for expressing different aspects of the past (simple past, periphrastic past tense, past perfect tense, and present perfect tense), and two forms for expressing the future (simple future and periphrastic future tense). Catalan has a marker for the indicative mood, one for the subjunctive and another for the imperative, apart from two morphological markers for expressing conditionals (simple and periphrastic). There are also the impersonal forms of the verb: infinitive, gerund and participle. There are three morphological markers for person in the singular and three more for the plural. This complex system of morphological marking is augmented by the existence of three conjugations, all of which have their own morphological paradigms. Together, these different functions give rise to 18 different indicative morphemes, six different morphemes to express conditionality, and 18 morphemes for expressing subjunctive. For each one of these different morphemes, there are six separate forms (three for singular and three for plural). Apart from that, there are nine different morphemes to express the impersonal forms of verbs. Summed up, this makes the verb morphology much more complex than in, for example, English.

Adjectives have the same morphological status as nouns. They possess morphological markers for gender and number. Furthermore, adjectives must agree with the noun they modify in gender and number (see examples 1 and 2).

(1) El gos negre.
The (masc. sing.) dog black (masc. sing.).
The black dog.

(2) Les cases grans.
The (fem. pl.) houses big (fem. pl.).
The big houses.

With respect to closed class words in Catalan, we will first consider the pronominal system. We differentiate tonic and atonic forms within this system, which makes the rather complex pronominal system of Catalan—where double pronouns are possible—even more complex. Tonic forms, which are independent morphemes at the surface level, serve the function of nominative, accusative, dative and ablative (*en, hi*). Atonic pronouns (clitics), which express accusative or dative, do not have independent morphological forms, but are added to the end of the verb they go with instead. Dative pronouns can be used emphatically, which leads to a reduplication of the dative pronoun after the explicit form of the dative, if and only if the explicit form is placed before the verb (see example 3), which is not its canonical place.

(3) Als concursants $\textbf{els}_{\text{dative}}$ $\textbf{hi}_{\text{dative emphatic}}$ donen diners.
To the contestants (dative pl.) to them (dative pl. + emphatic) they give money.
They give money to the contestants.

Articles and pronouns have to agree with the noun they modify in number and gender (see example 4).

(4) Les noies maques.
The (fem. pl.) girls pretty (fem. pl.).
The pretty girls.

An important morphological feature of Catalan is the possibility of contracting closed class elements, for reasons of syllabic simplification. First, articles in their singular form are contracted before nouns with a vocalic onset (examples 5 and 6). Second, articles with a vocalic onset become contracted if they are preceded by a preposition with a vocalic offset (examples 7 and 8). Third, two pronouns are contracted if the offset of the first and the onset of the second are vocalic (example 9) or if the resulting contraction of one of them gives rise to a syllabic simplification (example 10).

(5) L'home (*el$_{\text{masc. sing.}}$ home).
The (masc. sing.) man.

(6) L'herba (*la$_{\text{fem. sing.}}$ herba).
The (fem. sing.) grass.

(7) als$_{\text{prep. + art.}}$ amics (*a$_{\text{prep.}}$ els$_{\text{art. masc. pl.}}$ amics).
To the friends.

(8) Del$_{\text{prep. + art.}}$ peix (*de$_{\text{prep.}}$ el$_{\text{art. masc. sing.}}$ peix).
Of the fish.

(9) Anar-se'n$_{\text{pron. + pron.}}$ (*anar-se$_{\text{reflexive}}$ en$_{\text{ablative}}$).
Go away from.

(10) Dóna-ls-hi$_{\text{pron. + pron.}}$ (*Dóna-los$_{\text{accusative masc. pl.}}$ hi$_{\text{dative masc. sing.}}$).
Give them to him.

On the syntactic level, the following aspects should be mentioned as structurally important in Catalan: Catalan is a pro-drop language, meaning that the subject may be absent at the surface level in cases where it can be omitted. The basic word order of Catalan is SVO, although typologically it may be considered a language with a relatively free word order (Moreno-Cabrera, 1997). Nevertheless, this basic word order may be changed freely if the intrasyntagmatic structure of the phrases is not altered. In Catalan, the following phrases are possible: noun phrase (NP), verb phrase (VP), adjectival phrase (AP), adverbial phrase (AdvP) and prepositional phrase (PP).

Noun phrases consist of a determiner, a noun and possibly an adjective, in that strict order (example 11). If the adjective position is taken by a subordinate clause, this subordinate clause must be placed in the adjective position (example 12).

(11) Els cotxes nous.
The (masc. pl.) cars new (masc. pl.).
The new cars.

(12) Els cotxes que es fabriquen a França.
The (masc. pl.) cars which are made in France.
The cars which are made in France.

A verb phrase in Catalan is usually formed by a verb and, depending on its valency, a direct, an indirect and/or a circumstantial complement. The canonical order is as stated above, although the different complements of the verb, which are themselves NPs and have a rigid internal structural order (see above), can be moved as a whole to any place in the clause (*cf.* free word order above). Examples 13 through 15 exemplify this possibility of free ordering of constituents for a ditransitive verb (*portar* "bring").

(13) El Pare Noel porta regals als nens al desembre.
Santa Claus brings presents to the kids in December.

(14) Als nens porta regals el Pare Noel al desembre.
To the kids brings presents Santa Claus in December.
It's to the kids that Santa Claus brings presents in December.

(15) Al desembre, el Pare Noel porta regals als nens.
In December, Santa Claus brings presents to the kids.

Prepositional phrases are constructed with a preposition and a following NP or an infinitival phrase (see example 16 and 17).

(16) Sota la cadira.
Under the chair.

(17) Carn per menjar.
Meat for eat (inf.).
Meat for eating.

Aphasic Manifestations in Catalan

There is little literature on aphasia in Catalan. The very few published papers (Peña-Casanova & Bagunyà-Durich, 1988; Junque et al., 1989) do not describe case reports but are concerned with more general topics such as lesion localization or rehabilitation. This may have various causes, the most important of which seems to be sociolinguistic, alluded to above. As a matter of fact, nearly all speakers of Catalan are Catalan-Spanish bilinguals. This has led to a common practice of studying language deficits in the major language, Spanish, and transposing the results into the language not studied, in this case Catalan.

Another reason for the scarcity of studies is the lack of testing materials in Catalan. Although there are general neuropsychological tests containing rather extensive language testing sections, such as the *Barcelona Test* (Peña-Casanova, 1990), all these tests are validated and standardized in Spanish-speaking populations and Catalan versions, when available, consist of mere translations of the Spanish materials without any attention to language-specific factors in Catalan. The standard language tests, whether those with the classical syndromic approach, such as the *Boston Diagnostic Aphasia Examination* (Goodglass & Kaplan, 1972), or those that take a cognitive approach such as the *PALPA* (Kay, Lesser & Coltheart, 1992), have only been adapted for Spanish (Garcia-Albea & Sánchez Bernardos, 1986; Valle & Cuetos, 1995) and can therefore not be used on Catalan populations. The one exception to the rule is the *Bilingual Aphasia Test (BAT)* (Paradis, 1989), for which a Catalan version exists. Nevertheless, no normative data have been published on this test so that interpretation is generally done on an intuitive basis, taking into account the general syndromic classification scheme regarding fluent vs. non-fluent output, naming, repetition and associated disorders of reading and writing.

These two facts—the sociolinguistic reality of bilingualism in Catalonia and the scarcity of testing materials—pose a dilemma for neuropsychologists confronted with a Catalan speaker who has suffered a cerebral insult causing aphasia. They have to test the patient in a language other than his native language and then extrapolate data on the native language, Catalan, based on this evaluation. Normally, this process of extrapolation is based upon an informal translation of the Spanish test materials directly into Catalan.

Due to the above-mentioned facts, aphasia classification and aphasic symptom descriptions in case reports or unpublished presentations to local meetings rely on the classical syndromic approach (Basso & Cubelli, 1999; Damasio, 1998; Lecours & Lhermitte, 1979) and its description of symptoms.

Subject and Procedures

For the purposes of this research, we studied a Catalan aphasic who presented with Broca's aphasia in the chronic phase which had developed from near mutism in the acute and subacute phases. The patient was evaluated in the acute phase with the language subtests of the *Barcelona Test* and in the chronic phase once again with the *Barcelona Test* and the Catalan version of the *BAT*. The main focus of this study is the patient's spontaneous language output.

By studying his spontaneous language as well as the description of the picture story from the *BAT*, we will try to find out how the structure of Catalan can elucidate the types of errors made by the patient. We also compare the findings for spontaneous language output with the results of the pertinent subtests of the *BAT* in order to consolidate or refute our hypotheses based on the observation of spontaneous language.

Case report: MMR, male, 76 years of age, with only one year of formal education, suffered from a CVA of the left middle cerebral artery (MCA) which provoked an aphasic syndrome classified as Broca's aphasia.

His spontaneous language output in the acute phase consisted of a controlled verbal stereotypy of the least marked syllable type (CV) in Catalan ['tə]. Repetition was severely impaired due to the articulatory disturbance. Naming was functionally preserved in both visual and verbal modalities, apart from articulatory errors. The target, however, was always deducible. Comprehension was relatively well preserved. The patient made errors on five-step commands but obtained reasonable scores for his age and education in the complex verbal material subtest (open-ended yes/no questions). Reading and writing were severely compromised, although these language components were difficult to evaluate due to the patient's very low educational level. Reading comprehension was disrupted moderately, especially for non-words (*tumi* for *midu*, *dasomida* for *basomida*). Writing to dictation revealed literal paragraphias due to substitution (*sinagu* for *sinapo*), omission (*tama* for *togamo*) and metathesis (*saflo* for *lafo*).

In the chronic phase, MMR's spontaneous language improved from the controlled verbal stereotype ['tə] to non-fluent, anarthric speech (see Appendix for a transliteration of MMR's spontaneous speech on the *BAT*).

With regard to the *Barcelona Test,* the following findings are noteworthy: during evaluation of MMR's spontaneous language, various articulatory and syllabic simplification strategies were observed. Repetition got better in the chronic phase but reflected the same articulatory difficulties observed in spontaneous speech. Naming was still preserved, with a certain improvement in the articulatory deficits. In oral comprehension, MMR obtained ceiling scores. His reading and writing capacities remained unchanged.

Due to the improvement in the patient's linguistic capacities, we tested him with the Catalan version of the *BAT.*

Spontaneous language was assessed via an open-ended conversation about the patient's language skills in Catalan, his job situation prior to the brain damage and his family. Apart from that, the description of the picture story in the *BAT* is considered as spontaneous language output. Comprehension of the examiner during spontaneous speech was preserved.

Although naming scores on both the *Barcelona Test* and the *BAT* showed ceiling effects, some lexical difficulties could be observed in spontaneous language. MMR nearly always omitted verbs when they could be inferred from the context (example 18) and showed a clear tendency to overuse copula verb forms (see Appendix). Furthermore he also had difficulties, although to a minor degree, in producing proper names, which he replaced by empty expressions (example 19). (T= target sentence; G= gloss; ET= English equivalent of the target; DS= defective sentence; E= examiner; P= patient.)

(18) T: E: Fins quan va anar al col.legi? P: Jo? Jo hi vaig anar fins als set anys.
G: E: Until when did you go to school? P: I? I there went (1st pers. sing. past) until (prep. *fins* + prep. *a* + art. masc. pl.) seven years.
ET: P: Me? I went to school until I was seven years old.

DS: P: Jo? Als set anys.
G: P: I? ∅ (prep. *a* + art. masc. pl.) seven years.

(19) T: E: On va néixer? P: A Barcelona. E: On viu? P: A la Barceloneta. E: On treballava? Al port.
G: E: Where were you born? P: In Barcelona. E: Where do you live? P: In the Barceloneta. E: Where did you work? P: At the port.

DS: E: On va néixer? P: Aquí. E: On viu? P: Aquí. E: On treballava? A tot arreu.
G: P: Here. P: Here. P: Everywhere.

With respect to morphology, we observed difficulties in MMR's spontaneous language for closed class elements (pronouns, prepositions and articles) as well as for open class elements (verb morphology, NP agreement). Pronouns are used excessively in nominative case (see Appendix) and are misused in the accusative (example 20 for omission and example 21 for substitution), dative (example 22 for omission) and ablative forms (example 23).

(20) T: L'anglès a mi no m'agrada.
G: English to me (dative pron.) I don't like it.
ET: I don't like English.

DS: Anglès no, ∅ no m'agrada.
G: English no, ∅ I don't like it.

(21) T: L'he perdut tot.
G: It (accusative pron.) I have lost (1st pers. sing. past) all.
ET: I have lost it all.

DS: Hi he perdut tot.
G: It (dative pron.) I have lost (1st pers. sing. past) all.

(22) T: Als fills en català a tots.
G: To (dative pron.) the children in Catalan to all.
ET: I [speak] in Catalan to all my children.

DS: … i ∅ ∅ fills català a tots.
G: and ∅ (prep.) ∅ (dative pron.) children Catalan to all.

(23) T: Jo hi vaig dues vegades.
G: I there (ablative pron.) go two times.
ET: I go there twice.

DS: Vaig dos veces.
G: Go (1st pers. sing. pres.) ∅ (ablative pron.) two times (Spanish).

Regarding prepositions, we observed a tendency towards omission (example 22). The only preposition used was *a*, which serves many functions in Catalan: information about dative (*a tu* "for you"), direction (*a Barcelona* "to Barcelona"), intention (*a rentar-la* "to wash it") and location (*a casa* "at home"). MMR generally uses this preposition correctly, and it serves as a placeholder for other prepositions (example 24). When two prepositions are required by the context, one of them is omitted and the one present is always *a* (example 18).

(24) T: Sempre en castellà.
G: Always in Spanish.

DS: Sempre a castellà.
G: Always to Spanish.

Articles also tend to be omitted (example 25), although they do appear. They are always omitted, however, in the context of PPs (example 26). When they are used, agreement with the noun is sometimes violated (see below).

(25) T: La meva dona.
G: The (sing. fem.) my wife.
ET: My wife.

DS: Meva dona.
G: ∅ (art. sing. fem.) my wife.

(26) T: Al lavabo.
G: To the (prep. + art.) toilet.
ET: To the toilet.

DS: A lavabo.
G: To ∅ (art.) toilet.

Apart from the fact that these three classes of function words were generally omitted and, if used, misused, we also observed violations of agreement at the level of NP concerning these function words (example 27 for article-noun agreement, example 28 for pronoun-noun agreement).

(27) T: L'home.
G: The (contracted form masc. sing.) man.
ET: The man.

DS: La home.
G: The (fem. sing.) man.

(28) T: Aquesta noia se les mira totes.
G: This (fem. sing.) girl herself (refl.) at them (fem. pl.) looks all (fem. pl.).
ET: This girl looks at all of them.

DS: Aquesta noia se lo mira totes.
G: This (fem. sing.) girl herself (refl.) at it (neutral sing.) looks all (fem. pl.).

At the level of open class elements, one type of error concerned agreement between noun and adjective (example 29); these errors usually involved a violation of number agreement.

(29) T: Doscents quilos.
G: Two hundred (masc. pl.) kilos (masc. pl.).
ET: Two hundred kilos.

DS: Doscent quilos.
G: Two hundred (masc. sing.) kilos (masc. pl.).

The use of verb morphology is severely reduced in MMR's spontaneous speech; he has a tendency to overuse the present indicative (example 30) and impersonal forms of the verb (infinitive and gerund) (example 31).

(30) T: Jo vaig néixer aquí.
G: I was born here.
ET: I was born here.

DS: Jo neix aquí.
G: I am born (3rd pers. sing. pres.) here.

(31) T: No parava, treballava dia i nit.
G: No stopped (1st pers. sing.), worked (1st pers. sing.) day and night.
ET: I never stopped, I used to work night and day.

DS: No parar, dia i nit treballant.
G: No stop (inf.), day and night working (gerund).

Simple clauses concatenated with conjunctions are the most abundant type of syntactic construction (example 32) in MMR's spontaneous speech. The basic construction used involves a pronoun in nominative case followed, occasionally, by a verb and an ablative construction. This type of construction without a verb results in agrammatic clauses in Catalan. [$\text{Pronoun}_{\text{nominative}}$ $_{\text{VP}}$[(V) PP]]. MMR's few attempts to produce subordinate clauses resulted in agrammatic constructions (example 33). Occasionally, errors in subject-verb agreement were observed (example 34). A communicative strategy used by MMR in order to mitigate his lack of syntactic resources is the use of emphatic devices such as reduplication and intonation (example 35).

(32) T: L'home va corrents i crida a tothom.
G: The (masc. sing.) man runs and shouts to everybody (neutral pl.).
ET: The man runs away and shouts out to everybody.

DS: La home i corre i crida a totes.
G: The (fem. sing.) man and runs and shouts to all (fem. pl.).

(33) T: Jo era un dels que eren més forts.
G: I was one of those (prep. + art.) who were more strong.
ET: I used to be one of the strongest.

DS: Jo dels que més forts.
G: I of those who more strong.

(34) T: Els medicaments no li van bé.
G: The (masc. pl.) medications not to her go well.
ET: The medications do not work on her.

DS: Medicament no van bé.
G: ∅ (art. masc. pl.) medication (masc. sing.) no work (pl.) well.

(35) T: I allí només es parlava català.
G: And there only was spoken Catalan.
ET: And there, only Catalan was spoken.

DS: I allí català! Català! Català!
G: And there Catalan! Catalan! Catalan!

We can sum up MMR's spontaneous language deficits as follows: at the lexical level, he showed a preference for copula verbs over full verbs and an anomia for proper names.

Regarding the morphology of closed class elements, pronouns were generally misused in their accusative, dative and ablative forms although nominative forms were generally correctly used. Nominative forms were used much more frequently than in normal speech. As for prepositions, MMR used one preposition preferentially (*a*) and systematically omitted articles when they followed a preposition. In general, articles tended not to be present.

With respect to verb morphology, MMR clearly overused indicative and impersonal forms. Agreement errors were observed at the intrasyntagmatic level (noun-adjective agreement, determiner-noun agreement, pronoun-noun agreement), as well as at the intersyntagmatic level (subject-verb agreement).

At the syntactic level, a reduction of productive resources was observed, which led to an overuse of simple clauses united by conjunctions, and errors whenever he tried to form complex clauses, a phenomenon rarely observed in MMR's discourse. Given that all speakers of Catalan are bilingual—in this case in Catalan and Spanish—it was not surprising to observe some intrusions from Spanish into MMR's Catalan output (example 36), mainly at the lexical level.

(36) T: Dues vegades.
G: Two times.
ET: Twice.

DS: Dos veces.
G: Two (Spanish) times (Spanish).

The next step was to compare these results for MMR's spontaneous language output with his linguistic behavior on the pertinent subtests of the *BAT.* Lexical errors were only observed on the antonym subtests (2/5), where MMR produced synonyms instead of antonyms. The error rate increases to 3 out of 5—in fact, MMR always chooses the last item heard—when the antonyms have to be morphological equivalents. MMR's syntactic competence was assessed with the grammaticality judgment and construction of phrases subtests. On the first of these two subtests, MMR made errors only on ungrammatical phrases, three of which he judged to be grammatical. With regard to the construction of phrases subtest, MMR proved incapable of forming clauses containing complex NPs or of using the prepositions in PPs correctly. Verbs, once again, are used in their infinitive form. This lack of syntactic competence on the production side is confirmed by a rather peculiar impairment of the comprehension of syntactically complex material. MMR made errors on 20% of passive sentences (OVS), to which he generally responded with the less marked syntactic structure (SVO). Sentences constructed in VSO order elicited errors every time (100%); once again, the patient produced sentences of the standard SVO type.

Discussion

As mentioned at the beginning of the Case Report, MMR is considered to be a typical Catalan-speaking Broca's aphasic. As with descriptions of Broca's aphasia in any other language (Menn & Obler, 1990), he presented with severe articulatory difficulties in the acute phase which improved in the chronic phase to the point that he was classified as non-fluent and anarthric. His comprehension scores were acceptable from the onset, at least for syntactically simple structures. He also presented a rather severe morphological and syntactic deficit.

Although categorized as a typical Broca's aphasic, MMR shows some peculiarities, especially regarding his morphological and syntactic deficits which, in our opinion, have to be attributed to his native language, Catalan.

Talking in the first place about the pronominal system of Catalan, we observed many errors in MMR's production, which generally took the form of omissions. As mentioned in the second section of the paper on the relevant features of Catalan, the language permits relatively free ordering of constituents within clauses. This, however, does not mean that anything goes. If an element is moved from its canonical position—e.g. complements of verbs are canonically placed postverbally—this has to be marked at the surface level by means of pronouns. These pronouns only serve a filler-function in order to justify the stylistic movement of the complement, which must obligatorily be present at the surface level. They do not serve any syntactic function, though. That is why MMR omits accusative, dative and ablative pronouns so often, when they serve the above-described emphatic function. He never omits them when they serve a referential function. This also explains the overuse of the nominative pronoun, as it is never used in this way.

MMR's overuse of the most frequent and semantically most productive preposition (*a*) indicates that he seems to know when to put a preposition in a phrase—meaning that the structural principles of the prepositional system are basically intact. Nevertheless, he seems to have a problem activating the correct prepositions. Once again, semantic reasons may be adduced to explain this phenomenon. In fact, the preposition in a PP in Catalan is inferable from the rest of the PP in the majority of cases; this makes prepositions vulnerable to a cerebral lesion that alters the linguistic competence of an individual. MMR maintains the logical order of his propositions and tends to construct very simple clauses, and this ordering principle allows him to omit "semantically less relevant information". The presence of the preposition *a* seems to be due to its frequency of use, which makes it less vulnerable to omission.

Articles are elements that are extremely important from a syntactic viewpoint in Catalan. Even proper names have to be introduced by the corresponding article. Nevertheless, the semantic information (masc./fem.; sing./pl.) is generally represented in the noun as well as in the article. This, once again, makes them irrelevant for expressing the basic meaning of a clause. The errors of agreement observed between specifiers and nouns seem to indicate that there may be some remnants of structural knowledge. We find it difficult to account for these agreement errors—only very few instances were observed—as MMR was not specifically tested for perseveration of specifier-noun agreement. The other intrasyntagmatic and intersyntagmatic agreement errors, on the other hand, seem to point towards an underlying deficit affecting agreement. This has to be interpreted in the light of the complexity of agreement in Catalan. Each morpheme has to express more than one function at a time, which makes them structurally more complex to compute.

The errors and substitutions in verb morphology pointed out in the text only reaffirm that there is a structural breakdown in the linguistic system. As the indicative and impersonal forms of verbs are much more frequently used, they must be preserved. Since these errors do not occur in isolation but in the context of sentence production, they can be explained in terms of Kolk and colleagues' adaptive theory of structural simplification (Hofstede & Kolk, 1994; Kolk & Heeschen 1992; Kolk, 1995). This theory predicts different possible sources of underlying deficits that undermine the patient's attempts to produce and/or comprehend sentences. Among the possible factors affecting sentence production, Kolk (1995) adduces temporal limitations in the normal dynamic flow of information processing, which produce asynchronies in the coordination of lexical retrieval and syntactic elaboration. If, as we assume, MMR's lexical knowledge is better preserved, these asynchronies will affect, to a greater extent, the syntactic elaboration of sentences, as well as their comprehension.

In fact, this is what we have observed in MMR's sentence production and comprehension (Kolk, van Grunsven & Keyser, 1985). The predominance of nominal productions in MMR's discourse could be interpreted as a structural adaptation to the fact that verbs necessitate a greater load of syntactic processing, which seems to be most affected in MMR's linguistic system. The use of syntactically easy copula verbs together with nouns permits him to create functional discourse, to some extent. As a result of this adaptation to limited resources, syntactically difficult structures such as negation or subordinate clauses are either not present in MMR's output or, if they are, are constructed erroneously. The presence of the same deficit in the comprehension of syntactically difficult structures (passives, negative sentences, and sentences of the VSO type which do not follow the canonical order) emphasizes this deficit at the syntactic level (Nespoulous et al., 1988).

One last but very relevant fact about MMR's case of Broca's aphasia and, more generally, all types of aphasia in Catalan is the presence of intrusions from the second language, Spanish. These intrusions may help to overcome phonotactic difficulties —remember that the phonotactic system of Catalan is much more complex than that of Spanish. In other cases, they seem to be strongly lexicalized elements that are used in the context of sentences with a high emotive content.

Address correspondence to: Dr. Jordi Peña i Casanova, Cap, Unitat de Neuropsicologia i Logopedia, Servei de Neurologia, Hospital Universitari del Mar, Passeig Marítim, 25-29, 08003 Barcelona, Spain. E-mail: peter_neus@maptel.es

References

Basso, A., & Cubelli, R. (1999). Clinical aspects of aphasia. In G. Denes & L. Pizzamiglio (Eds.), *Handbook of clinical and experimental neuropsychology*. Hove: Psychology Press.

Damasio, A.R. (1998). Signs of aphasia. In M.T. Sarno (Ed.), *Acquired aphasia* (3rd ed.). London: Academic Press.

Garcia-Albea, J.E., & Sánchez Bernardos, M.L. (1986). *La evaluación de la afasia y trastornos relacionados* (Spanish adaptation of Goodglass & Kaplan's Boston Aphasia Battery). Madrid: Ed. Panamericana.

Goodglass, H., & Kaplan, E. (1972). *The assessment of aphasia and related disorders*. Philadelphia: Lea & Febiger.

Hofstede, B.T.M., & Kolk, H.H.J. (1994). The effects of task variation on the production of grammatical morphology in Broca's aphasia: A multiple case study. *Brain and Language, 46*, 278-328.

Junque, C., Vendrell, P., Vendrell-Brucet, J.M., & Tobeña, A. (1989). Differential recovery in naming in bilingual aphasics. *Brain and Language, 36,* 116-122.

Kay, J., Lesser, R., & Coltheart, M. (1992). *PALPA: Psycholinguistic assessments of language processing in aphasia.* Hove: Lawrence Erlbaum.

Kolk, H.H.J. (1995). A time-based approach to agrammatic production. *Brain and Language, 50*, 282-303.

Kolk, H.H.J., & Heeschen, C. (1992). Agrammatism, paragrammatism and the management of language. *Language and Cognitive Processes, 7*, 89-129.

Kolk, H.H.J., van Grunsven, M.J.F., & Keyser, A. (1985). On parallelism between production and comprehension in agrammatism. In M.-L. Kean (Ed.), *Agrammatism*. New York: Academic Press.

Lecours, A.-R., & Lhermitte, F. (1979). *L'aphasie.* Montreal/Paris: Flammarion.

Menn, L., & Obler, L.K. (Eds.) (1990). *Agrammatic aphasia: A cross-language narrative sourcebook.* New York/Philadelphia: John Benjamins.

Moreno-Cabrera, J. (1997). *Universales y tipología lingüística.* Madrid: Síntesis.

Nespoulous, J.-L., Dordain, M., Perron, C., Ska, B., Bub, D., Caplan, D., Mehler, J., & Lecours, A.-R. (1988). Agrammatism in sentence production without comprehension deficits: Reduced availability of syntactic structures and/or grammatical morphemes? A case study. *Brain and Language, 33*, 273-295.

Paradis, M. (1989). *Bilingual aphasia test (Catalan version).* Hillsdale, NJ: Lawrence Erlbaum.

Peña-Casanova, J. (1990). *Programa integrado de exploración neuropsicológica "Test Barcelona"* (Manual). Barcelona: Masson.

Peña-Casanova, J., & Bagunyà-Durich, J. (1988). Bases anatomo-funcionals del llenguatge: Un model avançat. *Limits, 4,* 19-37.

Selkirk, E.O. (1982) The syllable. In H. Van der Hulst & P. Smith (Eds.), *The syntax of words.* Cambridge (Mass.): MIT Press.

Valle, F., & Cuetos, F. (1995). *EPLA: Evaluación del procesamiento lingüístico en la afasia* (adaptation of Kay, Lesser & Coltheart, 1992). Hove: Lawrence Erlbaum.

Yates, A. (1975). *Catalan.* Sevenoaks, UK: Hodder & Stoughton.

APPENDIX

INTERVIEW (T= target sentence; G= gloss; ET= English equivalent of the target; DS= defective sentence; E= Examiner; P= Patient)

1) T: E: Quins idiomes parla? P: L'anglès no m'agrada i a mi no m'agradaria, no, no i jo estic a casa. Aquí no! No, és que els altres no m'agraden. No volia. Quan treballava al moll sí, però no vull no, no.
G: E: What languages do you speak? P: The English I don't like and to me no would like, no, no and I am home. Here no! No, is that the others no to me like. No wanted (1st pers. sing.). When worked (1st pers. sing.) at the port yes, but no want (1st pers. sing.) no.
ET: P: I don't like English, and I wouldn't like to speak it, no, no, this is my home so I don't speak English here! I don't like other languages. I didn't want to. I did so when I was working at the port, but I don't want to speak it now, no.

DS: E: Quins idiomes parla? P: Anglès… no… no… no ja no m'agrada no no i jo no m'agradaria no no i jo... a casa! Aquí no! No, és que els altres no m'agraden. No volia, quan treballo al moll sí… no vull no, no.
G: P: ∅ (art. masc. sing.) English… no… no… no to me like no no and I no to me would like no no and I at home! Here no! No, is that the others to me don't like. No wanted (1st pers. sing.), when work (1st pers. sing. pres.) at the port yes… no want (1st pers. sing. pres.) no, no.

2) T: E: Quin és el seu idioma matern? P: A la mare li parlava en català i als fills també en català a tots.
G: E: What is your mother tongue? P: To my mother to her spoke in Catalan and to the children in Catalan to all.
ET: P: I used to speak Catalan with my mother and I also speak Catalan with all my children.

DS: P: Mare també en català i fills català a tots.
G: ∅ (prep.) ∅ (art.) mother also in Catalan and ∅ (prep.) ∅ (art.) children Catalan to all.

3) T: E: A què es dedicaven els seus pares? P: El meu pare i la meva mare eren de Cartagena i eren militars.
G: E: What was your parents' job? P: The (art. masc. sing.) my (pron. 3rd pers. masc. sing.) father and the (art. fem. sing.) my (pron. 3rd pers. fem. sing.) mother were from Cartagena and were (3rd pers pl.) soldiers.
ET: E: What was your parents' job? P: My father and my mother were from Cartagena and they were soldiers.

DS: P: Mare pare eren de Cartagena i militars.
G: P: ∅ (art.) ∅ (pron.) mother ∅ (art.) ∅ (conj.) ∅ (pron.) father were from Cartagena and soldiers.

4) T: E: Quin era l'idioma amb què parlava als seus amics? P: Si parlaven en castellà, jo els hi parlava en castellà. Si parlaven en català, jo els hi parlava en català.
G: E: What was that language you used to speak to your friends? P: If spoke (3rd pers. pl.) in Spanish, I to them spoke (1st pers. sing.) in Spanish. If spoke (3rd pers. pl.) in Catalan, I to them spoke (1st pers. sing.) in Catalan.
ET: E: What was the language you used to speak with your friends? P: If they spoke Spanish, I spoke Spanish, and if they spoke Catalan, then I spoke Catalan.

DS: P: Castellà? Jo castellà! Català? Jo català!
G: P: Spanish? I Spanish! Catalan? I Catalan!

5) T: E: Fins quan va anar al col.legi? P: Jo? Fins als set anys. El germà de la meva mare era capellà i allí es parlava només català.
G: E: Until when went (2nd pers. sing.) to the school? P: I? Until to the seven years. The brother of my mother was priest and there was spoken only Catalan.
ET: E: When did you leave school? P: Me? When I was seven years old. My mother's brother was a priest and there we only spoke Catalan.

DS: Jo? Als set anys… al… al… el germà de ma mare era capellà i allí només català! Català! Català!
G: I? ∅ (prep.) at the seven years… the… the… the brother of my mother was a priest and there only Catalan! Catalan! Catalan!

6) T: E: Què va fer després de deixar l'escola? P: Quan va acabar la guerra, ens van posar en un camió i cap a casa. El meu germà sí, parlava català, castellà, anglès, rus… era pilot d'avió.
G: E: What do (2nd pers. sing. periphrastic past) after leaving the school? P: When finished (3rd pers. sing.) the war, they us put (3rd pers. pl.) into a truck and to house. My brother yes, spoke (3rd pers. sing.) Catalan, Spanish, English, Russian… was (3rd pers. sing.) pilot of an airplane.
ET: E: What did you do after leaving school? P: When the war was over, they put us into a truck and sent us home. My brother used to speak Catalan, Spanish, English, Russian… he was a pilot.

DS: P: Acaba la guerra, un camió i a casa! Ma germà sí, català, castellà, anglès, rus… pilot d'avió.
G: P: Finishes the war, a truck and to house! My brother yes, Catalan, Spanish, English, Russian… pilot of airplane.

7) T: E: A què es va dedicar? P: Jo tenia molt de treball. Jo treballava a tot arreu: a la marítima… i un dia me'n vaig anar.
G: E: What was your job? P: I had plenty of work. I worked everywhere: at the navy… and one day I myself left.
ET: P: I had many jobs and worked everywhere: in the navy… but one day I left it all.

DS: P: Jo tenia molt de treball. Jo treballo, sí, a tot arreu. A la marítima… un dia es va… me'n vaig anar.
G: P: I had plenty of work. I work (1st pers. sing. pres.) yes, everywhere. At the navy… one day it did… myself left.

8) T: E: Sempre ha viscut a Catalunya? P: Sí, sí, sempre. Jo vaig néixer aquí. Si parlen en castellà, jo parlo en castellà. Si parlen en català, jo parlo en català Que no m'entens? Al carrer!
G: E: Have you always lived in Catalonia? P: Yes, yes, always. I was born here. If speak (3rd pers. pl.) in Spanish I speak in Spanish. If speak (3rd pers. pl.) in Catalan, I speak in Catalan. That no to me understand (2nd pers. sing.)? To the street!
ET: P: Yes, yes, I always did. I was born here. If they speak Spanish, I do speak Spanish. If they speak Catalan, I do speak Catalan. If you don't understand me, it's your business!

DS: P: Sí, sí tot. Aquí, aquí, jo neix aquí. Si a castellà, jo castellà. Si català, jo català. Que no me entiendes? A la calle!
G: P: Yes, yes all. Here, here I born (1st pers. sing. pres.) here. If to Spanish, I Spanish. If Catalan, I Catalan. That no to me understand (in Spanish)? To the street (in Spanish)!

9) T: E: Era bo el seu català escrit? P: L'he perdut tot.
G: E: Was your written Catalan good? P: It (dative pron.) have lost (1st pers. sing. past) all.
ET: P: I've lost it all.

DS: P: Hi perdut tot.
G: P: It (dative pron.) have lost (1st pers. sing. past) all.

10) T: E: Quants anys tenia quan va aprendre a parlar en català? P: Ui! Deu o així.
G: E: How old were you when you learned Catalan? P: Wow! Ten or like this.
ET: P: Wow! Ten or so.

DS: P: Ui! Deu aixins.
G: P: Ten like this.

11) T: E: Amb quina freqüència llegia? P: De tant en tant. Escriure'l no, no sempre en castellà. I ara no en sé ni en català ni en castellà ni res.
G: E: With what frequency did you usually read? P: Not very often. Writing it no, no, always in Spanish and now no it (accusative pron.) know in Catalan nor in Spanish nor nothing.
ET: P: Not very often. I never wrote (in Catalan) no, no, always in Spanish but now I don't know how to do it, neither in Spanish nor in Catalan nor in any other language.

DS: P:Banantan. Escriure? No, no, no. Sempre a castellà. I ara no sé. Ni català ni castellà ni res.
G: Not very often (paraphasic). Writing ∅ (accusative pron.)? No, no, no. Always to Spanish. And now no ∅ (accusative pron.) know (1st pers. sing. pres.) nor Spanish, nor Catalan, nor anything.

THE MEMBERS OF YOUR FAMILY

T: La meva dona la tinc aquí, aquí, …pagant. I la dona …de … va anar a Sant Boi. I hi va estar dues vegades, ingressada allí. Abans estava ingressada aquí. I ara teniem una baralla i una altra baralla… sempre! La meva dona està ingressada. Els medicaments no li van bé. Dia i nit jo la tenia que portar al lavabo, rentar-la… tot ho feia jo! Però és impossible ja! Em volia pegar i tot!
G: My wife she have (1st pers. sing. pres.) here, paying. And the wife... from… went to St. Boi. And there (ablative pron.) she was two times, admitted there. Before that was (3rd pers. sing. pres. perfect) admitted here. And now had (1st pers. pl. pres. perfect) a quarrel and another quarrel… always! The (art. fem. sing.) my (pron. fem. sing.) wife is admitted here. The medications not her do (3rd pers. pl. pres.) good. Day and night I her had to (1st pers. sing pres. perfect) carry to the toilet, wash her… all it (accusative pron.) did (3rd pers. sing. pres. perfect) I! But is impossible now! Me wanted (3rd pers. sing. pres. perfect) hit and all!
ET: I had my wife admitted to this hospital and have to pay for it. My wife was admitted to St. Boi [mental hospital] twice before that. And before that, she had been admitted to this hospital. And lately we've had one discussion after another without a break. Now

she's here again. The medications do not have any effect on her. Night and day I had to care for her, bring her to the toilet, wash her and so on. I did it all. But now that is not possible anymore! She wanted to beat me lately!

DS: Meva dona tinc aquí...pagant. I na dona... de... va a sa... sa... a Sant Boi i jo vai dos veces ingressada. Medicament no van bé. Jo dia i nit tinc que... jo... a lavabo a rentar-la... tot jo! Impossible ja! Em vol pegar i tot!
G: My (poss. pron. 3rd pers. sing.) wife have (3rd pers. sing. pres.) here ... paying. And na (neologism) wife... from... went to San... San... to Sant Boi and I go two times admitted. Medicament no do good. I day and night have to... I... to the toilet, wash her... all I! Impossible now! Me wants (3rd pers. sing. pres.) to beat up and all!

WHAT'S YOUR JOB LIKE?

T: Jo era un dels més forts. Carregava dos cents quilos i movia quatre o cinc... dues tones... pom! Pom! No parava dia i nit treballant. Volies descansar? Sí, vés a la porra! Res! A treballar?
G: I was (1st pers. sing. pres. perfect) one of the most strongest. Carried (1st pers. sing. pres. perfect) 200 kilos and moved (1st pers. sing. pres. perfect) four or five... two tons... pom! Pom! Did not stop (1st pers. sing. pres. perfect) day and night working. Wanted (2nd pers. sing. past) to rest? Yes, go to hell! Nothing! To work!
ET: I was one of the strongest. I carried 200 kilos and moved four or five... two tons... pom! Pom! I never stopped and worked all day and night. If you wanted to take a break, don't even think about it! Go on working.

DS: Jo era un dels més forts... dos cent quilos i... a cinc... quatro o cinc... dos tonelades... Pom! Pom! No parar dia i nit treballant. Vols aguantar-te? Sí! A porra! Res! A treballar.
G: I was (3rd pers. sing. pres. perfect) one of the most strongest... 200 kilos and... to five... four (Spanish) or five... two tons... pom! Pom! No stop day and night working. Want (2nd pers. sing. pres.) hold on yourself? Yes! To hell! Nothing! To work.

BAT PICTURE STORY

T: L'home corre i crida. Aquesta noia se les mira totes.
G: The (art. masc. sing.) man runs and shouts. This girl herself them looks all.
ET: The man runs and shouts. This girl looks at all of them.

DS: La home i corre i crida. Aquesta noia se lo mira totes.
G: The (art. fem. sing.) and runs and shouts. This girl looks it all.

Manifestation of aphasic symptoms in Czech

Helena Lehečková

Dpt. of Slavonic and Baltic Languages, University of Helsinki, Finland

Abstract—Czech is a strongly inflecting language with a great number of different grammatical forms for each inflected word. Aphasia is always manifested in a certain impairment of the morphosyntactic structure. I have analysed spontaneous speech from 18 motor aphasics and discovered the typical manifestations of agrammatism in Czech: (a) omission of some grammatical words (mainly prepositions, auxiliaries and pronouns); (b) concentration of errors in some grammatical categories (especially case, tense and person); (c) overuse of certain forms of grammatical categories (masculine gender, singular number, nominative case, 3rd person, present tense, indicative mood, active voice and imperfective aspect). The forms most available to aphasics tend to correlate with the earliest acquired forms and the most frequent ones.

Key words: Czech, agrammatism, omissions, substitutions, acquisition, frequency

1. Czech language in normal use

Czech is a Slavonic language. It belongs to the West Slavonic group and it is spoken by 10 million native speakers, mostly living in the Czech Republic. Czech was a literary language as early as the 14th century. Owing to its very long and complicated historical development it is full of irregularities, double forms and stylistic variants. There is an unusually big difference between the written and spoken varieties: the literary language, which is codified in grammars and dictionaries, is spoken only in most official contexts, while normal oral communication is usually realized in common spoken language, which is a widespread interdialect, or regional dialects, or possibly in a combination of all three varieties.

1.1. Typological description of relevant aspects of Czech grammar

Czech is a strongly inflecting language. The typical structure of inflected word forms consists of one stem plus one ending.

STEM	+	ENDING

Exceptionally, the ending may be realized as a zero (e.g. in the nominative singular of some masculines, or in the genitive plural of some feminines and neuters). However, the zero ending may require changes in the stem. Thus, from the point of view of the language system, the stem is not a free morpheme although it may sometimes function as such.

One ending incorporates several grammatical meanings:

(1) *mužům*
men:M.D.PL
to men

STEM	+	ENDING
muž		*ům*
man		M.&D.& Pl.

The noun ending *-ům* expresses gender (masculine), case (dative) and number (plural).

Different parts of speech have their own paradigms:

(2) *těm dvěma mladým mužům*
those: M.D.PL two:M.D.PL young:M.D.PL men:M.D.PL
to those two young men

Different endings:	The same grammatical function:
-ěm	
-ema	MASCULINE DATIVE PLURAL
-ým	
-ům	

Even within one part of speech, one grammatical function can be expressed by many different endings (e.g. lst person singular present of verbs):

One function:	Many forms:			
3rd SG. PRESENT	-e	*nes*	*-e*	(he) carries
	-ne	*tisk*	*-ne*	(he) presses
	-je	*kry*	*-je*	(he) covers
	-í	*pros*	*-í*	(he) asks
	-á	*řík*	*-á*	(he) says

On the other hand, one grammatical ending can have several grammatical functions:

Many functions:	One form:			
M. ANIM. ACC. PL.	-y	*pán*	*-y*	men
M. ANIM. INSTR. PL.		*pán*	*-y*	
M. INANIM. NOM. PL.		*hrad*	*-y*	castles
M. INANIM. ACC. PL.		*hrad*	*-y*	
F. GEN. SG.		*žen*	*-y*	woman
F. NOM. PL.		*žen*	*-y*	
F. ACC. PL.		*žen*	*-y*	
F. VOC. PL.		*žen*	*-y*	
N. INSTR. PL.		*měst*	*-y*	towns

These two features are important for the description of aphasia in Czech:
(a) In principle, a mere stem without any ending is a non-word.
(b) There is no one-to-one correspondence between form and function.

1.2. Grammatical description of Czech

Compared to other languages, Czech grammar offers numerous possibilities for breakdown. Let us consider, for example, the category of grammatical gender. The typologically different languages Czech (inflecting), English (isolating) and Finnish (agglutinating) differ considerably in their realization of this grammatical category, and thus offer quite different sites for potential errors.

Explicit expressions of gender in different grammatical categories:

			CZ	ENG	FIN
1	nouns	lexical	-/+	-/+	- /+
2		derivational	+	(-)	-
3	adject.		+	-	-
		possessive adj.	+	-	-
4	numer.		+	-	-
5	pron.	attributes	+	-	-
6		1st/2nd pers. pron. 3rd pers. pron.	- +	- +	- -
7	verbs	pres./fut. ind. act. 1st/2nd person 3rd person	 - -	 - -/+	 - -
8		past/condit./pass. 1st/2nd person 3rd person	 + +	 - -/+	 - -
9		gerund	+	-	-

It is obvious that there is almost no space for making errors in grammatical gender in Finnish and there are restricted possibilities for doing so in English. In Czech, on the other hand, almost every inflected form is marked for gender and is thus liable to error.

1.2.1. Morphology

Czech morphology is very rich both in grammatical categories and their different realizations.

Nominal categories:	gender, number, case
Verbal categories:	person, number, tense, mood, voice, aspect, (gender)

a) GENDER.

There are 3 genders: masculine (M) animate (MA) and inanimate (MI), feminine (F), and neuter (N). Every noun belongs to one of the three possible genders (masculine, feminine, neuter). Within masculines the subcategory of animacy is differentiated:

(4)	*český pracovník*	-	*čeští pracovníci*
	Czech worker:MA.N.SG	-	Czech workers:MA.N.PL
(5)	*český slovník*	-	*české slovníky*
	Czech dictionary:MI.N.SG	-	Czech dictionaries:MI.N.PL

In names of human beings the division into masculines and feminines follows the biological division into males and females; in inanimates the distribution is arbitrary. There is no one-to-one correspondence between the formal characteristic of the word and its gender (e.g. nouns ending in a consonant are mostly masculine, but some of them are feminine, nouns ending in -e are either feminine, or neuter, rarely also masculine).

Gender in adjectives, pronouns, numerals and nominal verb forms is assigned by agreement with the head noun:

(6)MA: *Ten náš starý pacient byl vyléčen.*
that:MA our:MA old:MA patient:MA was:MA cured:MA
Our old patient there was cured.

(7)F: *Ta naše stará pacientka byla vyléčena.*
that:F our:F old:F patient:F was:F cured:F
Our old patient there was cured.

(8)N: *To naše staré auto bylo opraveno.*
that:N our:N old:N car:N was:N repaired:N
Our old car there was repaired.

b) NUMBER.

There are 2 numbers: singular (SG), and plural (PL). In nouns number is marked by reference, in other parts of speech by agreement.

c) CASE.
There are 7 cases: nominative (N), genitive (G), dative (D), accusative (A), vocative (V), locative (L), and instrumental (I).

d) PERSON.
There are 3 persons: 1st, 2nd, and 3rd. Person is expressed primarily in verb endings and only secondarily, for emphasis, by personal pronouns. If not emphasized, subject pronouns are not used.

e) TENSE.
There are 3 tenses: present (PRES), past (PAST), and future (FUT). The set of only three tenses is made more complex by the Slavonic aspect (e.g. the present form of a perfective verb refers to a future event). The present is expressed by simple conjugated forms. The past consists of an auxiliary (present tense of "to be") and a past participle that agrees with the subject in gender and number. The future tense is formed by an auxiliary (future of "to be") and the imperfect infinitive.

f) MOOD.
There are 3 moods: indicative (IND), imperative (IMP), and conditional (COND). The imperative is expressed morphologically in the 2nd person singular and plural and in the 1st person plural, and analytically in others. The conditional is expressed by a combination of the conjugated enclitic auxiliary *by* and a past participle that agrees with the subject in gender and number.

g) VOICE.
There are 2 voices: active (ACT), and passive (PASS). There are two forms of the passive: the auxiliary "to be" and a passive participle that agrees with the subject in gender and number, or a reflexive form of the verb with a completely suppressed subject.

h) ASPECT.
There are 2 aspects: imperfective (IMPF), and perfective (PF). Aspect expresses the way in which the an action is presented (e.g. stress on the process or result of the action, repetition or uniqueness of the action, telicity etc.). Almost all verbal lexemes exist in two aspectual forms: imperfective and perfective. The imperfective expresses the verbal action in general terms, as a process, while the perfective typically specifies completion of an act.

The structure of noun phrases (NP) and verb phrases (VP):

NP	=	STEM	+	ENDING							
				gender:	MA	MI	F	N			
				number:	SG	PL					
				case:	N	G	D	A	V	L	I

VP	=	STEM	+	ENDING				
				gender:	MA	MI	F	N
				number:	SG	PL		
				person:	1st	2nd	3rd	
				tense:	PRES	PAST	FUT	
				mood:	IND	IMP	COND	
				voice:	ACT	PASS		
				aspect:	IMPF	PF		

Inflected words take their grammatical forms as follows:

i) *Nouns*. 14 declensions are differentiated (6 for masculines, 4 feminines, 4 neuters) in so-called regular nouns, plus special declensions for nouns of foreign origin and irregular nouns. Even in regular nouns there are many exceptions influencing both the stem and the endings.

ii) *Adjectives*. 3 declensions (so-called hard, soft and possessive ones).

iii) *Pronouns*. Pronouns are inflected according to their own paradigms. In oblique cases there can be as many as 3 forms (with possible stylistic variants) for each case: an unstressed form, a stressed form and a form used after prepositions:

(9)	*ho, jej*	*jeho*	*pro něho, něj*
	him (unstressed):M.A	him (stressed):M.A	for him:M.A

iv) *Numerals*. The cardinal numerals 1, 2, 3, 4 have the whole paradigm, while the others differentiate two forms only: basic form and oblique case. Ordinal numerals are inflected as adjectives.

v) *Verbs*. There are 5 conjugations but within them different subtypes have to be differentiated. This means that so-called regular verbs are conjugated according to 14 paradigms. In addition, there are many irregular verbs, which are usually the most frequent ones.

1.2.2. Syntax

The relations within a clause are mainly organized by the finite verb and its rection. Arguments can be attached to verbs either directly:

(10) *Petr dal Zuzaně růži.*
Peter:N gave Susan:D a rose:A.SG.
Peter gave Susan a rose.

or through prepositions:

(11) *Petr se díval na film o lásce.*
Peter:N REFL.PRON watched on:PREP a film:A.SG about:PREP love:L.SG.
Peter watched a film about love.

Czech has a so-called free word order. The inflectional system is so highly developed that there is little scope for ambiguity, and syntactic relations are practically always transparent. This does not mean complete freedom in building sentences, however. Word order inside phrases is fixed:

(12) *Jeho velmi zajímavý článek o afázii / bude publikován / v našem časopise.*
His very interesting article about aphasia / will be published / in our magazine.

Word order is mainly organized on the informational principle. Old information comes at the beginning, while new information is placed at the end of the sentence:

(13)	*Pacient*	*vyprávěl*	*lékaři*	*o své nemoci.*
	The patient	told	the doctor	about his illness.
(13a)	*Pacient*	*lékaři*	*o své nemoci*	*vyprávěl.*
(13b)	*Pacient*	*vyprávěl*	*o své nemoci*	*lékaři.*
(13c)	*Lékaři*	*o své nemoci*	*vyprávěl*	*pacient.*
(13d)	*O své nemoci*	*lékaři*	*pacient*	*vyprávěl.*

Enclitics, i.e. grammatical words lacking word stress, have a fixed place: they follow the first stressed constituent in the clause:

(14) *Já jsem mu to dala.*
I:N have him:D it:A given.
I have given it to him.

(14a) *Dala jsem mu to já.*
given have him:D it:A I:N.
It was me who gave it to him.

2. Czech language in aphasia

Apart from my own studies (cf. References), Czech has not been described from the neurolinguistic point of view, nor is it represented in the cross-language sourcebook on agrammatic aphasia (Menn & Obler, 1990). Thus the aim of this paper is not to give a detailed description of a particular case; rather it is an attempt to show some general tendencies common to all the cases considered.

Owing to the very complicated grammar of Czech, aphasia is always manifested by some kind of disruption of the morphosyntactic structure. Generally speaking, grammatical problems in language production occur in two main types:

a) omission of grammatical morphemes;

b) substitution of incorrect grammatical morphemes for correct ones.

I have argued (Lehečková, 1988b, 1995) that the distribution of these two types of symptom is bound not only to the site of lesion but also to the type of language. In isolating and agglutinating languages both free and bound morphemes can be omitted. In inflecting languages, on the other hand, only free grammatical morphemes are omitted. Bound morphemes are substituted because word stems cannot stand as separate items. As has been described for several languages (e.g. Kukkonen, 1982; Lapointe, 1983; Miceli et al., 1983; Grodzinsky, 1984, 1986; Badecker & Caramazza, 1985; Stemberger, 1985; Heeschen, 1985; Menn & Obler, 1990; Bebout, 1993; Niemi et al., 1994; De Blesser et al., 1995/6), aphasics do not omit morphemes if their omission would result in non-words. I have shown (e.g. Lehečková, 1988a) that this holds for Czech as well.

Grammatical relations in Czech are mostly expressed by bound morphemes. The typical structure of inflected words consists of a stem and an ending neither of which exists as a separate word. All aphasic patients, independently of the type of impairment, make mistakes in grammar. As long as the forms used by the patients are analyzable (intelligible), incorrect grammatical forms tend to be existing words of Czech. Morphological errors are mostly manifested as substitutions of incorrect elements for correct ones. Thus there is no clear-cut difference between agrammatism and paragrammatism.

In what follows I will call agrammatism all disturbances of the normal morphosyntactic structure of utterances. Agrammatism in this sense is present to a certain degree in all types of aphasia (Lehečková, 1989) and it affects more or less all language modalities. In the present paper I will concentrate on spontaneous oral language production.

2.1. Possible manifestation of agrammatism in Czech

When analyzing the language production of an aphasic we must first find out how it differs from normal language use. However simple this demand may seem, it is not so easy to meet, especially in a language so rich in different varieties as Czech is.

Both for the practical purposes of language testing and the re-education of speech on the one hand, and for the theoretical goals of linguistic studies on the other, we must be able to compare two structures of every utterance: (a) the deviant structure of the utterance produced by the aphasic, and (b) the correct structure of the same utterance.

This process means that we must know what the patient was aiming at. There are two problems in meeting this requirement. First, we must know what meaning the patient was trying to convey. Second, we must decide in which variety (code) he or she attempted to convey the meaning. The choice of variety, i.e. literary (standard) language, common spoken language, or a dialect, influences not only prosody and lexicon, but also morphology. Those elements that are of special interest in agrammatism (both bound and free grammatical morphemes) have different forms in literary (i.e. consciously learned) language, and in varieties of spoken language.

(15a)	*Stař-í*	*lid-é*	*mluv-í*	*o*	*t-ěch*	*nov-ých*	*středis-cích.*
(15b)	*Star-ý*	*lid-i*	*mluv-ěj*	*vo*	*t-ěch*	*nov-ejch*	*středis-kách.*
(15c)	*Star-é*	*lid-e*	*mluv-ijó*	*o*	*t-ech*	*nov-éch*	*středis-koch.*
	Old	people	speak	about	those	new	centres.

(15a) is literary language, (15b) is common spoken language, (15c) is a possible dialect. It is obvious that inflected words can get different endings in different varieties and what is correct in e.g. common Czech is wrong in literary language.

To make the situation even more complicated, the choice of variety is not binding, i.e. one can fairly freely switch from one code to another. Different codes can be combined even within one utterance: (16a) is literary language, (16b) is common spoken language, (16c) is a possible combination of the two:

(16a) *s bílými okny*
(16b) *s bílejma voknama*
(16c) *s bílýma oknama*
with white:N.I.PL windows:N.I.PL

These facts constitute a problem in evaluating the material of language impairments. For a statistical analysis the errors must be counted, although it is not always clear where the error lies:

(17) *Malý kniha leží na stole.*
small:M.SG book:F.SG lie:3SG./PL. on table

The ungrammatical sentence (17) can either mean:

(17a) *Malá kniha leží na stole.*
small:F.SG book:F.SG lies:3SG on table
A small book lies on the table.

where the feminine form of the adjective was replaced by masculine (in literary language), or

(17b) *Malý knihy ležej na stole.*
small:M./F./N.PL books:F.PL lie:3PL on table
Small books lie on the table.

where plural was replaced by singular in the noun and the verb (in common spoken Czech) or

(17c) *Malé knihy leží na stole.*
small:M./F.PL books:F.PL lie:3SG./PL on table
Small books lie on the table.

where plural was replaced by singular in the adjective as well as the noun, and the feminine form of the adjective was replaced by masculine (in literary Czech).

It is not only substitution of incorrect forms for correct ones but also omitting that makes it difficult to interpret errors. The same incorrect utterance can be counted both as substitution and omission:

(18) *Ty vařit.*
you cook:INF

can be taken to be a replacement of the finite verb by an infinitive:

(18a) *Ty vaříš.*
you cook:2SG.PRES

or to be the omission of the auxiliary of the future tense:

(18b) *Ty budeš vařit.*
you will:2SG.FUT cook:INF

In interpreting the material obtained from spontaneous speech one can, of course, use the context and assume that the same variety is used throughout the text. In the present error analysis, the intended forms were assumed to be in the same variety as the immediate context and to be as close as possible to the target form, with a minimum number of deviant features. Nevertheless, the interpretation of the material is a problem that must be borne in mind when drawing conclusions. The results are influenced by the way we interpret the corpus, and thus the statistical analysis cannot be authoritative as far as absolute numbers are concerned. What it can provide are relative numbers showing certain tendencies in aphasic language use.

2.2. Agrammatism in aphasic subjects — review of previous cases

In general, agrammatism manifests itself in the avoidance of some grammatical elements and the overuse of others. It has been shown that while English agrammatism is characterised by omission of grammatical elements, in other languages agrammatism may be manifested in a different way, mainly by substitutions (Lehečková, 1987; Paradis, 1988; Niemi & Laine, 1989; Menn & Obler, 1990; Grodzinsky, 1990; Kolk & Heeschen, 1992; De Blesser et al., 1995/6; Lukatela, Shankweiler & Crain, 1995; Nilipour & Paradis, 1995; Tesak & Niemi, 1997).

In my investigations of aphasia in Czech, I tried to find out if all the forms from the set of permissible inflectional configurations are equally likely to be used, or if there is any preference in using some forms instead of others.

The questions studied were: (a) Are the erroneous forms existing forms of the same grammatical category? and (b) If so, which forms usually replace the others?

Material

As a linguist based in Finland, I have not been in permanent touch with Czech aphasic patients. Their choice and diagnosis (including the determination of the type of aphasia) have been made by speech pathologists and neurologists with whom I have been co-operating. I have not seeked to classify deficits. My aim has been to capture the type of language errors that occur in aphasia and to characterize them linguistically.

I studied a total of 35 Czech aphasics whose clinical diagnosis was the following: 17 cases were classified as motor aphasia, 14 as mixed aphasia with a predominant motor constituent, 2 as mixed aphasia with a predominant sensory constituent and 2 as amnesic aphasia. As the types of aphasia were represented unevenly in the material, I concentrated mainly on motor aphasia.

The material analysed in the synoptic study (Lehečková, 1988a) consisted of recordings of spontaneous speech from 17 motor aphasics. I met each patient during one of his or her rehabilitation sessions and had a talk with them. The conversation was recorded. The tasks performed by the patients were: (a) speaking about their illness; (b) speaking about their profession; (c) telling a story (Red Riding Hood); and (d) describing a picture (a family sitting at the breakfast table in the kitchen).

If the patient spoke spontaneously I did not interrupt, otherwise I asked questions to keep up the conversation. The amount of material obtained from different patients was uneven. Depending on the severity of impairment, each interview yielded 5-20 minutes of recordings. Although the type of errors in different patients did differ as to quantity, there were similarities as to manifestation.

When analysing the recordings I compared the patients' utterances with correct structures in the variety of common spoken language. It is the usual code for the conversational situation and it was the variety the patients approached most closely. Only one patient systematically used literary language, and so his utterances were related to the grammatical structure of literary Czech.

In the study, two types of relation between the patient's utterance and the norm were left without further analysis: (a) if the uttered form was unrecognisable (it was a non-existent word) or unanalysable (it was used without context and thus was grammatically ambiguous: e.g. *hodný holka* could be interpreted as N.SG *hodná holka* "good girl" or N/A.PL *hodný holky* "good girls"); and (b) if the uttered form was identical with the norm. It would certainly deserve further analysis because what patients do correctly is of no less interest than the description of their errors. However, for the purpose of this report I have concentrated on the analysis of errors.

In analysing the material, I used the minimal reconstruction procedure, i.e. correction toward those elements that "add least" to what the patient really said (cf. Menn & Obler, 1990).

The quantitative characteristics of the corpus can be found in Lehečková (1988a). The percentage of grammatically correct clauses varied in 17 patients from 15% to 83% (median 48%).

As spoken language is not codified, correctness had to be evaluated intuitively, on the basis of acceptability in common speech and comprehensibility for the conversation partner. Spoken language has not been studied enough to allow straightforward decisions about what is right and what is wrong in it. The first transcriptions of normal conversations (cf. Müllerová, Hoffmannová & Schneiderová, 1992) look surprisingly "abnormal" if compared to the standard language, and yet they are fully functional. Only after extensive corpora of spoken Czech have become available will it be possible to base the analysis of abnormalities on a more accurately determined spoken norm.

With the norm lacking, it is easier to identify substitution errors than omissions. While substitutions of grammatical elements occur seldom in normal language use, omissions of both grammatical and content words are frequent. Owing to the shortage of comparable material it is sometimes difficult to evaluate the difference between ellipsis and omission. In my corpus 38% of errors were classified as omissions and 62% as substitutions.

2.2.1. Omissions

There was not a single case in the material where a bound grammatical morpheme was omitted and a pure stem used. Sometimes a patient seeking for the correct form did use a stem (or the first syllable) only, but it was always with rising intonation and a pause. He repeated it until he found some ending and produced a stem plus an ending form:

(19) *žen- žen- ženou*
žen- žen- ženou:F.I.SG
woman

What was omitted were free grammatical morphemes: prepositions and auxiliaries. Omissions of pronouns were not very apparent because Czech predicates do not need pronominal subjects (the person is indicated by the verb ending). Surprisingly enough, content words, especially verbs, were omitted more often than grammatical words. Out of all the omissions in the corpus 30% were omissions of grammatical words and 70% were omissions of content words. Verbs were omitted both in their finite forms and as infinitives (i.e. the auxiliary was present but the infinitive of a meaning-bearing verb was missing, which is just the opposite of what would be expected). In some cases obligatory arguments of verbs were omitted, too.

2.2.2. Substitutions

Most grammatical errors were caused by substitutions of incorrect forms for correct ones. In the analysed material there were 205 errors caused by substitution. 98% of the erroneous forms were existing forms of the same category. Only 5 non-existing grammatical forms were found (2 were regular plural forms of irregular words). For the distribution of errors in different patients see Lehečková (1988a).

The present study aims at the generalisation of the type of aphasic errors in Czech. In what follows I will thus sum up my previous results and present them from two new points of view: (a) the distribution of errors among different grammatical categories; and (b) the distribution of errors among different forms within each grammatical category.

Ad a) Distribution of errors among different grammatical categories:

GENDER:	11%
NUMBER:	11%
CASE:	32%
PERSON:	13%
TENSE:	15%
MOOD:	15%

VOICE:	1%
ASPECT:	2%

The surprisingly high percentage of errors in mood results from the fact that the patients often tried to use the imperative in Red Riding Hood. In other tasks only the indicative was used.

Ad b) Distribution of errors among different forms within each grammatical category:

GENDER:	M	replaced F	in	61 %	of errors
	M	replaced N	in	26 %	of errors
	F	replaced N	in	13 %	of errors
NUMBER:	SG	replaced PL	in	100 %	of errors
CASE:	N	replaced non-N	in	58 %	of errors
	non-N	replaced non-N	in	40 %	of errors
	non-N	replaced N	in	2 %	of errors
PERSON:	3rd	replaced 1st	in	68 %	of errors
	3rd	replaced 2nd	in	21 %	of errors
	1st	replaced 2nd	in	11 %	of errors
TENSE:	PRES	replaced PAST	in	61 %	of errors
	PRES	replaced FUT	in	33 %	of errors
	FUT	replaced PRES	in	6 %	of errors
MOOD:	IND	replaced COND	in	89 %	of errors
	IND	replaced IMPER	in	11 %	of errors
VOICE:	ACT	replaced PASS	in	100 %	of errors
ASPECT:	IMPF	replaced PF	in	100 %	of errors

Examples:

GENDER:

(20) Target: Moje doktorka říká
Gloss: My (nom. sg. fem.) doctor (nom. sg. fem.) says (3rd pers. sg. pres.)
Target English equivalent: My doctor (female) says

Defective utterance: *Můj doktorka říká*
Gloss: My (nom. sg. masc.) doctor (nom. sg. fem.) says (3rd pers. sg. pres.)

(21) Target: Malá holka
Gloss: Little (nom. sg. fem.) girl (nom. sg. fem.)
Target English equivalent: Little girl

Defective utterance: *Malý holka*
Gloss: Little (nom. sg. masc.) girl (nom. sg. fem.)

(22) Target: Hloupý zvíře
Gloss: Stupid (nom. sg. neuter) animal (nom. sg. neuter)
Target English equivalent: Stupid animal

Defective utterance: *Hloupej zvíře*
Gloss: Stupid (nom. sg. masc.) animal (nom. sg. neuter)

(23) Target: Dobrý zdravý jídlo
Gloss: Good (nom. sg. neuter) healthy (nom. sg. neuter) food (nom. sg. neuter)
Target English equivalent: Good healthy food

Defective utterance: *Dobrá zdravý jídlo*
Gloss: Good (nom. sg. fem.) healthy (nom. sg. neuter) food (nom. sg. neuter)

NUMBER:

(24) Target: Mám dva chlapce
Gloss: Have (1st pers. sg. pres.) two (acc. masc.) boy (acc. pl. masc. anim.)
Target English equivalent: I have two boys

Defective utterance: *Mám dva chlapec*
Gloss: Have (1st pers. sg. pres.) two (acc. masc.) boy (nom. sg. masc. anim.)

CASE:

(25) Target: Nezná mýho muže
Gloss: Know (3rd pers. sg. pres.) my (acc. sg. masc. anim.) husband (acc. sg. masc. anim.)
Target English equivalent: She does not know my husband

Defective utterance: *Nezná mųj muž*
Gloss: Know (3rd pers. sg. pres.) my (nom. sg. masc. anim.) husband (nom. sg. masc. anim.)

PERSON:

(26) Target: Já musím hodně spát
Gloss: I must (1st pers. sg. pres.) much sleep (inf.)
Target English equivalent: I must sleep much

Defective utterance: *Já musí hodně spát*
Gloss: I must (3rd pers. sg. pres.) much sleep (inf.)

(27) Target: Karkulko, musíš tam
Gloss: Red Riding Hood (voc. sg. fem.), must (2nd pers. sg. pres.) there
Target English equivalent: Red Riding Hood, you must go there

Defective utterance: *Karkulko, musí tam*
Gloss: : Red Riding Hood (voc. sg. fem.), must (3rd pers. sg. pres.) there

(28) Target: Pepo, ty nikdy nemáš čas
Gloss: Pepa (voc. sg. masc.), you never have (2nd pers. sg. pres.) time (acc. sg. masc. inanim.)
Target English equivalent: Pepa, you never have time

Defective utterance: *Pepo, ty nikdy nemám čas*
Gloss: Pepa (voc. sg. masc.), you never have (1st pers. sg. pres.) time (acc. sg. masc. inanim.)

TENSE:

(29) Target: Bylo to 11. dubna 1980
Gloss: Is (3rd pers. sg. past neuter) it (nom. sg. neuter) 11 April 1980
Target English equivalent: It was April 11th 1980

Defective utterance: *Je to 11. dubna 1980*
Gloss: Is (3rd pers. sg. pres.) it (nom. sg. neuter) 11 April 1980

(30) Target: Zítra bude obědvat
Gloss: Tomorrow will (3rd pers. sg. fut.) eat (inf.) lunch
Target English equivalent: Tomorrow he will eat lunch

Defective utterance: *Zítra obědvá*
Gloss: Tomorrow eat (3rd pers. sg. pres.) lunch

MOOD:

(31) Target: Karkulko, jdi rovnou
Gloss: Red Riding Hood (voc. sg. fem.), go (2nd pers. sg. imper.) directly
Target English equivalent: Red Riding Hood, go directly!

Defective utterance: *Karkulko, jde rovnou*
Gloss: Red Riding Hood (voc. sg. fem.), go (3rd pers. sg. pres. ind.) directly

VOICE:

The passive is a rare form in spoken Czech and it never occurred in the speech of aphasics. In cases where a passive should have been used it was replaced by the active:

(32) Target: Vlk bude zastřelen
Gloss: Wolf (nom. sg. masc. anim.) will (3rd pers. sg. fut.) shot (pass. participle masc. sg.)
Target English equivalent: The wolf will be shot

Defective utterance: *Vlk zastřelí*
Gloss: Wolf (nom. sg. masc. anim.) will shoot (3rd pers. sg. fut. act.)

ASPECT:

In this category substitution is not as obvious as in others because aspect is often chosen on semantic grounds (i.e. both aspects are possible grammatically but they have different meanings). If aspect was used ungrammatically, imperfective replaced perfective:

(33) Target: Dcera koupila drahý auto
Gloss: Daughter (nom. sg. fem.) bought (3rd pers. sg. past pf.) expensive (acc. sg. neuter) car (acc. sg. neuter)
Target English equivalent: My daughter bought an expensive car

Defective utterance: *Dcera kupovala drahý auto*
Gloss: Daughter (nom. sg. fem.) bought (3rd pers. sg. past impf.) expensive (acc. sg. neuter) car (acc. sg. neuter)

On the basis of the results of this study we can conclude that the characteristic features of agrammatism in Czech are: (a) the omission of some grammatical words (mainly prepositions, auxiliaries and pronouns); (b) the concentration of errors in some grammatical categories (especially case, tense and person); (c) the overuse of certain forms of grammatical categories (masculine gender, singular number, nominative case, 3rd person, present tense, indicative mood, active voice and imperfective aspect).

2.3. A new case study

The patient MT (born 1945, female, right-handed, computer maintenance person) suffered a haemorrhage in the left parietal region with right sided hemiparesis and mixed aphasia in February 1997. The haematoma was aspirated. Angiography revealed a residual arteriovenous malformation (AVM) which was irradiated by Gamma Knife in April 1998. MRI in figures 1 and 2 document the location and the extent of the lesion.

The patient had been given speech therapy since November 1997. An amelioration of hemiparesis and aphasia was observed during the rehabilitation.

I examined the patient in February 1999. She was diagnosed for residual hemiparesis on the right side, agraphia, alexia and expressive aphasia. Her sight and hearing, as well as her orientation in time and space, were normal. The patient still could not write with her right hand. She used her left hand in compensation, but only for a short time before she got tired. She had difficulties with reading, especially long words. She had special problems with the letters *v* and *t*, and she could not differentiate the letters *a* and *e*. Her spontaneous speech was relatively fluent, though slow in rate. The impairment of grammatical structure was mild. The patient often noticed that she had made a mistake and tried desperately to correct herself. If she had not succeeded she expressed her dissatisfaction:

(34) Target: Mohla bych vás poprosit o laskavost? Ale něco tam chybí, ne? Já jsem pak taková nešt'astná.

Gloss: Could (1st pers. sg. cond. fem.) you (acc.) ask (inf. pf.) for kindness (acc.sg. fem.)? But something there is missing, no? I am then so unhappy

Target English equivalent: Could I ask you for something? But something is missing there, isn't it? I am so unhappy then.

Defective utterance: *Mohl bych vás prosit --- laskavost? Ale něco tam chybí, ne? Já jsem pak taková nešt'astná.*

Gloss: Could (1st pers. sg. cond. masc.) you (acc.) ask (inf. impf.) (PREP omitted) kindness (acc. sg. fem.)? But something there is missing, no? I am then so unhappy

The patient had occasional word-finding difficulties, especially with members of automated sequences:

(35) *Jak se to řekne: angličtina, němčina ... jo, jazyky!*
How do you call it: English, German ... yes, languages!

(36) *Bylo to pondělí, úterý, ... ne, středa*
It was Monday, Tuesday, ... no, Wednesday

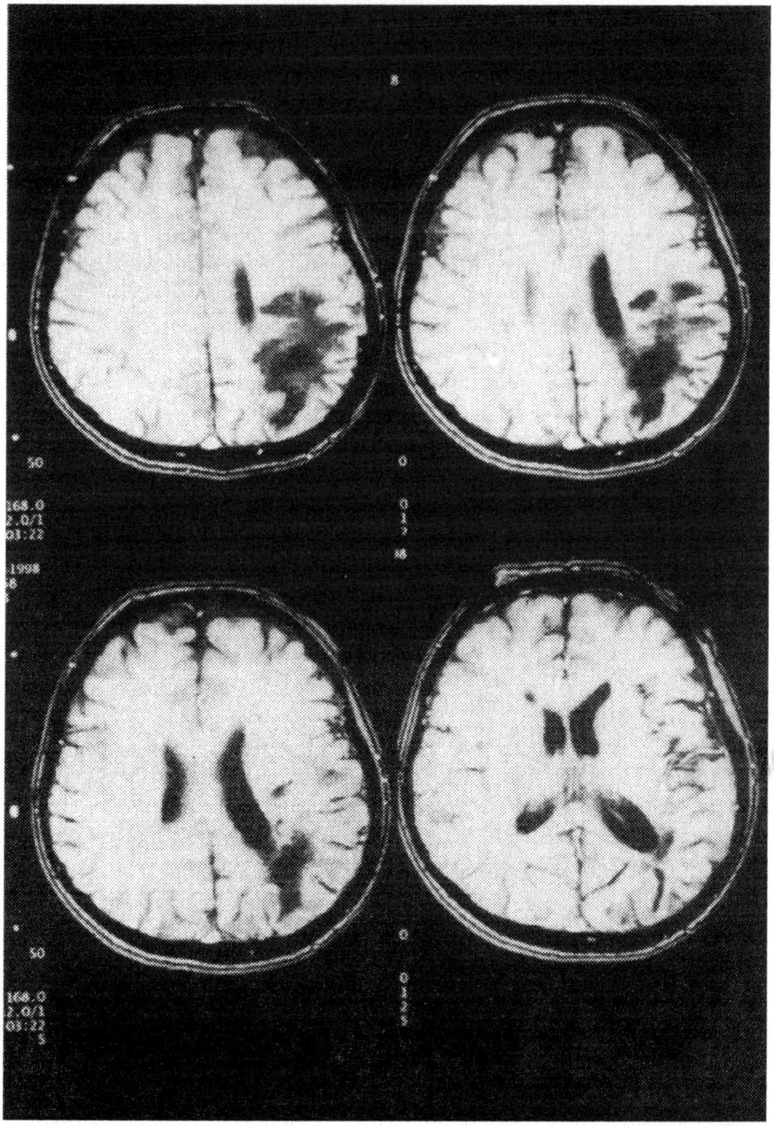

Figure 1. T1 weighted axial MRI sections representing the posthaemorrhagic lesion in the left parietal lobe. The small residual AVM was in the lateral wall of the posthaemorrhagic cyst.

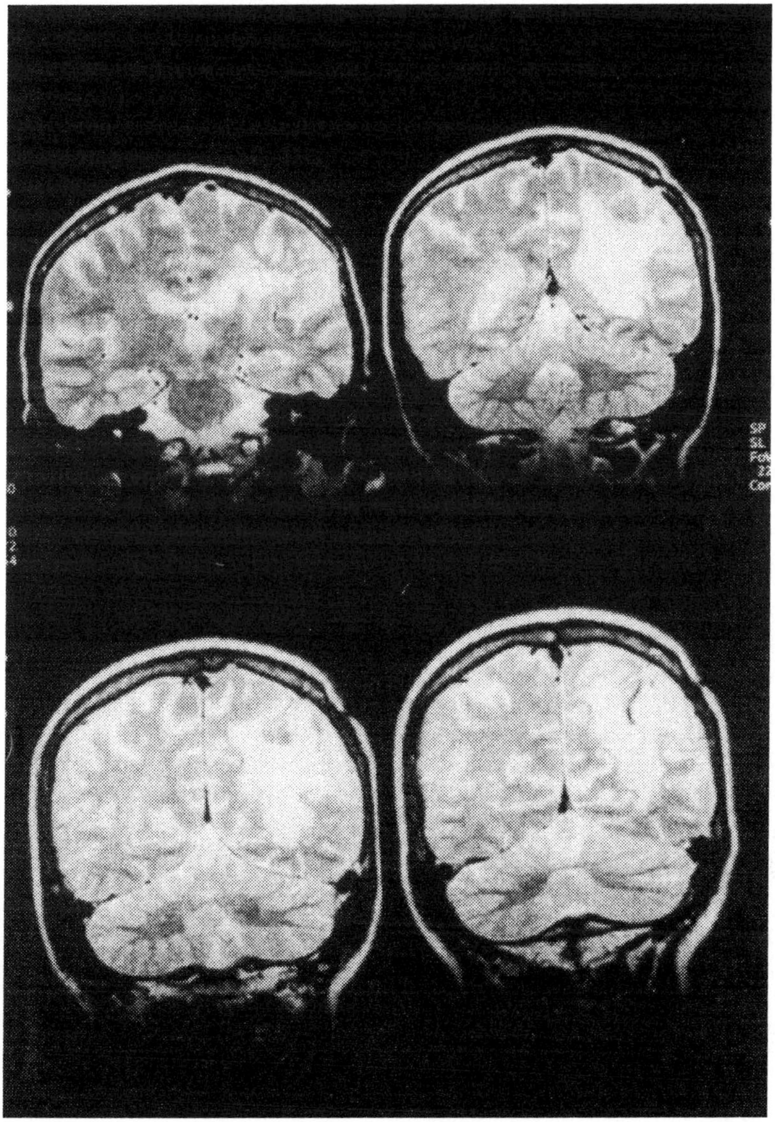

Figure 2. T2 weighted coronar MRI sections of the same lesion as in Figure 1. The lesion extends subcortically from cortex to the lateral ventricle.

(37) *Byl to pondělí,... ne, leden*
It was Monday, ... no, January

(38) *Chci deset, patnáct, ... ne, dvacet deka*
I want ten, fifteen, ... no, twenty decagrammes

Material
I met the patient in one session, our conversation was recorded. I asked her about her illness, about her work and about her hobbies. The analysed material comprises 824 clauses containing 4 126 words. The average number of words per clause (5) is rather high, because the repetitions were counted as separate words.

Of the total 824 clauses 89 were erroneous, i.e. 11% of clauses were ungrammatical. Among the errors 70% were classified as omissions, and 30% were substitutions.

2.3.1. Omissions

Omitted item:	Number of cases:	Percent of errors:
FINITE VERB in PRES	22	33 %
INFINITIVE	9	13 %
FINITE VERB in PAST	7	10 %
PAST PARTICIPLE	7	10 %
PREDICATIVE ADJECTIVE	6	9 %
NOUN after PREPOSITION	3	5 %
FINITE VERB in FUT	1	2 %
Content words		82 %
PRO/NOUN in OBJECT	6	
PRO/NOUN in SUBJECT	3	
PREPOSITION	3	

It is interesting to note that 82% of omissions are such that the omitted element is a content word, not a grammatical one. Curiously enough, there were no auxiliaries missing in the corpus, while infinitives and participles after auxiliaries were omitted in several cases.

Examples:

(39) Target: Nemůžu to vyslovit a někdy prostě to (nevyslovím ?), ale mám pocit, že teď mluvím dobře
Gloss: Cannot (1st pers. sg. pres.) it (acc. sg. neuter) pronounce (inf. pf.) and sometimes simply it (acc. sg. neuter) not pronounce (1st pers. sg. pres.), but have (1st pers. sg. pres.) feeling (acc. sg. masc. inanim.), that now speak (1st pers. sg. pres.) well

Target English equivalent: I can't pronounce it and sometimes I don't pronounce it, but I feel that now I speak well

Defective utterance: *Nemůžu to vyslovit a někdy prostě to ---, ale mám pocit, že teď mluvím dobře*
Gloss: Cannot (1st pers. sg. pres.) it (acc. sg. neuter) pronounce (inf. pf.) and sometimes simply it (acc. sg. neuter) (FINITE VERB omitted), but have (1st pers. sg. pres.) feeling (acc. sg. masc. inanim.), that now speak (1st pers. sg. pres.) well

(40) Target: No, tak jsem ukázala, když jsem nemohla vůbec mluvit, tak jsem jí ukázala tohleto
Gloss: well, so have shown (1st pers. sg. past fem.), when couldn_t (1st pers. sg. past fem.) at all speak (inf. impf.), so have (1st pers. sg.) her (dat. fem.) shown (past partcipře fem.) this (acc. sg. neuter)
Target English equivalent: Well, so I have shown it, when I couldn't speak at all, so I showed it to her

Defective utterance: *No, tak jsem ---, když jsem nemohla vůbec ---, tak jsem jí ukázala tohleto*
Gloss: well, so have (1st pers. sg.) (PAST PART. omitted), when couldn't (1st pers. sg. past fem.) at all (INF. omitted)), so have (1st pers. sg.) her (dat. fem.) shown (past partciple fem.) this (acc. sg. neuter)

(41) Target: Tak jsem furt chodila do nemocnice, když to přišlo
Gloss: So have (1st pers. sg.) all the time gone (past part. fem.) to hospital (gen. sg. fem.), when it came
Target English equivalent: So I used to go to the hospital when it occured

Defective utterance: *Tak jsem furt chodila do ---, když to přišlo*
Gloss: so have (1st pers. sg.) all the time gone (past part. fem.) to (NOUN omitted), when it came

(42) Target: Když z tý operace se probudím
Gloss: When after that (gen. sg. fem.) operation (gen. sg. fem.) wake (1st pers. sg. fut.)
Target English equivalent: When I wake up after the operation

Defective utterance: *Když --- tý operace se probudím*
Gloss: When (PREP omitted) that (gen. sg. fem.) operation (gen. sg. fem.) wake (1st pers. sg. fut.)

2.3.2. Substitutions

Replacing item:	Replaced item:	Number of cases:
PRES	PAST	4
NOM	LOC	4
NOM	ACC	2
NOM	GEN	2
SG	PL	2
MASC	FEM	2
3SG.	1SG	2
1SG	2SG	1
IND	COND	1
INDEF. PRON	FINITE VERB	4
		24 uncorrected errors
2SG	1SG	1
NEUT	MASC	1
INFINITIVE	PAST PARTIC	1
		3 self-corrected errors

On the whole, the impairment was milder than in the patients described in 2.2. There were only 27 substitutions, out of which 3 were self-corrected. Interestingly enough, the self-corrected errors do not correspond to the substitution hierarchy presented in 2.2.2., while the uncorrected errors do follow it.

(43) Target: Když mám dál
Gloss: When have (1st pers. sg. pres.) forward
Target English equivalent: When I have to continue

Defective utterance: *Když máš - mám dál*
Gloss: When have (2nd pers. sg. pres.) - have (1st pers. sg. pres.) forward

(44) Target: A tak se menoval potom Ringo
Gloss: And so was called (3rd pers. past. masc.) Ringo (nom. sg. masc.)
Target English equivalent: And so he was then called Ringo

Defective utterance: *A tak se menovalo - menoval potom Ringo*
Gloss: And so was called (3rd pers. sg. past neuter) - called (3rd pers. sg. past. masc.) Ringo (nom. sg. masc.)

(45) Target: Vždyt' jsem to takhle používala
Gloss: Have (1st pers. sg.) it (acc. neuter) like this used (past part. fem.)
Target English equivalent: I did use it like that

Defective utterance: *Dyt' jsem to takhle používat - používala*
Gloss: Have (1st pers. sg.) it (acc. neuter) like this use (inf.) - used (past part. fem.)

The majority of the substitution errors were existing forms of the same category, and as to the order of substitution they showed the same tendency as described in 2.2.2. The number of errors was nevertheless too small to yield an analogous table of distribution among different forms. The only difference from 2.2.2. was the use of indefinite pronouns instead of finite verbs (which sometimes occurs even in normal spontaneous speech):

(46) Target: Tak to mě tak rozzlobilo
Gloss: So it (nom. sg. neuter) me (acc.) annoyed (3rd pers. sg. past neuter)
Target English equivalent: So it annoyed me

Defective utterance: *Tak to mě tak tohleto*
Gloss: So it me so like this

(47) Target: No tak tohleto vidím, todleto tadyhle vidím
Gloss: So this see (1st pers. sg. pres.), this here see (1st pers. sg. pres.)
Target English equivalent: Well I can see this, I see this here

Defective utterance: *No tak tohleto tak, todleto tadyhle*
Gloss: Well so this so, this here

There were no problems with word order (which is fixed only as far as unstressed words are concerned). The patient even used rather complicated constructions, i.e. conditional, subordination. None of the grammatical substitutions was used systematically.

Examples:

(48) Target: Stalo se to v říjnu
Gloss: Happened (3rd pers. sg. past neuter) it (nom. sg. neuter) in October (loc. sg. masc.)
Target English equivalent: It happened in October

Defective utterance: *Stalo se to říjen*
Gloss: Happened (3rd pers. sg. past neuter) it (nom. sg. neuter) (PREP omitted) October (nom. sg. masc.)

(49) Target: Včera jsem byla sama doma
Gloss: Yesterday was (1st pers. sg. past fem.) alone at home
Target English equivalent: Yesterday I was alone at home

Defective utterance: *Včera sem sama doma*
Gloss: Yesterday am (1st pers. sg. pres.) alone at home

(50) Target: To jsou zase čísla

Gloss: Those are (3rd pers. pl. pres.) again numbers (nom. pl. neuter)
Target English equivalent: Those are numbers

Defective utterance: *To je zase čísla*

Gloss: That is (3rd pers. sg. pres.) again numbers (nom. pl. neuter)

(51) Target: To je pes mýho muže a mě

Gloss: It is dog (nom. sg. masc.) my (gen. sg. masc.) husband (gen. sg. masc.) and me (gen.)
Target English equivalent: It is my husband's and my dog

Defective utterance: *To je pes mýho muže a já*
Gloss: It is dog (nom. sg. masc.) my (gen. sg. masc.) husband (gen. sg. masc.) and I (nom.)

(52) Target: Co se mně bude líbit, tak si přečtu, a co ne, tak bych to zase vrátila

Gloss: What me (dat.) will please (3rd pers. sg. ind. fut.), so read (1st pers. ind. fut.), and what not, so would it again return (1st pers. sg. cond. fem.)
Target English equivalent: What will please me I will read, and what not, I would return again

Defective utterance: *Co se mně bude líbit, tak si přečtu, a co ne, tak bych to zase vrátím*
Gloss: What me (dat.) will please (3rd pers. sg. ind. fut.), so read (1st pers. ind. fut.), and what not, so would (1st pers. sg. cond.) it again return (1st pers. ind. fut.)

The biggest grammatical problem in the spontaneous speech of this patient seems to be the use of a preposition with a noun phrase. Either the preposition or the noun were omitted, or the noun was in a wrong case (nominative singular). The material contained 68 occurrences of the combination PREPOSITION + NOUN, out of which 46 were correct and 22 incorrect. The error rate (32%) is much higher than in other categories (median 11%).

Interestingly enough, in grammatical tests that were administered in written form during the next session, there were no preposition errors at all. The patient was asked to fill in correct prepositions and case forms of nouns given in the nominative singular, in written sentences. She succeeded 100%, even though after hesitation:

(53) Target: Vesnice byla po zemětřesení úplně zničena

Gloss: Village (nom. sg. fem.) was (3rd pers. sg. past fem.) after earthquake (loc. sg. neuteer) completely destroyed (pass. part. fem.)
Target English equivalent: The village was completely destroyed after the earthquake.

Defective utterance: *Vesnice byla za - na - ee - po zemětřesení úplně zničena*

Gloss: Village (nom. sg. fem.) was (3rd pers. sg. past fem.) behind - on - ee - after earthquake (loc. sg. neuter) completely destroyed (pass. part. fem.)

3. Generalisation of the type of errors

The analysis of spontaneous speech of Czech motor aphasics showed that: (a) the morpho-syntactic structure of language production is impaired in all patients; (b) grammatical errors result from both omissions and substitutions; (c) free grammatical morphemes are only omitted, not substituted; (d) bound grammatical morphemes are only substituted, not omitted; (e) morpho-syntactic errors caused by substitutions are more frequent than those caused by omissions of grammatical morphemes; (f) grammatical words are omitted less than content words; (g) in substitutions the replacing forms are existing grammatical morphemes, mainly belonging to the same grammatical category (e.g. one case ending substituting for another); (h) the richer a category is in forms, the more it is liable to errors; (i) there is a clear hierarchical order in the substitution of some grammatical forms for others.

Comparison of results from 2.2. and 2.3.:

		The sum of 17 motor aphasics:	The new patient (MT):
Clauses:	grammatical	48%	89%
	ungrammatical	52%	11%
Errors:	omissions	38%	70%
	substitutions	62%	30%
Omission:	grammatical words	30%	18%
	content words	70%	82%
Substitution:	case	32%	30%
	tense	15%	19%
	mood	15%	4%
	person	13%	15%
	gender	11%	11%
	number	11%	7%
	aspect	2%	
	voice	1%	
	other		14%

Czech is not represented in Agrammatic aphasia: a cross-language narrative sourcebook (1990); thus my study offers an opportunity to compare the generalizations made on the basis of 14 different languages with results from a new language. Czech data confirm the conclusion drawn by Menn & Obler (1990, p.1381) that "the simpler the paradigm, the fewer the erros". The majority of errors appeared in case, tense and person, which have the most extensive paradigms (cf. 1.2.1.), while two-member categories (aspect and voice) were mostly used correctly. On the other hand, my data do not support the hypothesis (Menn & Obler, 1990, p.1381) that "locally controlled grammatical morphemes are better preserved than those which are more globally controlled". There were fewer errors in gender and number (mainly controlled by agreement) than in case and tense (mainly controlled locally). However, it must be borne in mind that unlike some of the previously described languages, Czech expresses grammatical categories by bound grammatical morphemes, not function words. Obler acknowledges (personal communication, 2000) that Menn and Obler observed this local / global distinction at the sentence level, where negative markers and introductory words (such as "Well") tended to be spared. Thus further specification is required for their formulation of these phenomena.

The results of this study showed that there is a hierarchy in grammatical forms with respect to their availability for aphasic patients. The overused forms of grammatical categories seem to be the most resistant in aphasia. However, it is useful to bear in mind Goldstein's statement that brain-damaged patients' spontaneous behaviour never reflects the deficit itself, but rather the patients' reactions to the deficit (cf. Heeschen, 1985). Thus the above-mentioned results mean that some forms are more available than others. They may be used deliberately as a means of compensation for the deficit (Kolk & Heeschen, 1990). If patients feel that the word they are trying to use needs some grammatical form which they are not sure about, they react by choosing the form that is most easily available.

I wanted to find out if there is any connection between the forms best preserved in aphasia and those first acquired by children, as well as those most frequently used by normal speakers. The questions I studied were: (1.) Does the order of substitution correlate with order of acquisition? (2.) Does the order of substitution correlate with frequency of use?

3.1. Correlation with acquisition

In Pačesová (1979) the order of form acquisition in Czech children is stated as follows:

Gender:	F	M	N				
Number:	SG	PL					
Case:	N.SG	N.PL	A	G	L	D	I
Person:	3SG	3PL	1SG	1PL			
Tense:	PRES	PAST	FUT				
Mood:	IND	IMPER	COND				
Voice:	ACT	PASS					
Aspect:	IMPF	PF					

The set of forms acquired first differs from the most frequent replacing ones only in the category of gender. That children first acquire feminine forms results from the facts that: (a) children imitate the speech of their mothers and other female care-takers; (b) they prefer open syllables of the form C+V; (c) they use the ending *-a*, which is typical for feminines, most productively.

My findings support the well-known hypothesis suggested by Jakobson (1942) that the earlier a grammatical form is acquired by children the more resistant it is against impairment in aphasia. However, one systematic exception can be observed: children first learn suffixes and infixes, and only after that do they start to use prefixes (cf. Slobin, 1978). In agrammatism, on the contrary, the most impaired part of the word is the end, that is grammatical suffixes, while prefixation is less affected.

3.2. Correlation with frequency

I compared the most frequent replacing forms of grammatical categories with those most frequently used in normal language. The quantitative analysis of contemporary Czech (Těšitelová, 1985) showed that the order of frequency of grammatical categories is:

Gender:	M	F	N			
Number:	SG	PL				
Case:	N	G	A	L	I	D
Person:	3SG	3PL	1SG	1PL		
Tense:	PRES	PAST	FUT			
Mood:	IND	COND	IMPER			
Voice:	ACT	PASS				
Aspect:	IMPF	PF				

This analysis was based on written texts, which makes the results hardly comparable with my findings, but the concrete numbers are of little importance for our purpose anyway. What is of interest here, is the hierarchy of frequency, which appears to be clearly marked.

It is obvious that the most frequent replacing forms in aphasia are indeed those which are the most frequent in normal language use. This, of course, can be taken as a general tendency only. It is probable that the frequency of certain grammatical forms and their availability to aphasics depend also on the semantics of the word (e.g. names of places occur much more often in the locative than other nouns).

3.3. Conclusion

The order of substitution in Czech aphasia tends to correlate with order of acquisition and with frequency of use. The only difference appearing in the category of gender may mean that resistance to impairment in aphasia is more influenced by frequency than by early acquisition.

The dominant replacing forms in language impairment:	M	SG	N	3SG	IND	ACT	IMPF
The earliest acquired forms in language development:	F	SG	N	3SG	IND	ACT	IMPF
The most frequent forms in normal language use:	M	SG	N	3SG	IND	ACT	IMPF

This set of forms obtained by 3 different criteria seems to be primary in relation to the others. Further studies will be needed to verify their priority. Whatever the nature of the priority, the investigation reported here may contribute to the discussion about the basic forms of grammatical categories in morphologically rich languages.

Acknowledgements

I am most grateful to Milada Mimrová, Dagmar Mimrová and Jitka Stejskalová for allowing me to work with their patients and providing me with their documentation. I am indebted to Vilibald Vladyka from the Stereotactic Neurosurgery and Radiosurgery Department at the Homolka Hospital for the MRI documentation and its interpretation.

Address correspondence to: Dr. H. Lehečková, Slavistiikan ja baltologian laitos, PL 4 (Vuorikatu 5 B), 00014 Helsingin Yliopisto, Finland. E-mail: leheckov@cc.helsinki.fi

References

Badecker, W. & Caramazza, A. (1985). On considerations of method and theory governing the use of clinical categories in neurolinguistic and cognitive neuropsychology: The case against agrammatism. *Cognition*, *20*, 97-125.

Bebout, L. (1993). Processing of negative morphemes in aphasia: An example of the complexities of the closed class / open class concept. *Clinical Linguistics and Phonetics*, *7*, 161-172.

Crystal, D. (1981). *Clinical linguistics*. Wien: Springer Verlag.

De Blesser, R., Bayer, J. & Luzzatti, C. (1995/6). Linguistic theory and morphosyntactic impairments in German and Italian aphasics. *Journal of Neurolinguistics*, *9*, 175-185.

Dressler, W. U. & Stark, J.A. (Eds.) (1988). *Linguistic analyses of aphasic language*. New York: Springer-Verlag.

Grodzinsky, Y. (1984). The syntactic characterization of agrammatism, *Cognition, 16*, 99-120.

Grodzinsky, Y. (1986). Language deficits and the theory of syntax. *Brain and Language*, *27*, 135-159.

Grodzinsky, Y. (1990). *Theoretical perspectives on language deficits*. Cambridge, MA: MIT Press.

Heeschen, C. (1985). Agrammatism versus paragrammatism: A fictious opposition. In Kean (Ed.), *Agrammatism* (pp. 207-248). Orlando, Florida: Academic Press.

Jakobson, R. (1971). Towards a linguistic classification of aphasic impairments. *Selected Writings II*. The Hague: Mouton.

Jakobson, R. (1971). Kindersprache, Aphasie und allgemeine Lautgesetze. *Selected Writings I*. The Hague: Mouton.

Kean, M.L. (Ed.) (1985). *Agrammatism*. Orlando: Academic Press.

Kolk, H. & Heeschen, C. (1990). Adaptation symptoms and impairment symptoms in Broca's aphasia. *Aphasiology, 4,* 221-231.

Kolk, H. & Heeschen, C. (1992). Agrammatism, paragrammatism and the management of language. *Language and Cognitive Processes*, *7*, 89-129.

Kukkonen, P. (1982). *Nuoren aivoinfarktipotilaan kieliopillisia vaikeuksia: tapaustutkimus motorisesta afasiasta*. Helsinki: Pro gradututkielma.

Lapointe, S.G. (1983). Some issues in the linguistic description of agrammatism. *Cognition*, *14*, 1-39.

Lehečková, H. (1984). Neurolingvistika: předmět, metody a historie. *Slovo a slovesnost*, *45*, 154-157.

Lehečková, H. (1985a). Využití lingvistiky při rehabilitaci afázií. *Ceskoslovenská otolaryngologie*, *34*, 116-120.

Lehečková, H. (1985b). Jazykové aspekty typologie afázií. *Slovo a slovesnost*, *46*, 119-126.

Lehečková, H. (1986). Agramatismus v afázii. *Slovo a slovesnost*, *47*, 138-147.

Lehečková, H. (1987). Basic forms of grammatical categories: An evidence from agrammatism. In Lilius & Saari (Eds.), *The Nordic languages and modern linguistics* 6 (pp. 217-224). Helsinki: Yliopistopaino.

Lehečková, H. (1988a). Linguistic theories and the interpretation of agrammatism. *Clinical Linguistics and Phonetics*, *2*(4), 271-289.

Lehečková, H. (1988b). The influence of language type on the manifestation of agrammatism. In Koivuselkä-Sallinen & Sarajärvi (Eds.), *Proceedings of the 3rd Finnish conference of neurolinguistics* (pp. 63-72). Joensuu: Joensuun yliopistopaino.

Lehečková, H. (1989). A comparison of grammatical errors in motor and sensory aphasia. *Proceedings of the 21st congress of the international association of logopedics and foniatrics*, Praha, vol. 1, 82-84.

Lehečková, H. (1995). Typ jazyka a projevy fatických poruch v morfologii a syntaxi. *Acta Universitatis Carolinae - Philologica* 1, Slavica Pragensia XXXVII, 92-97.

Lehečková, H. (1997). Jazyk, komunikace a řečové poruchy. In Kulišták, P., Lehečková, H., Mimrová, M. and Nebudová, J. *Afázie* (pp. 125-175). Praha: Triton.

Lehečková, H. (1999a). Linguistic errors in impaired and imperfect language. In Nenonen and Järvikivi (Eds.) *Languages, minds, and brains* (pp. 91-101). Studies in Languages 34. University of Joensuu, Faculty of Humanities. Joensuu: Joensuun yliopistopaino.

Lehečková, H. (1999b). Use and misuse of gender in Czech. In Rissanen, Nevalainen and Saari (Eds.), *Gender in grammar and cognition*. II.: Manifestations of Gender (pp. 749-771). Trends in Linguistics, Studies and Monographs 124. Berlin: Mouton de Gruyter.

Lukatela, K., Shankweiler, D. & Crain, S. (1995). Syntactic processing in agrammatic aphasia by speakers of a Slavic language. *Brain and Language*, *49*, 50-76.

Menn, L. & Obler, L. (1990). *Agrammatic aphasia. A cross-language narrative sourcebook.* Amsterdam /Philadelphia: John Benjamins Publishing Company.

Miceli, G., Mazzucchi, A., Menn, L. & Goodglass, H. (1983). Contrasting cases of Italian agrammatic aphasia without comprehension disorder. *Brain and Language, 19,* 65-97.

Müllerová, O., Hoffmannová, J. & Schneiderová, E. (1992). *Mluvená čeština v autentických textech.* Jinočany: H&H.

Niemi J. & Laine, M. (1989). The English language bias in neurolinguistics: new languages give new perspectives. *Aphasiology, 3,* 155-159.

Niemi, J., Laine, M. & Tuominen, J. (1994). Cognitive morphology in Finnish: foundations of a new model. *Language and Cognitive Processes, 9,* 423-446.

Nilipour, R. & Paradis, M. (1995). Breakdown of functional categories in three Farsi-English bilingual aphasic patients. In Paradis (Ed.), *Aspects of bilingual aphasia* (pp. 123-138). Elsevier Science Ltd.

Ouhalla, J. (1993). Functional categories, agrammatism and language acquisition. *Linguistische Berichte, 139,* 182-196.

Pačesová, J. (1979). *Řeč v raném dětství.* Brno: Univerzita J.E. Purkyně.

Paradis, M. & Libben G. (1987). *The assessment of bilingual aphasia.* Hillsdale, N.J. and London: Lawrence Erlbaum Ass.

Paradis, M. (1988). Recent developments in the study of agrammatism: their import for the assessment of bilingual aphasia. *Jounal of Neurolinguistics, 3,* 127-160.

Paradis, M. (1998a). Acquired aphasia in bilingual speakers. In Taylor Sarno (Ed.), *Acquired aphasia,* 3rd edition, (pp. 531-549). San Diego: Academic Press.

Paradis, M. (Ed.) (1998b). *Pragmatics in neurogenic communications disorders.* Oxford: Pergamon Press.

Slobin, D.I. (1978). Developmental psycholinguistics. In Dingwall (Ed.), *A Survey of linguistic science* (pp. 298-410). Stamford, Connecticut: Greylock Publishers.

Stemberger, J.P. (1985). Bound morpheme loss errors in normal and agrammatic speech. *Cognitive Neuropsychology, 1,* 281-313.

Tesak, J. & Niemi, J. (1997). Telegraphese and agrammatism: a cross-linguistic study. *Aphasiology, 11* (2), 145-155.

Těšitelová, M. (1985). *Kvantitativní charakteristiky současné češtiny.* Praha: Academia.

Manifestations of Aphasia in Persian

Reza Nilipour[*] and Shahla Raghibdoust[**]

[*]*University of Social Welfare and Rehabilitation Sciences and School of Intelligent Systems, IPM, Iran.*
[**]*College of Rehabilitation, Tehran University of Medical Sciences*

Abstract—The general characteristics and specific language deficits of seven native speakers of Persian who became aphasic (with three different etiologies) are discussed. Three major linguistic deficits related to site and size of lesion and to individual differences emerge from the data: breakdown of the verb, deletion of free grammatical morphemes, and substitution of bound grammatical morphemes. Four types of language-specific agrammatic deficits are described: (a) substitution of a filler verb */budan/* 'to be' as a default for all kinds of verbs, including transitive active verbs; (b) substitution of the polymorphemic infinitive for the contextually proper inflected form of the verb; and (c) tendency to omit the *ezafe* linking morpheme */-e/* and the NP-internal conjunction */va/* 'and'.

Keywords: aphasia, Persian, agrammatism, inflection, substitution, typology.

Introduction

Although aphasiological and neurolinguistic studies on Persian are in their infancy, a number of systematic case studies have been reported in the literature during the past decade or so, from which we can extract some major features of Persian agrammatic language for the purpose of cross-linguistic comparison. Apart from the case studies reported here, there has been no documented report in the neurolinguistic literature on Persian aphasiology, not even in the cross-language source book on agrammatic aphasia (Menn & Obler, 1990), until recently (Nilipour, 2000). The major aim of this paper is not to give a comprehensive description of Persian aphasiology, but rather to attempt to depict the general characteristics of agrammatic language in Persian. It is also an attempt to show the general trend of aphasic deficits in different types of aphasia in Persian. With these aims in mind, we first present a short description of three published aphasia cases (Nilipour, 1988, 1989; Nilipour & Ashayeri, 1989), then we describe two unpublished cases (Raghibdoust, 1999) and, in the final part, we present two newly published cases (Nilipour, 2000) of agrammatic aphasics and their grammatical violations, compared with subject control data.

All aphasic data reported here are based on systematic assessments with the same standard aphasia test, *The Bilingual Aphasia Test* (the BAT, Farsi Version). Based on these results, the cases have met the general clinical characteristics of four types of aphasia syndromes: Broca's aphasia (MG, RL, HB, and MN), conduction aphasia (PA), transcortical motor aphasia (TB) and transcortical sensory aphasia (AS). With respect to etiology, they are of three kinds: cerebrovascular accident (CVA) (PA, MG and RL), trauma (AS, HB and MN) and arteriovenous malformation (AVM) (TB).

The grammatical violations and deficits of two patients (HB and MN) reported here are matched with control data based on the descriptive framework of the *Cross-Language Aphasia Study* (Menn & Obler, 1990: ch. 2) and may be used for cross-language comparison purposes. In five other patients (PA, TB, AS, MG and RL), the reported aphasic deficits and grammatical violations are based on the results of the general assessment as well as the BAT post-test analysis (Paradis & Libben, 1987) of the connected speech samples elicited from each patient during the evaluation procedure.

1. Persian grammar in normal use

BASIC TYPOLOGY

Persian is an Indo-European language, belonging to the Iranian branch of the Indo-Iranian group. Typologically, it is an SOV language with a rather rich morphology. But it is an atypical SOV language in the sense that it has prepositions rather than postpositions. The word order is rather loose and the order of all major constituents of the sentence may vary for pragmatic purposes. The subject may be optionally omitted since the verb is inflected for person and number. Direct object and indirect object are marked with postposed */râ/* and preposed */be/* markers respectively. Adjectives follow the head noun and auxiliaries follow the main verb, but modals precede the main verb. Arabic, an unrelated Semitic language, is a major source of loan words. Arabic nouns typically retain their Arabic plural forms, making them irregular in Persian.

There is no gender in Persian, and hence no gender agreement. There is also no number agreement for adjectives in prototypical noun phrases (N + ADJ). But there is subject-verb agreement with respect to person and number.

MORPHOLOGY

THE NOUN

Persian has two major types of word formation: compounding and derivation. In compounding, two or more stems are joined to make a single lexical item (example 1); in derivation, a new lexical item is made using a stem plus bound derivational elements such as suffixes and prefixes (example 2). A combination of the two means is also possible, that is, compounding of stems plus a derivational suffix or prefix (example 3). These patterns of word formation are applicable to all major lexical categories.

1. */âb mive/*	*/ruz nâme/*	2. */xaste-gi/*	3. */dandân peze_g-i/*
water fruit	day letter	tired-ness	tooth physician-*i*
fruit juice	newspaper	tiredness	dentistry

Derivational morphemes are a good source of new lexical items by being attached to the present and past stems of the verbs:

4. */xor-âk/* = present stem + */âk/*	food
5. */xor-e_/* = present stem + /e_/	dish
6. */xord-an-i/* = past stem + Infm + */-i/*	edible

Definite nouns are generally unmarked in Persian, while indefinite nouns are marked with the suffix */-i/*. A noun denoting a specific direct object may also be followed by the specific direct object marker */râ/*.

Nouns are pluralized by adding the plural morpheme (*/-hâ/* as unmarked morpheme for all nouns, */-ân/* as marked morpheme for some animate nouns) to the singular base form:

7.	*/zan-i/*	*/zan-hâ/*	*/zan-ân/*	*/medâd-i/*	*/medâd-hâ/*
	a woman	the women	the women	a pencil	the pencils
8.	*/deraxt/*	*/deraxt-hâ/*	*/deraxt-ân/*		
	tree	trees	trees		

9. */deraxt-hâ râ bor-id-and/*
   tree-s 'the' cut-ed-they
   They cut the trees.

THE VERB

Persian verbs are either simple or compound. The verbal element is derived from a base form called the infinitive, consisting of the past stem plus an infinitive suffix. Each verb has a past stem and a present stem. The present stem of regular verbs is derived from the past stem by deleting the past marker:

Simple verb		PRES. STEM	PAST STEM
Regular Verb			
10.	*/xor-d-an/*	*/xor/*	*/xor-d/*
	eat-PAST- Infm		
	to eat		
Irregular Verb			
11.	*/âmad-an/*	*/â/*	*/âmad/*
	came-Infm		
	/did-an/	*/bin/*	*/did/*
	saw-Infm		

Compound verb

A compound verb consists of a noun or adjective followed by a verbal element.

12. */zamin xordan/*
    ground to beat
    to fall down
13. */xolâse kardan/*
    summary to do
    to summarize

The past stem yields the forms of the past tense (both simple and progressive) and the present stem yields the present, future and imperative. Every verb is conjugated for person and number by adding the personal endings to the present or past stem.

Two major verb prefixes are used to mark aspect: */mi-/* indicates the duration and progression of the action, and */be-/* is affixed to the verb in subjunctive and imperative forms.

14.

	PRESENT		PAST	
	mi-xân-am	I am reading /	*xând-am*	I read
	PROG-read-I	I read	read-PAST-I	
	mi-xân-i	you are reading	*xând-i*	you read
	mi-xân-ad	he/she/it reads	*xând*	he/she/it read
	mi-xân-im	we read	*xând-im*	we read
	mi-xân-id	you read	*xând-id*	you read
	mi-xân-and	they read	*xând-and*	they read

15. */sib mi-xor-i/*
apple PROG-eat-you
Are you eating the apple? / Do you eat the apple?

16. */sib râ be-xor/*
apple-the IMP-eat
Eat the apple.

PRONOUNS

The personal pronouns have six independent forms for first, second and third person, singular and plural, without any sex distinction. Aside from the independent personal pronouns, there are personal inflectional endings attached to the verb that denote the person and number of the subject. Pronominal enclitics (*-m, -t, -_, -mân, -tân, -_ân*) are attached to the preceding word, functioning as attributes.

17. */man sib-a_ râ xord-am/*
I apple-his OBJ ate-I
I ate his apple.

18. */u sib-am râ xord/*
he apple-my OBJ ate
He ate my apple.

There are also demonstrative pronouns (*/in/* 'this' and */ân/* 'that') as well as reflexive pronouns functioning as independent attributes:

19. */in ketâb râ be-xân/*
this book-the read
Read this book.

20. */ketâb-e xod-am râ be u dâd-am/*
book-of myself OBJ to he gave-I
I gave him my own book.

SYNTAX

OBJECT MARKER

The syntax of Persian is characterized by certain grammatical morphemes, notably */râ/* as postposed direct and */be/* as preposed indirect object markers. The postposition */râ/* is used primarily as the direct object marker, as well as marking the specificity of the object.

21. *\/pul be man be-deh/*
money to me IMP-give-you
Give me some money.
22. */pul râ be man be-deh/*
money OBJ to me IMP-give-you
Give me the money.

PREPOSITIONS

Persian has eight basic prepositions. They can be divided into two categories according to meaning: (1) those used to express spatial relationships, and (2) those used to express other syntactic relationships:

23. */az/* 'from', */be/* 'to', */dar/* 'in', */bâ/* 'with', */tâ/* 'as far as' or 'until'
24. */bâ/* 'with', */barâye/* 'for', */joz/* 'except', */bi/* 'without'

EZAFE (LINKING) MORPHEME

The *ezafe* morpheme */-e/* is used to link a head noun to its complements or modifiers; it can often be translated as 'of', e.g. */eyd-e now ruz/* 'holiday of new day' (New Year's Day). The *ezafe* construction is the universal type of attributive construction in Persian; i.e. it allows various lexical items to be combined as noun attributes, such as nouns, adjectives, pronouns (personal, reflexive, interrogative and demonstrative) and ordinal numbers. If a lexical item has several modifiers, they are placed one after another following the modified word, each pair connected with an *ezafe* marker */-e/*.

25. */kif-e siyâh-e bozorg-e pedar-e pir-e to/*
bag-of black-of big-of father-of old-of you
Your old father's large black bag.

Word order in an *ezafe* construction chain is highly significant. The modified item is always directly followed by the qualitative modifier, then by the modifier of possession:

26. */divâr-e siyâh-e otâq/*
wall-of black-of room
The black wall of the room.

ORTHOGRAPHY

Persian is written from right to left, but numbers are written from left to right. The script was originally borrowed from Arabic but has been modified to some extent. The 32 characters include 28 Arabic characters plus four additional ones representing four Persian phonemes not found in Arabic. In most cases, there is no graphemic representation for short vowels (e, a, o), but long vowels do have a graphemic representation. There is rarely a one-to-one correspondence between consonantal phonemes and characters due to the major differences between the Persian and Arabic phonological systems.

2. Aphasic symptoms in Persian

A. Subjects, with general assessment and connected speech samples

A summary of the grammatical violations in the speech of five native speakers of Persian who became aphasic as a result of three different etiologies is given below. Their general background information is given in Table 1. (For detailed information on the general linguistic performance, deficits and etiology of TB, PA, and AS, see Nilipour (1988, 1989) and Nilipour and Ashayeri (1989); for the two unpublished case studies, MG and RL, see Raghibdoust (1999).)

Table 1. General background information on five aphasics

	TB	PA	AS	MG	RL
Age	26	48	49	32	49
Sex	M	F	M	F	M
Occupation	Student	Clerk	Surgeon	Housewife	Businessmn
Years of education	15	15	22	10	8
Native language	Persian	Persian	Persian	Persian	Persian
Other languages	English	English	German & English	Azari	Azari
Handedness	R	R	R	R	R
Etiology	AVM	CVA	Trauma	CVA	CVA
Lesion side	L & R	L	L	L	L
Lesion site	L. temporo-parieto-occipital R. temporal	Fronto-temporal	Fronto-temporal	Frontal	Fronto-temporal
Post-onset assessment	22 months	48 months	2 months	18 months	18 months
Aphasia type	Transcortical motor	Con-duction	Trans-cortical sensory	Broca's	Broca's

A.1 Review of three published cases

CASE ONE: TB

TB is reported to have relatively good comprehension and repetition; based on the assessment, he was diagnosed as having transcortical motor aphasia (Nilipour, 1988). Overall, his deficits may be summarized as general disruption of the VP and lexical access limitations. In terms of specific language deficits, his grammatical violations may be grouped into four categories. The following examples for each category are taken from his elicited samples of connected speech.

Deletion of obligatory free morphemes (preposed */be/*, postposed */râ/* particles and prepositions)

1. */pesar [be] doxtar ne_un mi-deh-ad/*
   boy [to] girl show PROG-giving-he
   The boy is showing [the birds] [to] the girl.

2. */mardom do nafar [râ] bord-and/*
   people two persons [OBJ] took-they
   People took two persons.

Incorrect subject-verb agreement

3. */ânhâ parande bud/* (singular verb for plural subject)
   they bird was
   They was bird.

4. */se tâ ba_e mord* [SG]/ (singular verb for plural subject)
   three kid died [SG]
   Three kid died.

5. */ân ne-mitun-e xub bud-and/* (plural verb for singular subject)
   he cannot well became-PL
   He could not become well.

Verb or clause deletion

6. */ba?dan ye doxtar* [V]/
   then one girl
   Then a girl…

7. */doxtar goft-e_ ke* [V]/
   girl said-she that [V]
   The girl said that…

8. */mi-re be xânum* [V]/
   PROG-goes-he to lady [V]
   He goes to the lady…

Substitution of the nominal or verbal element of a compound verb by an empty pronoun or irrelevant noun

9. */ba?dan _iz kard-e_/*
   then thing did-he
   Then he did something.

10. */in ne-mi-tune aslan dast bo-kon-e/*
    this cannot at all hand SUB-do-he/
    He cannot hand "move" at all.

CASE TWO: PA

PA is reported to suffer from impaired repetition (at the sentence level) and limited, slow oral production. Consequently, she was diagnosed with conduction aphasia (for further details, see Nilipour (1989) and Nilipour and Paradis (1995)).

It is reported that her performance is relatively similar in both languages and the final recovery pattern was parallel recovery. Remarks concerning her linguistic deficits and grammatical violations are based on the general assessment and connected speech samples in Persian. The violations were task-specific in both languages and they were manifested at the sentence level in both repetition and reading aloud. PA's grammatical violations in the two languages had different manifestations as a result of the languages' different structural properties. In English, free grammatical morphemes were deleted in obligatory contexts, but in Persian there were different types of errors. Some examples of her linguistic deficits in Persian are given below.

Verb breakdown

The verb was the most affected element of the sentence. Substitution and/or omission of the inflectional morphemes in the target verb resulted in a change in tense from present to past in 12 different sentences.

11. Target: */doxtar pesar râ hol mi-deh-ad/*
    girl boy OBJ push is-giving-she
    The girl is pushing the boy.
    Patient:*/doxtar pesar râ hol dâd/*
    girl boy OBJ push gave-she
    The girl pushed the boy.

12. Target: */zan ân mard râ ne-mi-bus-ad/*
    woman that man OBJ not-is-kissing-she
    The woman is not kissing that man.
    Patient:*/zan ân mard râ bus-id/*
    woman that man OBJ kissed-she
    The woman kissed the man.

Omission of free grammatical morphemes

13. Target: */in sag ast ke gorbe râ gâz-a_ mi-gir-ad/*
    this dog is who cat OBJ bite-him PROG-take-she
    It is the dog who is bitten by the cat.

Patient:/*ân sag [0] [0] gorbe gâz-[0] gereft*/
that dog [is] [who] cat bite-[him] took-she
This [is] the dog the cat bit.

14. Target: /*xod-a_ râ zan mi-zan-ad*/
self-her OBJ woman is-beating-she
The woman is beating herself.
Patient:/*xod-a_ [râ] ân zan zad*/
self-her [OBJ] that woman beat-she
That woman beat herself.

In general, there were more omissions than substitutions of free grammatical morphemes. Bound morphemes and inflectional endings were more vulnerable to substitution.

CASE THREE: AS

The clinical picture of AS's performance can be summarized as fluent speech, poor comprehension, relatively good repetition and impaired writing, which is compatible with a diagnosis of transcortical sensory aphasia. The details of AS's residual capacities and deficits as well as his patterns of language recovery in Persian, German and English are provided in Nilipour and Ashayeri (1989) and Nilipour and Paradis (1995).

The data concerning the patient's performance in Persian include his spontaneous speech, descriptive speech and spontaneous writing. The elicited spoken and written speech samples in Persian, although cohesive and pragmatically sound, were structurally varied and complex, and involved a number of lexical and syntactic violations. His elicited spontaneous speech contained a total of 227 words, with an MLU of six words. The syntactic deficits in AS's speech included four instances of paragrammatism and three cases of omission of obligatory morphemes. His sample of descriptive speech included a total of 95 words and MLU of 6. The patient's grammatical violations at the VP level, in general, fall into the following classes:

Incorrect subject-verb agreement between first, second or third person

15. /*do pesare man hami_e gerye mi-kon-am*/
two son-of me always cry doing-I
My two sons I am always crying.

Verb breakdown

Substitution of the verb

16. /*ye dafe pâre od*/ (substituted for /*_ekast*/ 'broke')
suddenly tore off
It suddenly tore off.

17. /*ne_an mi-dâd-and ke pâ-_ ke ik dâst*/*
show is doing that leg-his
They were showing that his leg…
*semantic paraphasia substituted for the main lexical verb

Substitution of the verbal element of a compound verb

18. */se tâ ba_e râ negâh mi-dâr-and/* (substituted for */mi-kon-and/* 'are doing')
    three kids OBJ look PRG-have-they
    They are holding look the three kids.
19. */ba?d ye dafe _oru gereft-am/**
    then sudden begin took-I
    Then suddenly I took a begin.
    /gereft-am/ 'took-I' is substituted for */kard-am/* 'did-I'

The general trend in the deficits in AS's Persian was substitution of the verb, manifested as either subject-verb disagreement or substitution of the whole main verb or the nominal or verbal element of a compound verb.

A.2 Two new case studies

CASE FOUR: MG

MG is a right-handed native speaker of Persian, a housewife with high school education. She was 32 years old when she suffered an embolic CVA in 1996, leaving her with a right hemiplegia and complete muteness. Subsequent medical examinations and CT scans revealed a left frontal lobe lesion specifically affecting Broca's area.

MG was administered the standard Persian version of the BAT (Paradis et al., 1987) around one and a half years post-onset. At the time of evaluation, she showed noticeable improvement in all language modalities, particularly in production, as a result of an intensive speech therapy program.

BAT ASSESSMENT

Based on the results, her clinical picture matches the classical profile of a severe agrammatic aphasic. Her speech output was extremely nonfluent, halting and telegraphic, and was restricted to the production of a limited number of content words. Her comprehension, by contrast, was remarkably well preserved. She displayed a perfect performance on eight different comprehension tasks and near normal performance (80% or more) on six other comprehension tasks. MG's remarkably high level of performance on comprehension subtests stands in sharp contrast to her poor performance on production subtests. She failed completely at four production tasks and scored very low (10%) on three other tasks.

In addition, MG's high score on the grammaticality judgment subtest indicates that her ability to recognize the syntactic well-formedness of different sentence structures is very good. The results of MG's performance on comprehension and grammaticality judgment are consistent with the BAT characterization of Broca's patients, whereby comprehension and grammaticality judgment impairments do not necessarily co-occur with expressive agrammatism. Based on the results of the assessment, MG can be considered as a typical agrammatic patient with severely reduced expression, poor repetition and well-retained comprehension.

We also obtained a sample of MG's connected speech in order to more precisely characterize her language impairments. A post-test analysis of her connected speech confirmed that her speech was extremely laborious and telegraphic in nature. The elicited speech sample contained a total of 10 single-clause utterances, with complete deletion of VPs and omission of bound or free grammatical morphemes. As seen in the following examples taken from her elicited speech, nouns were the only elements used in the entire sample. They were all in the singular. No inflected verbs or infinitive forms, adverbs or adjectives were detected in MG's elicited speech.

20. Examiner: 'Where did you live when you were a child?'
Patient: */man [dar] Hamedan [zendegi mi-kard-am/*
I [in] Hamedan [living was-doing-I]
I Hamedan.

21. Examiner: 'Where have you traveled?'
Patient: */[be] Abadan [va] Haban [V]/*
[to] Abadan [and] Ahvaz [V]
Abadan Ahvaz.

22. Examiner: 'Did you go a long time ago?'
Patient: */bâ mâmân[-am] [be] Abadan [va] bâbâ [-âm] [V]/*
With mother[-my] [to] Abadan [and] father[-my] [V]
With mother Abadan, father.

CASE FIVE: RL

RL is a 49-year-old male right-handed native speaker of Persian with eight years of education. At the age of 47, RL suffered a CVA due to an occlusion of the left internal carotid artery. A CT scan revealed an extensive lesion in the left hemisphere involving the fronto-temporal lobe. He initially presented with severe aphasic symptoms and was characterized as having right hemiplegia as well as speech apraxia. However, his various linguistic abilities, particularly production, improved rapidly following regular speech therapy for one and a half years before the administration of the BAT. At the time of testing, RL was not able to use his right hand at all. However, he could walk unsupported, but very slowly.

BAT ASSESSMENT

Based on his BAT scores, RL can be characterized as a mild agrammatic aphasic with occasional word-finding problems in spontaneous speech and slightly impaired comprehension. His performance on nine comprehension tasks was intact and he achieved above-chance performance (60%–80%) on eight other tasks. By comparison, he passed only eight production tasks and failed or scored less than 30% on the rest. He obtained a perfect score on the grammaticality judgment test, demonstrating that his interpretation of complex sentences was significantly better than chance and that he did not rely solely on lexical semantics to assign syntactic relations. However, compared to MG and many other agrammatics, his production was less agrammatic.

To provide a better analysis of RL's language characteristics, we elicited a sample of his connected speech, a description of the history of his illness. The elicited sample comprised a total of 112 words in 34 different sentences. The sentences included 32 simple and two complex sentences involving the relative clause marker */ke/*. A post-test analysis of the data revealed that RL's elicited speech was not error-free, although, unlike typical agrammatic aphasics, he did not exhibit a strong tendency to omit function and inflectional items. Most noun phrases in elicited speech samples were single nouns, but *ezafe* constructions were also used three times. Deletion of an obligatory grammatical morpheme, which occurred only once, was restricted to */râ/*. No evidence of the deletion of prepositions was observed. Also, */râ/* was used inappropriately once. In addition, three cases of incorrect subject-verb agreement were found. In two contexts, the third person singular zero morpheme was substituted for the plural of the verb (*goft*–0 instead of *goft-and*; *umad*–0 instead of *umad-and*), while in one instance, the plural form was substituted for the singular verb (*goft-and* instead of *goft*-0). The following violations are taken from his elicited speech sample:

Deletion of grammatical morphemes

23. */un âqâ maqâzeye man [râ] dâ_t/*
    that man store-of me [OBJ] had
    That man had my store.

24. */un vaqt goft-am ke [az] injâ- man _iz kard/*
    then told-I that [from] here-my thing did
    Then I told that [from] here something was doing.

25. */hamâm-am-o gereft-am [va] raft-am/*
    shower-my-OBJ took-I [and] went-I
    I took my shower [and] went away.

There was also one instance of addition of the grammatical morpheme */râ/* as a direct object particle:

26. */raft-am unjâ râ/*
    went-I there OBJ
    I went there OBJ

Substitution of free grammatical morphemes

27. */dar hodude dah tâ doktor umad <u>ru-ye*</u> sar-am/*
    about ten doctor came on-of head-my
    About ten doctors came <u>on</u> my head.
    /ru-ye/ is substituted for */bâlâ-ye/* 'over'

Incorrect subject-verb agreement

In two obligatory contexts, a singular inflectional morpheme is used for a plural subject.

28. */dar hodude dah, ha_t...doktor umad[-and] ru-ye sar-am/*
    about ten, eight doctor came[-PL] on-of head-my
    About ten, eight doctors came[-PL] on my head.

29. */unvaqt goft[-and] _i-ye âqâ/*
    then said[PL] what-is sir
    Then asked[PL] 'what is it, sir.'

There is also one instance of plural inflection for a singular subject.

30. /*un âqâ goft-<u>and</u> eyb na-dâre*/
    that man said (PL) problem not-has
    That man said(PL) 'there is no problem.'

Verb substitution

There is one instance of an empty verb replacing the main lexical verb.

31. /*goft-am ke az in-jâm _iz kard*/*
    told-I that from my-here something did
    I said 'from here something did.'
    */*_iz kard*/ as an empty verb replaces /*âb mi-_ekad*/ 'water is drooling'
    There is also one instance of relative clause deletion.

32. /*goft-am ke ….*/
    told-I that …
    I said that …

B. Review of two published cases with the control data

The two patients reported in the following section became aphasic as a result of trauma. Both patients were assessed with the standard short version of the BAT (Paradis et al., 1987) and connected speech samples were elicited and analyzed with materials included in the CLAS protocol (Menn & Obler, 1990). Based on the results of these assessments, both patients were diagnosed as having Broca's aphasia and satisfied the CLAS I clinical standards for agrammatism: slow and halting speech, short and/or fragmentary sentences, and limited use of the syntactic and morphological resources of their native language. The performance of both patients and the disruptions in their speech are compared with matched control data. In this section, their most salient agrammatic features are briefly reviewed. The general background information on both patients and the control subject are given in Table 2. For details on each case, consult Nilipour (2000).

CASE SIX: HB

HB's comprehension and production were impaired, but his comprehension was relatively better preserved than his expression. His utterances were short, and his grammar was very restricted and simple.

All HB's utterances were single clauses, with or without a lexical verb. Omissions and substitutions occurred across all speech samples, but there were three times as many omissions as substitutions (86 vs. 30). About 70% of word deletion errors involved function words, and 74% of the deleted content words were lexical verbs. Most lexical verbs were replaced by /*ast*/ 'is'. HB omitted over 58% of grammatical morphemes in the required contexts, with about 35% correctly used and the remaining 7% incorrectly used (see Table 3).

Compared with the control subject, HB's performance is indicative of his poor access to lexical categories and complex syntax (cf. 4.2 vs. 8.6 for MLU and 185 vs. 377 for total words). His limited number of required contexts for all grammatical categories is further evidence of his simple syntax (144 vs. 328). He had especially poor access to prepositions and the *ezafe* morpheme /*-e*/, which are needed for complex NP structures, and he also made limited use of derivational and inflectional morphemes.

GRAMMATICAL VIOLATIONS

The verb phrase proved to be the most vulnerable constituent of the sentence at both the syntactic and morphological levels. In 36% of HB's utterances, the lexical verb was totally missing and in 28% of them the produced form (/*ast*/ 'is', /*hast*/ 'there is') was not relevant to the context, but instead functioned as a filler. There were two instances of the imperative /*bi-yâ*/ 'come', which consists of the subjunctive prefix followed by the bare stem and two instances of /*mi-xor-ad*/ 'is eating'), in the third person singular. In the matched control data, 86 lexical verbs were found.

Table 2. General background information on two aphasic patients and control

	HB	**MN**	**control AM**
Age	20	21	17
Sex	M	M	M
Occupation	Student	Student	Student
Years of education	10	11	11
Native language	Persian	Persian	Persian
Handedness	Right	Right	Right
Etiology	Trauma	Trauma	—
Lesion side	L	L	—
Lesion site	Fronto-temporal	Parietal	—
Post-onset assessment	20 months	10 months	—
Aphasia type	Broca's	Broca's	—

A typical NP was a single word or a compound word. The conjunction /*va*/ 'and' was missing from within NPs more than 50% of the time. Noun attributes and determiners were absent. A summary of HB's grammatical errors and their distributions and the matched control data is given in Table 3. The following examples taken from his connected speech represent his major grammatical violations.

Verb breakdown

Deletion of the main lexical verb

33. /*[man] do sâl [dar] jebhe [V]*/

[I] two year [in] war front [V]

Two years [in] the war front.

34. */mard zambil [V]/*
man basket [V]
The man [has] a basket.

Substitution of the verb
35. */zan zambil <u>ast*</u>/*
woman basket is
The woman is basket.
*/ast/ 'is' substituted for /dâr-ad/ or /mi-bar-ad/ 'is carrying'

Table 3. HB's distribution of grammatical errors and the matched control data

	Items	*Correct* N*	%	*Incorrect* N	%	*Omission* N	%	*Total* N	*Control Data*
1	Def. art.	0		0		0		0	0
2	Indef. art.	3	75	1	25	0		4	11
3	Preposition	3	13	3	13	18+6	74+100	30	36
4	Postp. */râ/*	0		0		5	100	5	9
5	LINK morph.	2+2	33+50	0		4+2	67+50	10	35
6	POSS. Morph.	0		0		4	100	4	10
7	Pronoun	2+2	33+100	0		4	67	8	12
8	DER morph.	2	50	0		2	50	4	10
9	CL. INTER. Conj. */va/*	4+8	45+47	0+2	18	5+9	55+53	28	30
10	PL. morph.	0+1	100	0		0		1	11
11	Infm. marker	0		0		0		0	4
12	PST. morph.	0		0		0		0	10
13	Inflect. Morph.	4	100	0		0		4	69
14	PROG. */mi-/*	2	100	0		0		2	50
15	IMP. */be-/*	2	100	0		0		2	7
16	NEG. morph.	0		0		1	100	1	3
17	Aux	0		1	33	2	67	3	11
18	CL. EXTER. Conj.	0		0		0		0	10
	Total	37	34.9	7	6.6	62	58	106	328

* The first figure in each column refers to the spoken data, and the second to the written data. When there is only one, it corresponds to the spoken data. The control data are only for spoken language.

36. */mard sobhâne <u>ast</u>/*
man breakfast is
The man is breakfast.

37. */mard dâne [ruye] zamin <u>ast*</u>/*
man seed [on] ground is
The man is seeds [on] the ground.
*/*ast*/ 'is' is substituted for */mi-pâs-ad/* 'is spreading'

Disruptions of grammatical items
The indefinite article was used incorrectly in 25% of the four obligatory contexts.

38. */[dar/ _âr_ambe âta_-i [V]/*
[on] Wednesday fire-art [V]
Wednesday a fire.

Prepositions were used correctly in 13%, incorrectly in 13% and deleted in 74% of the 30 obligatory contexts.
39. */dozd-i [dar] xâne ast/*
thief-a [in] house is
There is a thief [in] the house.

40. */âb [az] _ir ast/*
water [from] tap is
The water [from] the tap is.

The postposed particle */râ/* was absent from all obligatory contexts (0/5).
41. */dozd-i panjere [râ] bâz ast/*
thief-a window [OBJ] open is
A thief is (open) window.

The *ezafe* linking morpheme was absent from 67% of the six required contexts in spoken language.
42. */panjere[ye] xâne bâz ast/*
window-[of] house open is
The window [of] the house is open.

Possessive morphemes were deleted from all four required contexts.
43. */man be dast va sar[-am] xompâre [V]/*
I to hand and head[-my] shrapnel [V]
I hand and head shrapnel [*/xord/* 'hit'].

Pronouns were used correctly in 33% and deleted from 67% of the six obligatory contexts.
44. */[u] pâ ast/*
[he] foot is
[He] foot is. ('He runs away')

The clause-internal conjunction */va/* 'and' was also vulnerable and was deleted from 45% of the nine obligatory contexts in speech.
45. */dozd-i pul [va] sâ?at [râ] ast/*
Thief-a money [and] watch [OBJ] is
The thief is money [and] watch.

A general review of HB's linguistic performance indicates that the most salient disrupted major lexical category was the main lexical verb, which was either deleted (36%) or substituted (28%) in required contexts. Among grammatical items, prepositions (45% out of 24), the *ezafe* linking morpheme /*-e*/ (67% out of 6) and the clause-internal linking morpheme /*va*/ (55% out of 9 spoken contexts) were the most salient disrupted items (for details, see Table 3).

CASE SEVEN: MN

Based on the results of the assessment, MN's comprehension was much better preserved than his expression. Function words were more vulnerable to deletion than content words. As a result, 73% of the missing words were function words. Another major feature of MN's speech was the use of the infinitive rather than the contextually required inflected form of the verb.

A comparison of MN's linguistic performance and that of the control subject in parallel tasks indicates that his poor access to lexical categories and function words (10 vs. 19) resulted in the production of short, simple sentences (MLU 4.4 vs. 6.7).

Infinitive form of the verb

There were six instances of infinitive forms used for the contextually required inflected form of the same verb.

GRAMMATICAL VIOLATIONS

The verb phrase was more vulnerable to disruption than the noun phrase. In 22% of all instances, the verb was missing, and in 19% of them, MN provided the infinitive form of the verb where the context required an inflected form. There was only one instance of a VP with the auxiliary verb and three instances of the past tense. In the matched spoken control data, 15 instances of inflected verbs were observed, with no infinitives.

Noun phrase structure was simple at the syntactic level, but richer at the morphological level. The *ezafe* morpheme /*-e*/ appeared in four contexts to connect the elements of noun phrases. Prepositional phrases containing a preposition were used in six different instances, while prepositions were missing from seven other obligatory contexts out of 14. The distribution of MN's grammatical errors among different categories and the matched control data are given in Table 4. The following examples taken from his connected speech represent the most salient grammatical violations in his performance.

Verb breakdown

The verb was the most disrupted lexical category in both spoken and written data. It was used correctly in six spoken and one written out of 24 required contexts. The major verb-related problems were as follows:

Deletion of the verb

The verb was absent from five spoken and four written contexts.

46. /*juje[-hâ] bâ madar-a_ [-ân] [V]*/
    chick[-s] with mother-her[-s] [V]
    The chick[-s] with her[-s] mother [V]

Table 4. MN's distribution of grammatical errors and the matched control data

	Items	*Correct*		*Incorrect*		*Omission*		*Total*	*Control*
		N*	%	N	%	N	%	N	*Data*
1	Def. art.	9	100	0		0		9	2
2	Indef. Art.	0		0		0		0	0
3	Preposition	4+3	40+43	1	20	2+4	40+57	14	5
4	Postp. */râ/*	0		0		4+1	100	5	2
5	LINK morph.	0+2	100	0		0		2	5
6	POSS. Morph.	2+1	100+50	0		0+1	50	4	2
7	Pronoun	0+4	67	0		0+2	33	6	2
8	DER morph.	0+0		0		0+1	50	1	2
9	CL. INTER. Conj. */va/*	0		0		1+1	100	2	4
10	PL. morph.	0		0		5		5	4
11	Infm. Marker	0		1+6	100	0		7	0
12	PST. Morph.	2+2	50+100	0		2	50	6	0
13	Inflect. Morph.	2+1	40+33	1	20	2+2	40+66	8	16
14	PROG. */mi-/*	1+1	100	0		0		5	11
15	IMP. */be-/*	0		0		0+1	100	1	1
16	NEG. morph.	0+1	100	0		0		1	0
17	Aux	0		0+1	100	0		1	0
18	CL. EXTER. Conj.	0		0		0		0	4
	Total	35	47	11	13	29	39	74	60

* The first figure in each column refers to the spoken data, and the second to the written data. When there is only one, it corresponds to the spoken data. The control data are only for spoken language.

47. */man az sar, pâ [va] dast [V]/*
    I from head, leg [and] hand [V]
    I from head, leg [and] hand [V].

Broken-off form of the verb

A broken-off form of the verb, which is similar to the bare verb stem, was used in three spoken contexts.

48. */sâqe _eka[-st]/*
    branch break [past]
    The branch break

49. */man bâ mâ_in niru mi-âvar-d-an/*
    I with truck troops PROG-bring-d-Infm
    I to bringing troops with the truck

50. */man bisto do mâh xedmat kar-d-an bud-an/*
    I twenty-nd-two month service do-ed-Infm be-ed-Infm
    I to be to do service for twenty-two months.

Disruption of grammatical items

Prepositions were among the most disrupted grammatical items. They were deleted in 40% of spoken and 57% of written cases out of 14 required contexts.

51. */mard-e [râ] [dar] bimârestân xâb-un-d-an/*
    man-the [OBJ] [in] hospital hospitalize-ed-Infm
    The man hospital to hospitalize.

52. /[*man râ be] bimârestân [bor-d-and*]/
    [I OBJ to] hospital [took-they]
    The hospital.

The direct object marker was missing from four spoken and one written obligatory contexts.

53. */ba?dan zan-e âdam-e [râ] sedâ kard/*
    then woman-the guy-the [OBJ] call did-she
    Then the woman called the guy.

The conjunction */va/* 'and' was missing from one spoken and one written context.

54. */mard-e [va] juje[-hâ] bâ _âxe odâr.../*
    man-the [and] chick[-s] with branch fell
    The man [and] the chick[-s] fell with the branch.

The plural morpheme was absent from five obligatory contexts (see examples 46 and 54 above).

The infinitive marker was used inappropriately in seven different contexts as a result of substituting the infinitive for the contextually proper inflected form of the verb.

55. */[man] âmad-an [be] Ahvaz/*
    [I] come-Infm [to] Ahvaz
    To come Ahvaz.

The person-number inflectional morphemes were among the most disrupted grammatical items. They were used correctly only in five out of 25 required contexts. There were both substitutions and deletions of inflectional morphemes in obligatory contexts.

56. */[dar] kordestân bi-sim dâ_t/*
    [in] Kurdistan wireless had-he
    [in] Kurdistan he had wireless.

The progressive morpheme */mi-/* was used only in two required contexts, but was absent from contexts where the lexical verb was either deleted or replaced by an infinitive form.

3. Discussion and summary of the results

Four different types of aphasic syndromes in seven native speakers of Persian were briefly reviewed. They all showed relatively better comprehension than production except for AS, whose comprehension was more impaired than his production.

The pathological data suggested that they all had simplified syntax and suffered from some type of breakdown of the VP as manifested by deletion and/or substitution, and different degrees of NP disruptions, mostly manifested by the deletion of preposed and/or postposed particles (*/be/* and */râ/*) and prepositions. Based on the general characteristics of their deficits, they may be classified into four groups: (1) General agrammatic symptoms of Broca's aphasia in MG, RL, HB and MN accompanied by specific features such as substitution of a filler verb */budan/* 'to be' for all kinds of verbs by HB and substitution of the polymorphemic infinitive for the contextually proper inflected form of the verb by MN. (2) Task-specific agrammatic features in PA's speech, characterized by verb-tense substitution and deletion of free grammatical morphemes. (3) General grammatical violations accompanied by naming difficulties and substitution of empty words and semantic paraphasia in TB. (4) Paragrammatic symptoms in AS's speech, characterized by substitution of different parts of compound verbs.

The four agrammatic patients did not have the same linguistic profile on all measures, and represented varying degrees of severity of the same pathological phenomenon. Their symptomatic differences may be due to their pathological and individual differences. However, the same principles apply to all. Namely, the overall result of their agrammatic performance on various tasks was indicative of their tendency to simplify syntactic structures, omit grammatical morphemes and rely more on nouns than verbs. In particular, they failed to produce well-formed complex structures such as embedded structures and relative clauses. Moreover, they all had more difficulty in producing verbs than other lexical categories. These findings are comparable with the reported results in other languages (Menn & Obler, 1990).

However, the disruption of the verb had different manifestations across Persian aphasic subjects. The major types of verb breakdowns were as follows: (1) deletion and/or substitution of the lexical verb or of nominal or verbal elements of a compound verb; (2) deletion and/or substitution of inflectional morphemes; (3) substitution of the infinitive for the contextually proper inflected form of the verb; (4) substitution of a filler verb */budan/* 'to be' for the appropriate lexical verb; (5) incorrect subject-verb agreement; (6) broken-off verb forms producing partial words.

Disruption of the verb has already been reported in other languages (e.g. Italian (Miceli & Mazzucchi, 1990); Hindi (Bhatnagar, 1990)), but the data in Persian are suggestive of two major types of verb disruption which may be thought of as language-specific: (a) substitution of a filler verb 'to be' */budan/* as a default for all kinds of verbs, including transitive active verbs; (b) substitution of the infinitive for the contextually proper inflected form of the verb.

The substitution of the verb 'to be' for all kinds of verbs appears to be a new finding in aphasiological literature for two reasons: (1) common observation across languages reports more omissions of low-content verbs ('have', 'be') than of lexical main verbs, and also greater accessibility of rich main verbs (Menn & Obler, 1990: 1377); (2) substitution of 'be' has been reported only for intransitive verbs (Kegl, 1995). However, the data for at least one patient (HB) show the reverse trend. HB had a very strong tendency to substitute the low-content copula 'is' and existential 'there is' for a main lexical verb. Nevertheless, he substituted the verb 'to be' for all kinds of verbs, including transitive active verbs (for further details, see Nilipour (2000)).

HB's data are also suggestive of two more language-specific features: the tendency to omit the NP-internal conjunction */va/* 'and', and the use of the present tense as a default, despite its more complicated morphological form (for details, see Nilipour (2000)).

4. Conclusion

The overall linguistic performance of the Persian aphasic patients reviewed in this chapter is suggestive of certain universal and language-specific agrammatic features. Among universal features, the data from the four Broca's patients tend to show simplification of syntax, more reliance on canonical forms, resulting in less syntactic variation, and lesser accessibility of verbs as opposed to nouns. These general features are in line with data reported from other languages (Menn & Obler, 1990).

As for language-specific agrammatic features, the present data suggest greater vulnerability of the VP as opposed to the NP. The disruptions in NPs are manifested in the deletion of the *ezafe* linking morpheme */-e/* as well as deletion of the clause-internal conjunction */va/*, resulting in a simplified NP. Among free grammatical morphemes, the items most vulnerable to deletion were the postposed direct object marker */râ/* and prepositions.

With regard to disruption of VPs, the present data support an etiological distinction in Broca's aphasia. There is more deletion of the main lexical verb in severe cases with CVA etiology, as manifested in MG, whereas one finds language-specific substitutions for the main verb in severe cases of trauma, as seen in HB and MN. The manifestations of verb substitution take the form of low-content verbs such as */budan/* 'to be' substituted for all kinds of verbs, as manifested in HB, and the substitution of the polymorphemic infinitive form for the contextually proper inflected verb form, as manifested in MN. As the Persian data so far are limited to these cases, these conclusions will have to be verified by further research.

Address correspondence to: Reza Nilipour, Department of Speech Pathology, University of Welfare and Rehabilitation Sciences, Evin, Tehran 19834, IRAN.
E-mail: nilipour@karun.ipm.ac.ir

References

Bhatnagar, S.C. (1990). Agrammatism in Hindi: One case study. In L. Menn and L.K. Obler (Eds.), *Agrammatism: A cross-language narrative source book,* vol. 2 (pp. 975-1011). Amsterdam: Benjamins.

Kegl, J. (1995). Levels of representation and units of access relevant to agrammatism. *Brain and Language, 50,* 151-200.

Menn, L., & Obler, L.K. (Eds.) (1990). *Agrammatism: A cross-language narrative source book,* 3 vols. Amsterdam: Benjamins.

Miceli, G., & Mazzucchi, A. (1990). Agrammatism in Italian: Two case studies. In L. Menn and L.K. Obler (Eds.), *A cross-language narrative source book,* vol. 1 (pp. 717-816). Amsterdam: Benjamins.

Nilipour, R. (1988). Bilingual aphasia in Iran: A preliminary report. *Journal of Neurolinguistics, 3,* 185-232.

Nilipour, R. (1989). Task-specific agrammatism in a Farsi-English patient. *Journal of Neurolinguistics, 4,* 243-253.

Nilipour, R. (2000). Agrammatic language: Two cases from Persian. *Aphasiology, 14*(12), 1205-1242.

Nilipour, R., & Ashayeri, H. (1989). Alternating antagonism between two languages with successive recovery of a third in a trilingual aphasic patient. *Brain and Language, 36,* 23-48.

Nilipour, R., & Paradis, M. (1995). Breakdown of functional categories in three Farsi-English bilingual aphasic patients. In M. Paradis (Ed.), *Aspects of bilingual aphasia* (pp. 123-138). Oxford: Pergamon Press.

Paradis, M., & Libben, G. (1987). *The assessment of bilingual aphasia.* Hillsdale, NJ: Lawrence Erlbaum.

Paradis, M., Paribakht, T., & Nilipour, R. (1987). *The bilingual aphasia test (Farsi version).* Hillsdale, NJ: Lawrence Erlbaum.

Raghibdoust, S. (1999). Comprehension and grammaticality judgment in Persian-speaking agrammatics. Unpublished dissertation, Department of Linguistics, University of Ottawa.

Grammatical structuring in Broca's and Wernicke's aphasia in Finnish

Marja-Liisa Helasvuo*, Anu Klippi°, Minna Laakso‡

**Department of Finnish, University of Helsinki, °Department of Phonetics, University of Helsinki, ‡Centre for Cognitive Neuroscience, University of Turku*

Abstract—The purpose of this paper is to examine the linguistic problems of aphasic speakers of Finnish. The focus is on Broca's and Wernicke's aphasia. First, we present an overview of the special characteristics of the grammar of Finnish. Secondly, there is a discussion of previous studies on aphasic speakers of Finnish. Thirdly, we present an analysis of our data from conversation and picture description task by speakers with Broca's and Wernicke's aphasia. The analysis focuses on case marking, subject-verb agreement, word order and the expression of tense in the speech of Finnish aphasics. As a whole, many linguistic features are preserved both in Broca's and Wernicke's aphasia. Even the neologistic words in Wernicke's aphasia are appropriately inflected. However, our findings suggest that aphasic errors are not always systematic and furthermore, they may be context-dependent. For example, Broca's aphasics produced case marking and agreement patterns in some contexts correctly, whereas in some other contexts they were produced erroneously. The word order patterns were similar to those found in conversational discourse in general. However, it is sometimes impossible to give a definitive analysis of the word order or structure of a given grammatical construction. This is due to the fact that sentence structure is sometimes badly distorted both in Broca's and Wernicke's aphasic cases because of difficulty in finding lexical content words. We conclude with a comparison of our findings with previous studies of Finnish aphasics, proposing some methodological implications for further studies.

Keywords: Finnish, Broca's aphasia, Wernicke's aphasia, case marking, agreement, tense expressions, word order

1. Introduction

There are approx. 5 million speakers of Finnish, most of them living in Finland. The estimate of new aphasic cases per year is 3000-3500 persons (based on Siirtola 1985). The systematic study of aphasia was started in Finland some twenty years ago, and the research has been active ever since, although there are only a few scholars working in this research area.

The beginning of aphasia research has been closely related to the history of Finland: after the Second World War, there were about 3000 young soldiers with brain injuries in Finland. Thus, there was an acute need for rehabilitation, and a new rehabilitation clinic was established. Psychologist Niilo Mäki, a student of Kurt Goldstein and Adhemar Gelb in the late 1920's in Frankfurt-am-Main, was appointed the head of the psychological-pedagogical unit of the clinic. Mäki (1951) reported that he had about 480 aphasic patients in rehabilitation. He also gave some rough evaluation of the outcome of the rehabilitation: in 68-69 % of the aphasic cases, aphasic disorders practically disappeared, 30 % of the cases gained a good amount of help from the aphasia therapy and about 1-2 % of the cases did not benefit from the therapy. Unfortunately, Mäki did not report his cases in detail, and most of his work has not been reported at all.

The first linguistically-oriented studies on aphasia were published in the 1980's in Finland. Most of the studies focus on the linguistic features of agrammatism in Finnish Broca's aphasics (e.g. Kukkonen 1983, 1990, Niemi, Laine & Koivuselkä-Sallinen 1990), but observations on the lexical and grammatical features of Wernicke's aphasia were reported as well (e.g., Niemi & Koivuselkä-Sallinen 1987, Kukkonen 1993). The studies were either single-case studies, or they were based on a limited number of cases. Furthermore, there is a lot of variation in the speech samples used in these studies. There are studies based on data from storytelling, written materials and conversation.

The purpose of this paper is to provide a description of features of aphasic speech in Finnish with a focus on Broca's and Wernicke's aphasia. First, we will give an overview of the relevant characteristics of the language. Then, there will be a brief review of previous studies on aphasic speakers of Finnish. Finally, we will analyze certain morphosyntactic features of Finnish in aphasic expressions with the help of examples from conversation and picture description. As a conclusion, we will consider our findings in the light of the previous studies on Finnish.

2. Characteristics of Finnish

Finnish is a member of the Finno-Ugric language family. Just like the other members of this language family, Finnish is characterized by a rich morphology, both in terms of derivation and inflection. In this paper, we will focus on features of inflectional morphology, and their relation to certain syntactic patterns. We will first discuss nominal inflection. Then there will be a discussion of verbal markings, especially agreement and tense markers. Finally, we will take a brief look at word-order patterns.

Finnish has an elaborate case marking system with 15 cases. Basically, the object is distinguished from the subject through case marking: the object is marked either with the partitive or the accusative, whereas the subject stands in the nominative, which is unmarked and has no inflection. Consider ex. (1). (Transcription symbols and abbreviations used in the glosses are explained in Appendix 1.)

(1) Broca 2, Picture description (WAB)

M:	*mies (3.3)*	*luke-e*	*kirja-a.*
	man+NOM	read-3SG	book-PTV
	The man (3.3) is reading a book.		

In example (1), the subject argument (*mies* 'man') is in the nominative case, whereas the object argument (*kirjaa* 'book') is inflected in the partitive case. The partitive case marks it as the object of the clause. Note however, that no other interpretation of the relationship between the arguments is semantically possible: the book cannot read the man.

The locative cases can be used to convey quite concrete spatial meanings (ex. 2) as well as more abstract meanings (ex. 3).

(2) Wernicke 3, Conversation

S: *se* *on Mechelininkadu-lla.*
it is Mechelininkatu-ADE
It is on Mechelininkatu (name of a street in Helsinki).

(3) Wernicke 1, Conversation

H: *mei-llä* *ol-i* *(.)* *kurssi*
we-ADE be-PST+3SG course+NOM
We had a course.

In ex. (2), the speaker tells about her former place of work using – quite correctly - the adessive form of street name. Ex. (3) is an instance of a possessive construction, which is the grammaticalized way to express a possessive relationship in Finnish. In this construction, the possessor is expressed through an adessive noun phrase (*meillä* 'we+ADESSIVE') and the "possessed" is a nominative noun phrase (*kurssi* 'course') which comes after the copula.

In Finnish, the predicate verb agrees with the subject according to person and number. Finnish makes a three-way distinction in terms of person (1st, 2nd and 3rd) and a two-way distinction in terms of number (singular : plural; see ex. 4).

(4) Wernicke 1, Conversation

H: mä ol-i-n just lähte-ny tänne kato.
I be-PST-1SG just leave-PCP here see
I had just left to (come) here you see.

In ex. (4), the predicate verb *olin lähteny* 'had left' agrees with the subject *mä* 'I' in number (singular) and person (1st person). The agreement marker *–n* is attached to the auxiliary *ol-* 'be'.

Since the aphasia data mostly comes from the spoken variety, it is important to note that the colloquial agreement system differs slightly from the standard. In the colloquial language, the 1st person plural pronoun is most often used with a verb in the passive form instead of the verb form with the 1st person plural marker. Furthermore, the number distinction has been neutralized in the 3rd person, and the singular form is used for both singular and plural subjects (for a discussion of the colloquial system, see Helasvuo 2000). Ex. (5) illustrates the use of the 3rd person singular form in connection with plural subjects.

(5) Wernicke 1, Conversation

H: *ne-kin* *käy* *ilmeisest*
they-CLT visit+3SG obviously
They also go there obviously.

In ex. (5), even though there is a 3rd person plural subject *ne* 'they', the predicate stands in the 3rd person singular form. The 3rd person singular has been called the unmarked member of the agreement system (see Hakulinen & Karlsson 1979), since it is the form which is used when person distinctions do not apply (e.g. when there is a full clause functioning as the subject).

Finnish exhibits a tense system with four tenses, present, past, present perfect and past perfect. The present and past tense are both simple tenses, whereas the present perfect and the past perfect are periphrastic forms, consisting of the auxiliary *olla* 'be' and a participle of the main verb. There is no future form, the present tense being used for future reference. The present tense has no ending (i.e. it is unmarked), and it is the most frequent tense. The past tense is marked with an affix *–i*. One common usage for the past tense is in narrative contexts. In our data, we find that the unmarked tense, i.e. the present, is sometimes used in past contexts instead of the past tense. It is important to note that this is not pathological as such, as the present tense can be used in narrative contexts in normal speech also, but only for special effects: it can be used for dramatizing or highlighting some point (cf. the historical present). In our data, the complex tenses – the present perfect and the past perfect – are sometimes used without the auxiliary, i.e. the element which carries the markers for tense and person, thus leaving only the participle form. Consider ex. (6).

(6) Broca 1, Conversation

J:	*ih*	*ittet*	*se-n (0.3)*	*TEH-nyt.*
		self	it-ACC	do-PCP
		(I) myself done it.		

In ex. (6) the speaker is talking about a renovation project and showing pictures to the therapist. He refers to a storage shed shown in the picture, and explains that he has done it himself. However, he does not have the *olla*-auxiliary, which would carry the tense and person markers.

Finnish word order has been characterized as being relatively free, with "very few genuinely grammatical constraints" (Vilkuna 1989). This is certainly true if we look at word order from the perspective of single sentences or isolated fragments of texts: syntactic permutations rarely yield ungrammatical orderings. However, in a study based on data from conversational discourse, Helasvuo (2000) reports that the data show a relatively fixed Subject – Verb order, as over 90 % of subjects are preverbal. By contrast, Hakulinen et al's (1980) study on written Finnish shows that approx. 70 % of subjects precede the verb. Furthermore, it is important to note that full lexical subjects are a minority among subjects in the spoken data, as almost 80 % of all subjects are pronominal (Helasvuo 2000). These differences between the written and the spoken variety of Finnish are important to bear in mind when looking at the data from aphasics and when trying to determine the best way to make comparisons with normal data.

Helasvuo (2000) also shows that word order patterns are dependent on the type of subject: in clauses with pronominal subjects, the subject precedes the verb in over 95 % of the cases. In clauses with full lexical subjects there is more variation, but even there the preferred order is Subject – Verb. This fact may be relevant when evaluating the findings on aphasic data from different kinds of tasks. For example, it seems that lexical arguments are more frequent in elicited narratives based on pictures than in conversation.

3. Previous Finnish research on aphasia

The first Finnish aphasia studies with linguistic orientation aimed to analyze the linguistic characteristics of non-fluent aphasia (Kukkonen 1983, Kukkonen & Pajunen 1986). Niemi and his colleagues have conducted several studies focusing for instance on temporal delay and lexical retrieval in Finnish posterior aphasics (Niemi & Koivuselkä-Sallinen 1987), lexical deformations in posterior aphasia (Niemi, Koivuselkä-Sallinen & Laine 1987), grammatical disorders (Niemi 1988, I-II), syntax in Wernicke's aphasia (Niemi, Koivuselkä-Sallinen & Sarajärvi 1988), nonlexical grammatical deviations in "paragrammatic" aphasia (Niemi 1990), agrammatism in Finnish (Niemi, Koivuselkä-Sallinen & Laine 1990), and syntax and inflectional morphology in aphasia (Niemi, Laine, Hänninen & Koivuselkä-Sallinen 1990). A little later, Kukkonen (1990) published a study of phonological disturbances in aphasia and paragrammatism in Finnish (see also Kukkonen 1993). The latest approach in aphasia research in Finland deals with conversational speech (Klippi 1996, Laakso 1997, Laakso & Klippi 1999, Leiwo & Klippi 2000).

Aphasic morphosyntactic structures in Finnish

As was mentioned earlier, Finnish is characterized by a rich system of morphological affixes. This is a special characteristic of Finnish, which differentiates it from many more widely studied languages. Therefore, it is not surprising to find that the early linguistically oriented research reflected a keen interest in the study of morphosyntactic errors by Finnish aphasic speakers.

Grammatical errors connected to anterior aphasics have been studied by Kukkonen (1983), Kukkonen & Pajunen (1986) and Niemi, Laine, Hänninen & Koivuselkä-Sallinen (1990). These studies deal with the phenomenon of agrammatism and the problems related to this concept based on the Finnish materials. Kukkonen (1983) studied speaker N, basing her study on recorded materials from speech therapy sessions, as well as written exercises done by the patient and data from a one-hour interview with the patient. Speaker N had morphological difficulty. The examples analyzed by Kukkonen show that a form resembling the suggested basic form tends to substitute for other word-forms. N used forms that do not exist in the normal language. He also produced examples of unsystematic affix deletion. However, he did not choose a wrong variant of a given ending. According to Kukkonen, N simplified his speech production by dropping endings, although he knew their basic meaning, which is evidenced by examples where the endings are used hypercorrectly. Kukkonen is rather careful with her interpretation of these errors. She suggests two possible interpretations (p. 470): some parts of the inflection process might be dropped, thus resulting in the error, or the words may actually transfer from one inflection type to another.

Niemi & Koivuselkä-Sallinen (1983) studied a case of a Finnish posterior aphasic in naming and repetition tasks and in interview. Contrary to Kukkonen's findings, their data reveal that this aphasic speaker made paraphasic substitutions of suffixes: he had a tendency to use a special suffix *–ja,* which he attached to both verbal and nominal stems. Niemi and Koivuselkä-Sallinen (1983) analyze the *–ja*-suffix as a partitive ending, but we find this analysis questionable. It is true that one of the partitive endings in the plural is *–ja*, where the *–j-* stands for plural and *–a* for partitive, but the same suffix is also used as a derivational affix indicating the agent of the action indicated by the verbal stem, e.g. *opetta-ja* 'teach+AGENT SUFFIX = teacher'. Thus, the first case studies on aphasic morphosyntax suggest that whereas the anterior Broca's aphasic used base forms and omitted endings, the posterior aphasic used the appropriate base form but added an inappropriate suffix to it.

Niemi, Laine, Hänninen & Koivuselkä-Sallinen (1990) analyzed the speech of two agrammatic aphasics. Their data was based on interviews and spoken narratives, auditory comprehension, writing, and oral reading. The authors reached the conclusion from their results that these speakers did not delete endings in speech and the few instances of morphological errors were substitutions. The affixes were replaced by less marked ones in several instances. The linguistic problems of these speakers were mostly failures to produce the correct syntactic phrases, low use of coherent discourse, and dysfluency. Thus, both speakers were regarded as "syntactically" but not "morphologically" agrammatic.

Niemi, Koivuselkä-Sallinen & Laine (1987) studied the relationship between lexical deformations and morphosyntactic factors in posterior aphasia. Their results showed that the paraphasias appeared more often in the syntactically derived words than in the lexical ones. Accordingly, they suggested that morphosyntactic factors might interfere with word processing in posterior aphasia. In his further work, Niemi (1988, 1990) points out that syntax is connected to word formation processes in paragrammatism.

Sentence structure in Finnish aphasic speech

In her study of the Broca's aphasic case, speaker N, Kukkonen (1983) found that the grammatical subject is rare. Only 58 % of sentences had a subject. Kukkonen links this observation to Vygotsky's concept of inner speech in which the natural form is predication. Her interpretation is that N's speech resembles his inner speech.

In 1986, Kukkonen & Pajunen analyzed N's case in more detail and compared it to speaker A, who also had Broca's aphasia. Based on the spoken and written materials from speaker N and the mostly written materials from A, they made three claims. In the case of these aphasics, (1) case assignment is easier with concrete verbs than with abstract ones (i.e., lexical factors interfere with case assignment), (2) these agrammatic aphasics tend to use polysemic verbs in their prototypical meaning, and (3) agrammatic aphasics use syntactically simple basic sentences.

Niemi, Koivuselkä-Sallinen & Sarajärvi (1988) and Niemi (1990) studied the syntax of Wernicke's aphasics in narration. Niemi (1990) focused on the complexity of the subject constituents and word order. He found that in the data from speakers with Wernicke's aphasics, the subject preceded the verb in over 80 % of the cases, whereas in the data from speakers with Broca's aphasics, the percentage was 91.3 %. He compares this to Hakulinen et al.'s (1980) study on written Finnish, and suggests that his calculations reveal a bias towards canonical word order (Subject – Verb –order) in aphasic speakers. However, if we take data from the spoken variety as a source for comparison, we find that the word order patterns are quite similar in the data from the aphasic speakers, as over 90 % of the subjects precede the verb in conversational discourse (see above section 2 and Helasvuo 2000). In order to be able to evaluate the differences that Niemi found in the word order of Broca's aphasics as compared to the word order of Wernicke's aphasics, we should need to know the distribution of pronominal vs. full NP subjects in Niemi's two data sets.

According to Niemi (1990), the two Wernicke's aphasic speakers he studied used less complex subjects (e.g., embedded clauses in the subject NPs) in a narrative task than normal speakers in an interview conducted for dialectological research. When they tried to use embedded subjects, the resulting clauses were syntactically ill-formed. Niemi's conclusion was that both the low frequency and the structure of complex NPs in Wernicke speech show deviation, which is hard to account for using a lexical explanation alone.

Broca's vs. Wernicke's aphasia in Finnish

The previously mentioned studies, Niemi, Laine, Hänninen & Koivuselkä-Sallinen (1990) and Niemi (1990), did not establish qualitative differences in the linguistic deficits in Broca's and Wernicke's aphasia in Finnish. The researchers of these studies suggest a continuum of complexity of syntactic constructions with normal speakers at the one end and Broca's aphasics at the other end, while Wernicke's aphasics are between these two groups.

However, Kukkonen (1993) contradicted this proposal in her study "Paragrammatism in Finnish". She presented narrative data on Wernicke's aphasics and found that two of these speakers produced longer stories and more complex utterances than normal control speakers. The studied aphasic speakers made numerous morphological and syntactic errors, too. Her conclusion was that paragrammatism is not a homogeneous phenomenon and considerable variation could be found within the group.

4. Features of aphasic speech

In this section, we will analyze aphasic expressions in connection with certain morphosyntactic features that are characteristic of Finnish. We will focus on case marking, verbal agreement, tense expressions, and word order. Our database consists of conversations and picture description tasks with 4 speakers with Broca's aphasia and 5 with Wernicke's aphasia. Background information on the informants can be found in Appendix 2.

Case marking

Case assignment seems to be well preserved in our data. In Wernicke's aphasia, even neologisms and paraphasias are case marked appropriately. Ex. (7) illustrates this. It comes from a conversation between a speech therapist and a speaker with Wernicke's aphasia. The therapist has asked about the speaker's mother.

(7) Wernicke 3, Conversation

1 S: *joo: kyllä hän vieläkin asu-u kiiltolai-ssa.*
yeah sure s/he still live-3SG ?-INE
Yeah she sure still lives in *kiiltolaki* (neologism).

2 (0.6)

3 t: *asu-u-ks hän siinä SAma-ssa talo-ssa.*
live-3SG-Q s/he there same-INE house-INE
Does she live in the same house?

4 S: Ei sama-ssa mutta hän asuu (.) kiiltolahja-n (0.5) lai-lla.
NEG same-INE but s/he live-3SG ?-GEN top?-ADE
Not in the same (house) but she (he) lives on top (?) of *kiiltolahja* (neologism).

5 t: *mi-ssä [asu-u?*
what-INE live-3SG
Where does she live?

6 S: *[kiiltolahe-ssa.*
?-INE
In *kiiltolahti* (neologism).

In ex. (7), there are several examples of neologisms that are inflected appropriately. In line 1, the speaker produces a neologism *kiiltolaissa* (kiiltolaki-INESSIVE), and after a clarification question by the therapist (line 3), she modifies it to *kiiltolahjan lailla* (kiiltolahja-GENITIVE laki-ADESSIVE, line 4). After still another request for clarification (line 5), she produces *kiiltolahessa* (kiiltolahti-INESSIVE, line 6). The neologisms in lines 1 and 6 are clearly nominal, and semantically it is clear from the context that the neologisms refer to something that can be construed as a place. The neologism in line 4 is also used as a nominal element in a construction that could be a postpositional phrase where the nominal element is inflected in the genitive case (noun-GENITIVE + postposition). However, we cannot know for sure if the speaker intends it to be a place name and thus, a proper noun, or whether it is meant to be a common noun.

Our findings of correct case markings in the speech of Wernicke's aphasics are in contradiction with the finding of Niemi and Koivuselkä-Sallinen (1983), who found that the posterior aphasic case they studied made substitution errors on suffixes (see section 3 above). However, we find it possible that their findings on the posterior aphasic case might be due to perseveration. Namely, the patient used a special suffix *–ja* extremely frequently. For example, when asked to name and repeat the word *lentokone* 'airplane', the patient said *lentokone-ja* 'airplane+JA'.

In Broca's aphasia, it seems that case endings are used appropriately most of the time, and the morphophonological changes that some inflectional classes require in the stem are also correctly produced. However, some Broca's aphasic speakers show a tendency to use uninflected single noun phrases in contexts that require an inflected form. In the following example (8) the aphasic speaker produces an uninflected proper noun as an answer to a question. The target line is line 6.

(8) Broca 1, Conversation

1 E: *mi-ssä* *sä* *olit* *tö-i-ssä?*
what-INE you were work-PL-INE
Where did you go to work?

2 (1.3)

3 J: *mitä.*
what?

4 M: *mi-ssä* *sä* *olit,.*
what-INE you were
Where were you?

5 (0.6)

6 J: *Lemmikäinen.*
Lemminkäinen (name of a company in Finland).

Example (8) comes from a conversation between four aphasic speakers and a therapist. Before this sequence the therapist has suggested that they should interview J. In line 1, E asks where J used to work before he was taken ill. J does not seem to hear (or notice) the question as there is a fairly long pause (line 2) after which J asks "What?". M repeats the essential parts of the question (line 4), and J answers with an uninflected noun phrase, instead of an inflected noun phrase *Lemminkäisellä* 'Lemminkäinen+ADESSIVE' required by the form of the question. These uninflected expressions are very typical of this speaker, and in that sense his speech corresponds to the classical descriptions of omission of grammatical morphemes in agrammatic and telegraphic speech in other languages (Goodglass & Menn 1985, Kolk & Heeschen 1992). However, a closer look at the contexts in which these uninflected expressions occur reveals that they are restricted to certain sequential contexts. Namely, they appear as answers in question-answer sequences where the answering turn only consists of one phrase, or as topic-initiators introducing new topics. In longer utterances, the noun phrases are inflected correctly. Example (9) illustrates this. It comes from the same conversation as example (8).

(9) Broca 1, Conversation

1 t: *tarkotatko että ehdit olla kolme vuotta Suomessa.*
Do you mean that you managed to be three years in Finland.

2 (0.5)

3 J: *juu ei kun.*
yeah no but,

4 t: *vai.*
or

5 J: *juu ei kun, (1.3) ö- men-i-n, (0.7) tonne tonne*
yeah no but go-PST-1SG there there
yeah no but, (pause) er- I went (pause) there there

6 *hh. (1.2) katos, .hh (0.5) Valmeti-lle.*
look V.-ALL
hh. (pause) you see, to Valmet (name of a company in Finland).

In a longer answer, the same speaker J is perfectly capable of using the appropriate case ending. In line 5, he uses the verb *menin* 'I went', which requires a locative case argument in either the allative or the illative case, and in line 6 he produces the required argument *Valmetille* 'Valmet + ALLATIVE'. We could conclude that since J is capable of using the appropriate endings, the uninflected forms in the short, one-word answer sequences might be due to strategic adaptation (Heeschen – Schegloff 1999): because the appropriate case marker is already given in the preceding question, there is no immediate need for it in the answer. It is important to note, however, that this is a phenomenon that we do not find in conversational discourse by normal speakers.

Verbal agreement

In section 2, we mentioned that the 3rd person verb form has been called the unmarked member of the agreement opposition. It is not surprising to find then that in our data from Broca's aphasics, there are cases where a 3rd person verb form (i.e. the unmarked member of the system) is used in connection with a 1st person subject. Consider ex. 10.

(10) Broca 2, Conversation

M: *minä edisty-y koko ajan.*
I progress-3SG all time
I get better all the time.

In ex. 10, a 3rd person singular verb form is used in connection with a 1st person singular pronoun *minä* 'I'. Note that this kind of combination (1st person singular pronoun + 3rd person singular verb form) would not be acceptable in the normal spoken variety. This usage is not consistent as the same speaker uses the 1st person pronoun with the correct verb form a little later in the conversation (see ex. 11).

(11) Broca 2, Conversation

M:	minä	ole-n (.)	sairastunut.
	I	be-1SG	get ill-PCP
	I have (.) become ill.		

The incorrect usage of the 3rd person verb form in connection with the 1st person singular subject is mostly limited to cases where the verb is relatively infrequent and has high semantic content (such as *edistyy* 'progress' in ex. 10). Note that *edistyy* 'progress' is morphologically complex also: it is a reflexive derivative of the verb *edetä* 'go further'.

It is also worth noting here that in our data from aphasic speakers, 1st person subjects often appear together with cognitive verbs with which they form constructions that are produced as wholes, such as *em mä tiiä* 'I don't know', *em mä muista* 'I don't remember', *mää luulen* 'I think/guess', *mä aattelin* 'I think'. It is important to note that 1st person subjects tend to co-occur with cognitive verbs in the spoken language in general (see Helasvuo forthcoming for Finnish, Kang 1997 for French, Scheibman forthcoming for English). In English, there are several 1st person subject + verb constructions that have been further grammaticalized and are used as discourse markers (*I think, I guess, I don't know*, cf. also *you know*; see Östman 1981, Thompson & Mulac 1992, Kärkkäinen 1998, Bybee & Scheibman 1999). In our aphasia data, these 1st person subject + cognitive verb constructions are most often produced as chunks, with no pauses in between. They also show well-formed verbal agreement. Even in the most difficult cases of aphasia, these constructions are usually produced fluently. Example (12) comes from a speaker who has severe Broca's aphasia with great problems in finding words. Speaker P and his therapist are speaking about dogs that he used to have, and the therapist asks about the breed.

(12) Broca 4, Conversation

1 t: *onk se alunperin,. (0.7) paimenkoira.*
Is it originally (pause) a shepherd dog?

2 P: *(0.4) EEi.*
No.

3 t: *ei.*
No.

4 P: *sehän oo on tota,. (1.2) ääh,. (2.5) ööh, (1.7) mm, (0.9) mmm*
it is like,

5 (0.9)

6 t: *metsästys,.*
hunting

7 P: *em mä tiedä yhtään mut, (1.7)*
NEG I know at all but
I don't know at all but,

The therapist asks about the breed of the dogs the patient used to have whether they were shepherd dogs. P denies this, and tries to explain what kind of dogs they are (line 4). There are long pauses and particles that indicate word search (*tota, ääh, ööh, mm*). In line 6 the therapist offers the word *metsästys* 'hunting' that could form the first part of a compound *metsästyskoira* 'hunting dog'. P does not deny or confirm this, but just says that he doesn't know (line 7). The fluency of the utterance in line 7 is in sharp contrast with P's previous turn, which displays severe problems in finding the proper words and expressions.

Example (13) illustrates the use of cognitive verb constructions with 1st or 2nd person subjects in the data from Wernicke's aphasics. The speaker has been telling about his work and he has described the kinds of duties he has.

(13) Wernicke 1, Conversation

1 t: *mut kuuluuk siihe mitää muuta siihen työhön.*
Is there anything else to that job?

2 (2.5)

3 H: *no, siinä on sitte semmos-ta KAIkenlais-i-a*
well there is then kind.of-PTV all.kinds.of-PL-PTV
well, there is kind of all kinds of

4 *.hh (05) jo-ta vähän (.) jo konki pitäs pitäs öö*
that-PTV somewhat already ? should should
(inbreath) (pause) that somewhat already *konki* (neologism) should should er

5 *tommonen (1.0) hhh tuommos-i-a (3.2) tuommos-i-a*
that.kind.of that.kind.of-PL-PTV that.kind.of-PL-PTV
that kind of (pause) (outbreath) those kinds of (pause) those kinds of

6 *tuommos-i-a e:-n mä tiedä, mm ei ku*
that.kind.of-PL-PTV NEG-1SG I know no but
those kinds of I don't know, mhm no but

7 *läänee jos su-lta jotain py(r)msii ni kummenee*
? if you-ABL some ? so ?
läänee (neologism) if you some *pyrmsii* (neologism) so *kummenee* (neologism)

As an answer to the question by the therapist (line 1), speaker H produces a reply that is full of neologisms (line 4 *konki*, line 7 *läänee*, *pyrmsii* and *kummenee*) and elements that indicate word-searching problems (repetitions and repairs). In the midst of this sequence, however, the speaker produces the cognitive verb construction *en mä tiedä* 'I don't know' in line 6, which stands out as the part of the answer that immediately makes sense.

In the speech of Wernicke's aphasics, we did not find any clear instances where the verb was incorrectly inflected and yet did not agree with the subject. Even neologistic verb forms were in agreement with the subject. Consider ex. (14).

(14) Wernicke 1, Conversation

1 H: *Ai mi-stä me ollaan täälä öö lomenne[l-tu, just.*
PRT what-ELA we have here ?-PCP yes
Oh from what we have here *lomenneltu* (neologism), yeah.

2 t: *[Nii mitä*
Yeah what

3 *mitä me ollaa kaikke-e teh-ty ja mitä sä oot ollu myös*
what we have all-PTV do-PCP and what you have been also
what we have been doing and what you have been too.

In example (14), speaker H is using a neologism *lomenneltu*, which has the participle ending *–tu* and is part of the present perfect verb form *ollaan* +V-PCP 'have + PARTICIPLE'. The therapist recognizes the neologistic element as a present perfect form as she rephrases it with a low content, general verb *ollaan tehty* 'have done, have been doing' (line 3). However, our finding here is not consistent with previous findings on other languages. Researching an English-speaking posterior aphasic, Caplan, Kellar and Locke (1972) found that neologistic verb forms did not always approriately agree with the subject, although in some cases they did.

Tense expressions

Both Broca's and Wernicke's aphasics tell stories of past events in conversation. On the whole, Wernicke's aphasic speakers use the tense forms appropriately in their narration. In the following example (15) the aphasic speaker tells about his visit to see a doctor at the central hospital:

(15) Wernicke 5, Conversation

1 A: *Kyllä mä kerrankuule keskussairaala-s niin, ol-i-n*
yes I once listen central hospital-INE so be-PST-1SG
Sure once you see in the central hospital so I was

2 *tämä-n sok- sokerin (1.5) takia men-i-n yy (0.5)*
this-GEN sugar because.of go-PST-1SG
because of this su- sugar (pause) I went err (pause)

3 *kolome tuntia.KOLOme tuntia odot-i-n sitä.*
three hours three hours wait-PST-1SG it-PTV
three hours. THREE hours I waited for him.

In ex. (15), speaker A tells about his visit to the hospital and uses several past tense forms in his narration, *olin* 'I was' (line 1), *menin* 'I went' (line 2), and *odotin* 'I waited' (line 3).

In Broca's aphasia, however, auxiliaries in the periphrastic tense forms, the present perfect and past perfect, are often omitted, and participial verb forms are used without the auxiliaries (see ex. 16).

(16) Broca 1, Conversation

J: *tämä tämä. (4.6) ruostu-nut KAikki.*
this this rust-PCP all
This this, (4.6) (has become) rusted all.

In ex. (16), the speaker shows a photograph and tells how the things he has helped to build and renovate have become all rusty. He uses the participial form of the verb *ruostua* 'to rust, to become rusty', omitting the auxiliary *on,* which is required for the correct use of the present perfect.

Sometimes whole verbs are lacking and the reference to past time is conveyed with the use of an adverb. Ex. (17) illustrates this: speaker M is telling about herself when she went to school.

(17) Broca 2, Conversation

1 M: *minä,. (0.3) tunnollinen oppilas. (0.2) [tu tu nii.]*
I,. (0.3) conscientious pupil. (0.2) [tu tu yes.]

2 t: *[nii nii nii joo et,.]*
[yes yes yes yeah so,.]

3 M: *SILLO*
back then.

In ex. (17), the speaker characterizes herself with a nominal clause in line 1. In Finnish nominal clauses, the copula is expressed in all tenses, and it is the element which carries the tense marker. In ex. (17), however, the copula is omitted, and hence, there is no expression of the intended past time reference. The speaker receives a response from the therapist and after this she adds the time adverb *sillo* 'then' that makes the time reference more explicit.

Furthermore, Broca's aphasic speakers favor direct reported speech, which makes it possible to use the present tense in narration (see ex. 18).

(18) Broca 1, Conversation

J:	*Minä*	*sano-i-n*	*Tauno-lle (.)*	*pai*	*paa-t*	*suoja-an*
	I	say-PST-1SG	Tauno-ALL (.)		put+IMP-2SG	shelter-ILL
	I told Tauno, pu- put it into the shelter.					

In ex. (18), speaker J uses direct reported speech when telling about a past event, thus avoiding the complex modulations of deictic expressions required for indirect reported speech (e.g. you → s/he, imperative → conditional mood).

In the data from Broca's aphasics, reduplication is sometimes used to express aspect or mode of action described by the verb (Aktionsart). In a cross-linguistic perspective, aspect and mode of action are among those distinctions that can be conveyed inter alia through the use of reduplication (see Bybee et al. 1994: 166-174). In Finnish, reduplication has not been conventionalized as a grammatical marker. Consider ex. (19), where speaker M tells the therapist about her son who likes to sleep in the mornings, and it is very difficult for the mother to wake him up. The therapist asks how she manages to wake him up (line 1).

(19) Broca 2, Conversation

1	t:	*no millä sä sen saat sit,*		*(1.3)*	*[puhumalla.]*
		well how do you get him then, (1.3)			[by speaking.]
2	M:				[M MYöhästy.]
					be.late+PST+3SG
					w- was late.
3		(0.3)	MYöhästy.		
			be.late+PST+3SG		
		(0.3)	was late.		
4	t:	hmm. hmm. hmm.=			
5	M:	=m	MUistutus. (.)	Muistus.	
			note	note	
		= n- note. (.) note.			

In her answer to the question posed by the therapist, speaker M expresses iterative/frequentative aspect by repeating the verb *myöhästy* 'be late', instead of using the special suffix *–ele-* as in *myöhästele-* 'be in the habit of being late'. Also the noun *muistutus* '(teacher's) note' is repeated, thus conveying that the son had repeatedly received notes from the teacher. In the latter utterance the speaker accompanies her verbal expression by moving her hand forward twice on the table, which makes the recurring character of the events even more prominent.

Word order

According to Niemi (1990) aphasic speakers rely on canonical word order (Subject - Verb order). However, in our data from picture description tasks, word-order patterns were often peculiar. It is possible that this is due to the fact that the aphasic speakers attempted to produce whole sentences, whereas in conversation it was possible to use less complete and elliptical expressions, and there was also more time pressure. Consider ex. (20).

(20) Broca 2, Picture description

M:	*leija, (0.6)*	*leija, (0.2)*	
	kite	kite	
t:	*joo.*		
	yeah		
M:	*mies, (0.9)*	*leija-a*	*heittä-ä.*
	man	kite-PTV	throw-3SG
	man, (0..9) kite flies.		

In example (20), the speaker talks about a picture. She first introduces *leija* 'kite', which is also a focal element in the picture. Then she adds a noun phrase referring to the man *mies,* and after a pause she adds the object leijaa 'kite', now in the partitive case, and the verb *heittää* 'throws'. The verb-final word order may reflect the supposedly reduced processing capacity of verbal substance in both Broca's and Wernicke's aphasia.

In the data from Wernicke's aphasia, word order was often difficult to analyze, mainly because of word searching problems. Example (21) comes from a picture description task.

(21) Wernicke 3, Picture description

L:	*ma-*	*herra*	*juo*	*ja*	*meh-*	*mehnä*	*kahvi-a*	*juo.*
		sir	drink+3SG	and		?	coffee-PTV	drink+3SG
	ma- sir drinks and meh- *mehnä* (neologism) coffee drinks.							

In example (21), the speaker refers to a man in the picture with the somewhat odd *herra* 'sir', which is in the nominative case and could thus act as the subject of the predicate verb *juo* 'drinks'. However, this transitive verb is not followed by a possible object argument, but instead, there is the coordinating conjunction *ja* 'and', after which a coordinated verb would be expected. There is a neologism *mehnä* which does not carry any clear verbal or nominal morphological markings. It is followed by *kahvia* 'coffee', which is inflected in the partitive case, marking it as an object argument. The predicate verb *juo* 'drinks' is then repeated. In sum, the utterance starts with a Subject – Verb construction and ends with a Object – Verb construction, but it is unclear how the intermediate part of the utterance should be analyzed.

In the data from Wernicke's aphasia, word searching problems may result in long repair sequences (see Laakso 1997). In their corrective attempts in finding an appropriate lexical form, the speakers resort to new constructions over and over again. It is often impossible to give a definitive analysis of word order in these sequences. Consider ex. (22).

(22) Wernicke 5, Conversation

A:	*Ja*	*se̲*	*on*	*se:*	*kummasiellä #*	*yy#*	*siellä #*	*yyy#*
	and	it	is	it	funny there	uh	there	uh

And it is it's funny there< #uh# there< #u:h#

#aa# #aav# asi-	*asioita*	*joskus y- .hhh (.)*	*mä*
	things	sometimes	I

th- th- thi- things sometimes uh .hhh (.) I

joskus ### (1.3)	*°(eniten)°*	*PAremmin*	*paremmin*	*saa-n,*
sometimes	most	better	better	get-1-SG

sometimes ### (1.3) get (most) better better,

In ex. (22), the speaker starts out with a characterizing clause *se on kumma siellä* 'it's funny there', after which one would expect a complementizer clause explaining what is funny. Instead, the speaker uses the noun *asioita* 'things', which is semantically very vague. This noun does not seem to relate to the preceding construction nor does it belong to the following structure. At the end of the second line, the speaker produces the 1st person singular pronoun *mä* 'I', followed by an adverb *joskus* 'sometimes', and several attempts to form a comparative form. Only after that is there a finite verb *saan* 'get-1SG'. In the whole sequence it is hard to tell where exactly one construction ends and a new one begins.

To conclude, it seems that word order patterns are clearly constrained by how the speaker finds the words to construct the sentences. Most clearly this is manifested by Wernicke's aphasic speakers. Furthermore, our data shows that the tasks the speakers are engaged with (picture description task vs. conversation) have an effect on word order patterns.

5. Summary and discussion

The goal of this paper has been to provide an overview of the characteristics of the linguistic problems in the speech of Finnish aphasics. In regard to the morphosyntactic features studied here, namely case marking, agreement, tense expressions and word order, it is surprising how many features have been preserved.

Regarding case marking, both Broca's and Wernicke's aphasics were able to use different case endings appropriately in a variety of constructions. Even the neologistic words in Wernicke's aphasia were appropriately inflected. This is in contrast to the findings of Niemi and Koivuselkä-Sallinen (1983) who found that the posterior aphasic speaker they studied made paraphasic substitutions of suffixes. Furthermore, Niemi, Laine, Hänninen & Koivuselkä-Sallinen (1990) studied two Broca's aphasic speakers who were categorized as moderately agrammatic. These speakers produced simple and short syntactic patterns, and neither of them deleted endings. Their few morphological errors were substitutions. Although Niemi et al. regard their results as tentative, they doubt the existence of "morphological" agrammatism in Finnish. They base this interpretation on the data they had and on their empirical observations of other Broca's aphasics. However, it is clear that their conclusions are not supported by data from the more severe forms of Broca's aphasia (cf. Kukkonen 1983, Kukkonen & Pajunen 1986). Our data show that some speakers with Broca's aphasia have a tendency to use uninflected noun phrases, which is in accordance with Kukkonen's (1983) findings. Kukkonen (1983) shows that her aphasic case N substituted some word forms with forms resembling the suggested base form. However, a close microanalysis of our data reveals that the uninflected forms are restricted to specific sequential contexts, namely, to one-word replies to questions or to one-word utterances initiating a new topic.

In regard to agreement patterns, speakers with Wernicke's aphasia used agreement morphology appropriately, and this was true of most of the Broca's cases as well. However, when using morphologically complex or less frequent verbs, some speakers occasionally combined a 1st person subject with a verb inflected in the 3rd person.

In the expression of tense distinctions, speakers with Wernicke's aphasia used the different tense forms correctly. In our data from Broca's aphasics, there were examples of all the different tense forms (except the past perfect, which is quite infrequent in the spoken language in general, see Helasvuo 1991). In the periphrastic tense expressions, however, the auxiliary was occasionally left out, leaving just the participle form of the main verb to express the time relationship. In predicate nominal clauses, the copula was sometimes missing, but in these cases the speakers used some other means to express the time relations, e.g. time adverbs.

With regard to word order we found that in our aphasia data from conversation, the word order patterns were similar to those found in conversational discourse in general, whereas in our material from picture description tasks, there were sometimes quite peculiar word orders. We suspect that this is due to the task at hand. This finding highlights the need to take into account the type of data when interpreting results.

It is important to bear in mind that in both Wernicke's and Broca's cases, sentence structure is sometimes so distorted because of word searching and repair attempts, that it makes it difficult to determine where one construction ends and another starts. In particular, this is true when we consider complex sentence structures in the data from Wernicke's aphasics. We have shown that the deviant structure of sentences in Wernicke's aphasia is caused by repetitive attempts to repair lexical difficulties (cf. ex. 22 above). We would therefore like to propose that the deviant structures are not due to an underlying syntactic deficit as e.g. Niemi (1990) has suggested. However, further research on sentence structure of Wernicke speakers is needed to verify this.

When trying to capture a broader picture of the characteristics of aphasic speech in Finnish, we cannot dismiss the possible effects of the methodology used in the studies, especially in the data collection. The Finnish aphasia studies can be categorized as single case studies and, as was mentioned earlier, the data collection has not been consistent. The data come from a variety of sources, namely from elicited materials, e.g. naming, repetition and picture description tasks, from written materials and from interviews and conversations. The crucial difference between these contexts is the time allotted to the speakers: in elicitation and narrative the speaker is usually allowed to use time freely, whereas in conversation there are always time limitations in turn taking. This may affect the productions of aphasic speakers, particularly in Broca's aphasia. Our empirical observations suggest that in a picture description task, aphasic speakers with Broca's aphasia tend to produce grammatically more complex utterances, although the pauses between the constituents may be very long, often several seconds. In conversational settings such long pauses are usually not possible without losing the turn. This may lead Broca's aphasics to the use of short, elliptic utterances (cf. Heeschen & Schegloff 1999).

This observation leads us to five conclusions regarding methodology: first, more research should be focused on comparing different types of data from the same speaker and secondly, when comparing different studies, the type of data should be taken into account when discussing the results. Thirdly, when comparing aphasic data with data from normal speakers, special care should be taken in choosing the normal data in order to make a fair comparison. *Inter alia*, if we have conversational data from aphasics, then the normal data should come from conversation as well.

Fourthly, a comparison of our data with previous studies on Finnish aphasics suggests that there is broad variation of aphasias within the classical aphasia categories. Although rough analysis of aphasic features links a speaker to a certain aphasia category, individual variation may be broad.

The relationship between Broca's and Wernicke's aphasia is clearly a very problematic one. Niemi and his colleagues (1990) have proposed a continuum of complexity of syntactic constructions, with Broca's aphasics at the one end and Wernicke's aphasics in the middle and normal speakers at the other end. However, Kukkonen (1993) has shown that there are counterexamples to this proposal. We find it difficult to evaluate the proposals, but it seems evident that there is a clear need for further research based on a careful microanalysis of the data. We also find that syntactic complexity varies according to the type of discourse under study, i.e. whether we have data from written materials, elicited narration, or conversation. Furthermore, our data from both Broca's and Wernicke's aphasia suggests that the most severe problems in both aphasia types are lexical-semantic or lexical-phonological, and that these problems inevitably interfere with the construction of sentences in aphasic speech. In particular, we find that word searching and repetitive attempts to repair the errors make the sentence structure distorted.

Fifthly, evolution of aphasia should be studied more carefully. We have known some aphasic speakers for years and our hypothesis is that aphasic speech may still change after several years from onset if the speaker is oriented towards developing his or her speech production. The number and nature of errors might be worth studying in a longitudinal perspective. There is a clear need for more longitudinal research on long-term changes in aphasic speech production.

Address correspondence to: Dr. Anu Klippi, Department of Phonetics, University of Helsinki, P.O. Box 35, Vironkatu 1 B, 00014 Helsinki, Finland. E-mail: anu.klippi@helsinki.fi

References

Bastiaanse, R., & Jonkers, R. (1998). Verb retrieval in action naming and spontaneous speech in agrammatic and anomic aphasia. *Aphasiology, 12*(11), 951-969.

Bybee, J., Perkins, R., & Pagliuca, W. (1994). *The evolution of grammar: Tense, aspect, and modality in the languages of the world.* The University of Chicago Press, Chicago.

Caplan, D., Kellar, L., & Locke, S. (1972). Inflection of neologisms in aphasia. *Brain, 95,* 169-172.

Goodglass, H., & Menn, L. (1985). Is agrammatism a unitary phenomenon? In M.-L. Kean (Ed.), *Agrammatism*, 1-26.

Heeschen, C., & Schegloff, E.A. (1999). Agrammatism, adaptation theory, conversation analysis: on the role of so called telegraphic style in talk-in-interaction. *Aphasiology, 13*(4-5), 365-405.

Helasvuo, M.-L. (1991). Who said what? A study of tense variation in Finnish spoken narratives. In Melvin Luthy (Ed.), *Proceedings of the Fourth Conference on Finnish Studies in North America.* UKAN, Helsinki.

Helasvuo, M.-L. (2000). *Syntax in the making: The emergence of noun phrases and clauses as syntactic units in Finnish conversation.* Amsterdam: Benjamins.

Helasvuo, M.-L. (forthcoming) Emerging syntax for interaction: Noun phrases and clauses as a syntactic resource for interaction. In E. Couper-Kuhlen & M. Selting (Eds.), *Interactional linguistics.* Amsterdam: Benjamins.

Kang, A. (1997). Interpreting *on*: A discourse-pragmatic perspective on the use of a French 'indefinite' pronoun in personal narratives. Manuscript. University of California, Santa Barbara.

Kärkkäinen, E. (1998). The marking and interactional functions of epistemic stance in American English conversational discourse. PhD Dissertation. Department of Linguistics, University of California.

Klippi, A. (1996). *Conversation as an achievement in aphasics.* Studia Fennica Linguistica 6. Helsinki: The Finnish Literature Society.

Kukkonen, P. (1983). Motorisen afasian lingvistisiä erityispiirteitä (Linguistic characteristics of motor aphasia). *Virittäjä, 4,* 462-481.

Kukkonen, P. (1990). *Patterns of phonological disturbances in adult aphasia.* Helsinki: The Finnish Literature Society.

Kukkonen, P. (1993). On paragrammatism in Finnish. *Nordic Journal of Linguistics, 16,* 123-135.

Kukkonen, P. & Pajunen, A. (1986). Rektio ja agrammatismi (Government and agrammatism). *Virittäjä, 1,* 22-45.

Laakso, M. (1997). *Self-initiated repair by fluent aphasic speakers in conversation.* Studia Fennica Linguistica 8. Helsinki: The Finnish Literature Society.

Laakso, M., & Klippi, A. (1999). A closer look at the "hint-and-guess" -sequences in aphasic conversation. *Aphasiology: Special Issue on Conversation Analysis, 4-5,* 345-363.

Leiwo, M., & Klippi, A. (2000). Lexical repetition as a communicative strategy in Broca's aphasia. *Aphasiology, 14* (2), 203-224.

Mäki, N. (1951). *Nordisk militärmedisinsk förenings förhandlingar* VIII, 64.

Niemi, J. (1987). Lexical deformations are sensitive to morphosyntactic factors in posterior aphasia. *Aphasiology, 1,* 52-57.

Niemi, J. (1988). Kieliopin tuottamisen häiriöt suomenkielisillä afaatikoilla I-II (Grammatical disorders in Finnish aphasics I-II). *Puheterapeutti,* 1, 7-9 and 2, 19-22.

Niemi, J. (1990). Nonlexical grammatical deviations in "paragrammatic" aphasia. *Folia Linguistica, 24,* 389-404.

Niemi, J. (1998). Modularity of prosody: autonomy of phonological quantity and intonation in aphasia. *Brain and Language, 61*, 45-53.

Niemi, J., & Koivuselkä-Sallinen, P. (1987). Temporal delay and lexical retrieval in narratives: aphasiological observations. *Journal of Communication Disorders 20,* 171-186.

Niemi, J., Koivuselkä-Sallinen, P., & Sarajärvi, L. (1988). Syntax in Wernicke speech: a quantitative analysis. In P. Koivuselkä-Sallinen & L. Sarajärvi, (Eds.), *Proceedings of the 3rd Finnish Conference of Neurolinguistics.* University of Joensuu: Kielitieteellisiä tutkimuksia 12, 73-79.

Niemi, J., Koivuselkä-Sallinen, P., & Laine, M. (1990). Quantitative analysis of syntax and inflectional morphology in aphasia. In J. Niemi & P. Koivuselkä-Sallinen (Eds.), *Joensuu Papers in Neuropsychology and Neurolinguistics,* vol. 3. Studies in Languages 19. Joensuu: University of Joensuu Press.

Niemi, J., Laine, M., Hänninen, R. & Koivuselkä-Sallinen, P. (1990). Agrammatism in Finnish: Two case studies. In L. Menn & L. Obler (Eds.), *Agrammatic aphasia: A cross-language narrative sourcebook.* Amsterdam: John Benjamins.

Östman, J.-O. (1981). *You know: A discourse functional approach.* Amsterdam: Benjamins.

Scheibman, J. (forthcoming): Local patterns of subjectivity in person and verb type in American English conversation. In J. Bybee & P. Hopper (Eds.), *Frequency effects and emergent grammar.* Amsterdam: Benjamins.

Siirtola, M. (1985). Afasian insidenssi, sairaidenkuva ja kuntoutusennuste. Turku: Kansaneläkelaitoksen julkaisuja 46. (in Finnish).

Tao, H. (1996). *Units in Mandarin conversation.* Amsterdam: Benjamins.

Thompson, S. A., & Mulac, A. (1991). A quantitative perspective on the grammaticization of epistemic parentheticals in English. In E. C. Traugott and B. Heine (Eds.), *Approaches to grammaticalization* (pp. 313-329). Amsterdam: Benjamins.

Appendix 1: Transcription symbols and glosses

1. Transcription symbols

The transcription symbols used are principally the same as in conversation analytic transcriptions (e.g. Levinson 1983, Atkinson & Heritage 1984, Button & Lee 1987).

Overlap and pauses

[ ]	beginning and end of overlap
(.)	micropause (less than 0.2 seconds)
(1.2)	measured pause (1.2 seconds)
=	two turns connected to each other without any pause

Intonation contour

.	falling
,	slightly falling
?	rising
,.	level

Breathing

.hhh	discernible inhalation
hhh.	discernible exhalation

Speech rate and emphasis

we::ll	prolongation of a part of a word
JUST	emphasized word or emphasized part of one
° °	silent voice

Others

puo-	incomplete word
#	creaky voice

2. Glosses

The morphemes have been indicated with dashes; in the case of fused morphemes, there is a plus sign in the glossing. The following form classes have been treated as unmarked and are not usually indicated in the glossing: nominative case and singular form in the nominal markings, present tense and active voice in the verbal markings.

Nominal markings

ACC	accusative
ABL	ablative
ADE	adessive
ALL	allative
ELA	elative
GEN	genitive
ILL	illative
INE	inessive
PTV	partitive
PL	plural

Verbal markings

1SG	first person singular person marking (likewise 2nd and 3rd)
1PL	first person plural person marking
IMP	imperative mood
PST	past tense
PCP	participle

NEG	negation verb

Other

Q	question clitic
CLT	other clitics
PRT	particle

Background information on the aphasic informants

Aphasia type, subject	*Sex*	*Age*	*Diagnosis*	*Lesion*	*Duration of illness*	*WAB AQ max. 100*	*Compr. max. 10*	*Repet. max 10*	*Severity max.5*
Broca 1, J	m	55	Inf.cer.	right temporo-parietal	2 yrs. 8 mos.	71.1	7.25	6.8	1—2
Broca 2, M	f	43	Inf.cer.	left temporal	13 yrs.	75	9.2	7.7	1—2
Broca 3, R	m	59	Inf.cer.	left frontotemporal	6 yrs.	79.1	9.85	8.7	2
Broca 4, P	m	39	Inf.cer.	left frontotemporal	3 yrs.	50.2	7.8	2.5	1—2
Wernicke 1, H	m	33	Inf.cer.	left temporal (large)	2 mos.	38.5	5.4	2	1
Wernicke 2, S	f	47	ICH	left temporal & left frontal	2 mos.	42.1	6.8	4.8	2
Wernicke 3, L	f	50	ICH	left temporal	9 mos.	45.2	6.3	1.8	2
Wernicke 4, I	m	66	Inf.cer.	left frontoparietal & parieto-occipital	3 mos.	45	3.6	2.8	2
Wernicke 5, A	m	63	Inf.cer.	left temporal	20 mos.	57.4	5.4	4.6	2

Table 1. Background information on the aphasic informants. (Inf.cer. = cerebral infarction, ICH = intracerebral haematome, WAB = Western Aphasia Battery, AQ = Aphasia Quotient, Compr = comprehension score, Repet = repetition score, Severity = severity of aphasia on BDAE Aphasia Severity Rating Scale with 1 = most severely aphasic – 5 = mildly aphasic.)

Manifestations of aphasia in Friulian

Franco Fabbro*°, Giovanni Frau°

* *Istituto Scientifico "E. Medea"* ° *University of Udine*

Abstract—Grammatical errors made by twelve aphasic patients (6 males and 6 females) with Friulian as native language (L1) have been studied. All patients were bilinguals, with Italian as second language (L2). L2 was generally learnt at kindergarten or in primary school. Seven (58%) patients showed a parallel recovery of the two languages, three patients (25%) showed a greater recovery of L1, while two patients (16%) showed a greater recovery of L2. The most frequently made grammatical error in Friulian was the omission of the second obligatory pronoun, a typical feature of that language. In Italian, the percentage of omitted pronouns was very low as in this language pronouns are only rarely obligatory. It is thus evident that when the Friulian language system is placed under stress by an aphasic insult, it is especially its production system of obligatory pronouns which tends to break down.

Key words: Friulian aphasia; obligatory pronouns; inflectional morphology; bilingual aphasia; languages recovery, Romance languages

1. Linguistic features of Friulian

In the rich and diversified landscape of Romance languages, Friulian is acknowledged as having its own autonomy. Its peculiar distinctive features derive from historical and linguistic events that determined the isolation of Friuli, in particular during the Middle Ages, a period which was fundamental for the consolidation of Romance languages (Gregor 1975, Frau 1984).

1.1 Linguistic features of Friulian

I. *Phonetics*. The following are the most typical features of Friulian phonetics: 1. The presence, unusual for Romance languages, of a double series of long tonic vowels and short tonic vowels, which are in phonological opposition (for example, *lât* 'gone' vs. *lat* 'milk', *crôt* '(I) believe' vs. *crót* 'frog', *mîl* 'honey' vs. *mil* 'one thousand', etc.); 2. Characteristic pre-palatal occlusive sounds *cj* and *ç* which are phonemes in Friulian (compare, for example, *cjòc* 'drunk' and *çòc* 'log'); 3. Palatalization of Latin *ca* and *ga* into *cja* e *gja* (e.g., *cjan* 'dog' and *gjat* 'cat', derived from Latin words *canem* and *gattum*); 4. Preservation of Latin –s in final position in plurals of nouns and adjectives (*rose* –> *rósis* 'flowers', *frut* –> *fruts* children') and in the second person of the verb [e.g., *tu tu àmis* '(2nd person, singular) you love', *vuàltris o amàis* 'you love' (2nd person, plural)].

II. *Lexicon*. The Friulian lexicon shows: 1. A considerable number of words of Latin origin which in ancient times (maybe already in regional Latin of Aquileia) acquired different meanings from those of other Romance languages. 2. Some words in Friulian have a Celtic origin and are derived from the variant of Latin spoken in Aquileia (a Friulian city of the Roman Empire). 3. Other words are derived from German languages – probably dating back to the Roman, the Gothic, and the Longobard periods – German spoken in the Middle Ages and modern German. 4. A similar contribution, though of secondary importance, came from Slavic languages.

III. *Morphosyntax*. Friulian is a richly inflected language. It differs for example from English under some crucial aspects: nouns and adjectives are marked for gender and number, and verbs for person, aspect and mode. The root of inflected words is specified by a phonological form which – like in English – corresponds to a word in that language. Many nouns in the masculine singular form are formed by combining the root of the word with a Ø affix (root + Ø): *frut* (boy) (MSG), *fruts* (MPL), *frute* (FSG), *frutis* (FPL). The same holds true for some adjectives in the masculine singular form: *brut* (MSG), *bruts* (MPL), *brute* (FSG), *brutis* (FPL). Other nouns and adjectives require that inflectional affixes be added to the root. For example, *biel* (beautiful), where the root *bie-* is not a word in Friulian, becomes *biel* (MSG), *biele* (FSG), *biei* (MPL), *bielis* (FPL).

Further, in Friulian there are many verbs which - unlike in Italian, French and Spanish - form some persons of the present tense, usually the first and the third persons singular, by combining the root of the verb with a Ø affix (root + Ø) such as, for example, the verbs '*cori*' (to run), '*viodi*' (to see), *tasê* (to be silent), etc., in the first and third persons singular:

Jo o còr (I run)
Tu tu coris (you run)
Lui al còr (he runs)
Jè e còr (she runs)
No o corin (we run)
Vualtris o coreis (you run)
Lôr e corin (they run)

Jo o viod (I see)
Tu tu viodis (you see)
Lui al viod (he sees)
Jè e viod (she sees)
No o viodin (we see)
Vuoaltis o viodeis (you see)
Lôr e viodin (they see)

Jo o tas (I am silent)
Tu tu tasis (you are silent)
Lui al tas (he is silent)
Jè e tas (she is silent)
No o tasin (we are silent)
Vualtris o taseis (you are silent)
Lôr e tasin (they are silent)

A peculiar feature of Friulian morphology is the constant use of pleonastic pronouns following subject pronouns for all persons (e.g., *jo o soi* 'I I am', *tu tu sês* 'you you are', *lui al è* 'he he is', *jê a jè* 'she she is"). In Friulian when the subject of a sentence is a noun, it must necessarily be followed by a pronoun, for example: '*Il cjan al còr in tal curtîl*' (The dog runs in the courtyard); '*Il frut al mangje le pome*' (The child is eating the apple). Unlike in English and Italian, in Friulian all full sentences contain an obligatory pronoun. For a more systematic study of the linguistic features of Friulian, the reader is referred to Francescato (1967), Iliescu (1972), Gregor (1975), Nazzi Matalon (1977), Rizzolatti (1981), Zannier (1983), Frau (1984), Marchetti (1985), and Haiman and Benincà (1992).

1.2 Sociolinguistic aspects

According to a recent survey, Friulian as mother tongue is still spoken by about 500.000 people in Friuli (in a population of 900.000 inhabitants), whereas the proportion of people with a passive competence is higher. All speakers of Friulian learn Italian at school as the language of instruction and speak Italian from at least 6 years of age. Friulian is also spoken abroad by some 20.000 people in Canada and 50.000 people in Argentina. All Friulian speakers in Italy are Friulian-Italian bilinguals, in Canada they speak English and Friulian and in Argentina they speak Friulian and Spanish. The Italian State has recently passed a bill laying down some rules for the safeguard of historical linguistic minorities, including Friulian (Bill N. 482 dated December 15, 1999). Friulian is officially granted the status of national language, even if only partially and confined to some sectors (for example, with regard to the education system, its use is limited and not compulsory).

2. Grammatical errors in aphasic patients

Many studies show that grammatical disorders typical of aphasia depend on the structure of each language. Their various manifestations are only trivially (and predictably) different in several languages. Grammatical disorders observed in aphasics speaking different languages are such only at the surface level, but their nature seems to have a universal character and follow the rule whereby aphasia can impair all grammar aspects of a language, even if at varying degrees of severity (Paradis 1988). Given this assumption, if inflectional morphology is vulnerable, a language with a rich inflectional system will show outstanding signs of agrammatism (Alajouanine 1968).

With regard to grammatical deficits, until the 1970s the literature on aphasia used to distinguish between two syndromes, namely: (1) agrammatism, characterized by the omission of free-standing grammatical morphemes, appearing in the context of short utterances (typical of Broca's aphasia) and (2) paragrammatism, characterized by the substitution of grammatical morphemes, appearing in the context of fluent speech (typical of Wernicke's aphasia). What characterizes a particular syndrome is the relative conspicuousness of a given symptom. Brancherau (1987) reported omissions and substitutions of both free-standing grammatical morphemes in the speech of agrammatic and non-agrammatic patients; however, agrammatics made more omissions than substitutions, while anomics, conduction and Wernicke's aphasics made more substitutions than omissions.

Many studies of clinical aphasiology attempted to define the linguistic features of agrammatism, as follows: (1) omission of free-standing grammatical morphemes (e.g. articles, prepositions, conjunctions, particles, pronouns, verb inflections, case markings); (2) omission or substitution of bound grammatical morphemes; (3) omission and occasional nominalization of verbs; (4) omission of the *copula*; and (5) reduction in mean utterance length. Agrammatics use a simplified register which is similar to baby talk or foreigner talk. In the speech of some agrammatic patients there is greater prevalence of omissions of free grammatical morphemes vs. omissions (or substitutions) of bound morphemes. No patient, however, has been reported to omit (or substitute, in rich inflected languages) only bound morphemes without omissions of free-standing grammatical morphemes (Paradis 1988).

Miceli et al. (1989) investigated the percentage of omissions vs substitutions of free-standing grammatical morphemes in some Italian agrammatic patients. Since their patients made both omissions and substitutions of free-standing grammatical morphemes, they drew the conclusion that the distinction between omission and substitution is arbitrary as it does not allow to clearly define the clinical category of agrammatism. The two authors suggested that agrammatism is a theoretical construct and not a natural category (Miceli and Mazzucchi 1990). Given the specific features of the Italian language, Miceli et al. (1989, Miceli and Mazzucchi 1990) defined agrammatism as a disorder of sentence production characterized by the omission of free-standing grammatical morphemes with or without substitution of bound grammatical morphemes (e.g. violations of determiner-noun agreement, violations of noun-adjective agreement, violations of subject-verb agreement).

2.1 Grammatical errors in bilingual aphasia.

A patient with "agrammatism" who speaks two languages rich in morphology (e.g., Friulian and Italian) shows similar grammatical errors in both languages. In contrast, patients who know a morphology-rich language and a morphology-poor language (Friulian and Chinese) will show a greater impairment of grammar in the language richer in morphology (cf. Paradis 1998). There are more contexts in Friulian than in Italian (particularly because of double subject pronouns) where agrammatic errors may be observed.

In order to discover the most salient errors in Friulian agrammatic patients, a group of twelve aphasic patients (6 males and 6 females), all right-handed (Briggs e Nebes, 1975), received a neuropsychological and neurolinguistic assessment. All patients were bilingual, with Friulian as native language (L1) and Italian as second language (L2), which was generally learnt at kindergarten or in primary school. All patients had learnt to read and write in Italian but not in Friulian. The language battery used for assessing language disorders was the *Bilingual Aphasia Test – BAT* (Paradis and Libben 1987; Paradis 1999) in the two versions, Friulian (Paradis and Fabbro 1993) and Italian (Paradis and Canzanella 1989). Some patients also received the Italian version of the *Aachener Aphasie Test - AAT* (Luzzati et al. 1992).

All patients were administered a battery of standardized neuropsychological tests for the assessment of orientation in time and space, attention, detection of agnosia, apraxia, verbal and spatial short-term memory deficits and verbal long-term memory deficits (Spinnler and Tognoni 1987). Furthermore, patients received a standard neurologic examination and neuroimaging study with CT scan or MRI to define the characteristics of the lesion (site, extent and type).

The analysis of grammatical errors made in Friulian and Italian was based on spontaneous speech samples and/or speech samples obtained from a story description (the BAT nest story description). Table 1 shows the patients' percentages of correct answers in the BAT linguistic levels both in L1 and L2. Table 2 shows the percentages of correct answers in the BAT linguistic skills. Appendices 1 and 2 describe some of the most significant grammatical errors made by the patients in Friulian (Appendix 1) and in Italian (Appendix 2). Table 3 reports the percentages of omissions, substitutions and additions of grammatical morphemes made by the first 4 patients in the two languages.

3. Case Reports

3.1 *Case 1 (KB)*

3.1.1 Clinical history. For clinical history and scores by Linguistic Skills and Levels (Tables 1 and 2) the reader is referred to Fabbro and Paradis (1995a).

3.1.2 Errors during spontaneous speech. In the BAT story description verbal fluency was in the normal range and similar in both languages (Friulian =125 words per minute; Italian =120 words per minute). In Friulian the most frequent errors were omissions of free-standing grammatical morphemes (KB generally omitted the second obligatory pronoun), whereas in Italian they were omissions of articles (see Appendices 1 and 2, and Table 3). This is probably due to the fact that in Friulian the subject is obligatory in all complete sentences and is formed by a noun plus a pronoun or by two pronouns (*Lui al* vai) (he he is crying), whereas in Italian pronouns can be omitted (*piange*; he cries), with the exception of some clitic pronouns which are obligatory ('*portami il gelato*', fetch me the ice-cream). The most frequent error made by KB in Friulian was omission of the second obligatory pronoun [*... e _ stin ancje a gustà e dopo _ lavin i plas e _ netin*, corrected sentence: ... *e o stin ancje a gustà e dopo o lavin i plas e o netin* (we stay for lunch. Then we wash the plates and we do the cleaning)].

3.2 *Case 2 (CB)*

3.2.1 Clinical history. For clinical history and scores by Linguistic Skills and Levels (Tables 1 and 2) the reader is referred to Fabbro and Paradis (1995b).

3.2.2 Errors during spontaneous speech. During the BAT story description the patient showed a reduced verbal fluency both in Friulian (90 words per minute) and Italian (80 words per minute). The most frequent grammatical errors were omissions of bound grammatical morphemes (pronouns, auxiliaries, full verbs) and substitutions of bound grammatical morphemes (see Table 3). In Friulan CB mainly omitted the second obligatory pronoun [_ *erin in tre fantatis* ___ *ladis là, e _ vin cjatât lavòr*, corrected sentence: *O erin in tre fantatis e o sin ladis là e o vin cjatât lavòr* (there were three of us, all girls, we went there and found a job)]. In Friulian CB made two violations in word order (see Appendix 1); this type of error is extremely rare both in Friulian and Italian (Miceli et al. 1989).

3.3 *Case 3 (EM)*

3.3.1 Clinical history. For clinical history and scores by Linguistic Skills and Levels (Tables 1 and 2) the reader is referred to Fabbro and Paradis (1995b).

3.3.2 Errors during spontaneous speech. EM's aphasia was more severe in Italian (40 words per minute) than in Friulian (80 words per minute). Verbal production in both languages was characterized by a massive omission of free-standing grammatical morphemes. In Friulian omissions of pronouns and auxiliaries prevailed, whereas in Italian omissions mainly concerned articles and auxiliaries (see Appendices 1and 2, and Table 3).

3.4 *Case 4 (OR)*

3.4.1 Clinical History. For clinical history and scores by Linguistic Skills and Levels (Tables 1 and 2) the reader is referred to Fabbro and Paradis (1995b).

3.4.2 Errors during spontaneous speech. OR was more fluent in Italian (140 words per minute) than in Friulian (130 words per minute). In both languages, OR mainly made omissions and, to a lesser extent, substitutions and additions of free-standing grammatical morphemes (see Appendices 1 and 2, and Table 3). The most frequent error made by OR in Friulian was omission of the second obligatory pronoun [*E vegnin vòt e jò __ jevât*, corrected sentence: *E vegnin vòt e jò o soi jevat (at 8 o'clock I got up)*]. In Italian OR made an error which so far had been considered impossible to make. He declined a verb according to the Friulian rule of root + Ø [*E dopo ha det si hai ragione*, correct sentence in Italian: *E dopo ha detto si hai ragione*; corresponding sentence in Friulian: *E daspò al à dit si tu as reson* (and then he said you are right)]. This error could be considered as a mixing phenomenon within a word (Italian root + Friulian inflectional affix which in the third person singular is equal to Ø).

3.5 *Case 5 (LM)*

3.5.1 Clinical history. For clinical history and scores by Linguistic Skills and Levels (Tables 1 and 2) the reader is referred to Fabbro et al. (1997).

3.5.2 Errors during spontaneous speech. LM's production in Friulian was fluent (160 words per minute), while it was in the normal range in Italian (130 words per minute). The patient made few errors which were similar in both languages (omissions and substitutions of free-standing grammatical morphemes) (see Appendices 1 and 2).

3.6 *Case 6 (PB)*

3.6.1 Clinical history. For clinical history and scores by Linguistic Skills and Levels (Tables 1 and 2) the reader is referred to Fabbro et al. (1997).

3.6.2 Errors during spontaneous speech. Verbal production was mildly slowed in Friulian (107 words per minute) and Italian, too (100 words per minute). The patient made few grammatical errors which in both languages consisted in substitutions of bound and free-standing grammatical morphemes, and also presented many repetitions of syllables and words with errors in word retrieval (see Appendices 1 and 2).

3.7 *Case 7 (RT)*

3.7.1 Clinical history. RT is a right-handed male, with Friulian as L1 and Italian as L2, and 5 years of primary school in L2. At the age of 51 he suffered a stroke which provoked an ischemic lesion in the left temporo-parietal region (documented by CT scan). Following the stroke the patient presented a paresis of the right limbs and transcortical sensory aphasia. For two years he received two weekly sessions of speech therapy, after which he received a neurolinguistic and neuropsychological follow-up. Intelligence was preserved. His short-term verbal memory span was reduced. He was neither apraxic nor agnosic, nor did he show attention deficits. His language skills were assessed with the BAT.

3.7.2 Scores by Linguistic Skills and Levels (see Tables 1 and 2). The number of correctly performed tasks was compared in the two languages by linguistic skills and levels using two one-way ANOVAs. In linguistic skills there were no significant differences between the two languages [$F(1,6) = 2.26$, $p = .18$], while linguistic levels in L1 were significantly more impaired than in L2 [$F(1,4) = 9.28$, $p < .04$].

3.7.3 Errors during spontaneous speech. RT showed aphasia with normal verbal fluency in both languages (L1=100 words per minute; L2=110 words per minute). Grammar errors were mainly substitutions of free-standing grammatical morphemes and they were more frequent in L2. The patient showed numerous cases of pathological mixing in both languages (Fabbro 1999) (see Appendices 1 and 2). During sentence production with mixing phenomena RT produced sentences in Italian without the final ending. For example, "Allora un uomo si, un uomo una signora *compain* una <u>don</u> si, un uomo una signora sta" [Then a woman, yes, a man a woman *the same (Friulian)* <u>woman</u> (word without ending) yes, a man, a woman is standing]. "*Tal ospedâl tal arbero si è ròt* un <u>ram</u>, un ramo si ruppe" [*At the hospital on the tree (Friulian)* a branch (word without ending) *broke (Friulian)*, a branch broke]. *Alore i* uccelli cadono. No si <u>cad</u> ... *no si just* <u>cad</u>" [*Then, the (Friulian)* birds fall to ground. No, they fall (word without ending) ... *no, right,(Friulian)* they fall (word without ending)]. La signora piange e *i* uccelli <u>piang</u> piangere <u>anc</u> e il merlo <u>piang</u> piange, perché *i* uccelli sono morti [The woman cries and *the (Friulian)* birds cry (word without ending) cry and the blackbird cries (word without ending) cries because *the (Friulian)* birds are dead]. This type of errors has never before been described in Italian aphasic patients (cf. Miceli and Mazzucchi 1990) and probably depends on mixing phenomena within words (cf. Case 4). As happens with loans from Italian, the patient only used the root of the Italian word truncating the word with a consonant, which is a typical feature of Friulian, whereas it hardly occurs in Italian.

3.8 *Case 8 (DC)*

3.8.1. Clinical History. OR is a 50-year old right-handed man with Friulian as L1 and Italian as L2; he received 13 years of schooling in Italian. In July 1999 he had an hemorrhagic stroke. One month later he was tested with the AAT and the BAT. The

AAT in his second language revealed 90% Broca's aphasia and 10% Wernicke's aphasia. Intelligence was preserved. His short-term verbal memory span was reduced. He was neither apraxic nor agnosic, nor did he show attention deficits. The neurological investigation detected a right hemiplegia. MRI revealed a lesion in the left basal ganglia and in the left semi-oval center.

3.*8.2 Scores by Linguistic Skills and Levels* (see Tables 1 and 2). The number of correctly performed tasks was compared in the two languages by linguistic skills and levels using two one-way ANOVAs. There were no significant differences between the two languages in linguistic skills [$F(1,6) = .97$, $p= .36$], nor in linguistic levels [$F(1,4)= .45$, $p<.45$].

3.*8.3 Errors during spontaneous speech.* The patient showed non-fluent aphasia in both languages (L1= 75 words per minute; L2= 65 words per minute), with many errors in word retrieval and tendency to jargonaphasia. In both languages grammar errors consisted in omissions and additions of free-standing grammatical morphemes in inappropriate contexts (see Appendices 1 and 2).

3.9 *Case 9 (LT)*

3.9.1 Clinical History. LT is a 54-year old right-handed woman with Friulian as L1 and Italian as L2. She received 5 years of schooling in Italian. In September 1999 she had an ischemic stroke. One month later she was tested with the AAT and the BAT. The AAT in Italian revealed 90% of anomic aphasia. Intelligence was preserved. She was neither apraxic nor agnosic. The neurological investigation detected a right hemiplegia. CT scan revealed an ischemic lesion in the left basal ganglia.

3.*9.2 Scores by Linguistic Skills and Levels* (see Tables 1 and 2). The number of correctly performed tasks was compared in the two languages by linguistic skills and levels using two one-way ANOVAs. There were no significant differences between the two languages in linguistic skills [$F(1,6) = 2.15$, $p= .19$], while linguistic levels in L2 were significantly more compromised than in L1 [$F(1,4)= 8.7$, $p<.05$].

3.*9.3 Errors during spontaneous speech.* Spontaneous speech was slowed in both languages (L1= 91 words per minute), with greater slowing in L2 (72 words per minute). In Friulian omissions of free-standing grammatical morphemes prevailed, whereas in Italian omissions and substitutions of free-standing grammatical morphemes were more frequent (see Appendices 1 and 2).

3.10 *Case 10 (VD)*

3.10.1 Clinical History. VD is a 78-year old right-handed woman with Friulian as L1 and Italian as L2. She received 8 years of schooling in Italian. In February 1999 she had an ischemic stroke. One month later she was tested with the AAT and the BAT. The AAT in her second language revealed 100% Wernicke's aphasia. Intelligence was preserved. The neuropsychologic examination revealed oro-facial and ideo-motor apraxia. Short-term verbal memory was reduced. The neurological investigation detected a right hemiplegia. CT scan revealed a left parieto-temporal ischemic lesion with cortical and subcortical involvement.

3.*10.2 Scores by Linguistic Skills and Levels* (see Tables 1 and 2). The number of correctly performed tasks was compared in the two languages by linguistic skills and levels using two one-way ANOVAs. In terms of linguistic skills the difference between the two languages was close to significance [$F(1,6) = 4.63$, $p= .07$], while there were no significant differences in linguistic levels between the two languages [$F(1,4)= 2.18$, $p<.21$].

3.*10.3 Errors during spontaneous speech.* Spontaneous speech was reduced in both languages (L1= 90 words per minute; L2= 80 words per minute). The most frequently made grammatical errors, especially in L2, were additions and substitutions of free-standing grammatical morphemes (see Appendices 1 and 2).

3.11 *Case 11 (LV)*

3.11.1 Clinical History. LV is a 54-year old right-handed man with Friulian as L1 and Italian as L2. He received 8 years of schooling in Italian. In November 1998 he had an ischemic stroke. Four months later he was tested with the AAT and the BAT. The AAT in his second language revealed 100% of global aphasia. Intelligence was preserved. The patient did not show agnosia, nor disorientation as to time and space. In contrast, LV presented ideo-motor and ideational apraxia. The neurological investigation detected a right hemiplegia. CT scan revealed a wide left parietal (cortical - subcortical) ischemic lesion.

3.11.2 Scores by Linguistic Skills and Levels (see Tables 1 and 2). The number of correctly performed tasks was compared in the two languages by linguistic skills and levels using two one-way ANOVAs. There were no significant differences between the two languages in linguistic skills [$F(1,6) = 3.23$, $p= .12$], whereas linguistic levels in L2 were significantly more impaired than in L1 [$F(1,4)= 17.9$, $p<.01$].

3.11.3 Errors during spontaneous speech. During the assessment of his spontaneous speech LV only spoke Friulian (pathological fixation on a language, cf. Aglioti and Fabbro 1993). Therefore, no spontaneous speech sample in L2 could be obtained. Production was hardly understandable owing to the presence of many verbal paraphasias and neologisms, whereas grammatical aspects of Friulian seemed to be less impaired (see Appendices 1 and 2).

3.12 *Case 12 AT*

3.12.1 Clinical History. AT is a 77-year old right-handed woman with Friulian as L1 and Italian as L2. She received 5 years of schooling in Italian. In July 1999 she had an ischemic stroke. One month later she was tested with the AAT and the BAT. The AAT in her second language revealed 96% Broca's aphasia. Intelligence was preserved. The neuropsychological examination did not show any signs of agnosia or apraxia, while verbal and spatial short-term memory and long-term memory were below the norm. The neurological investigation detected a right hemiplegia. CT scan revealed a left temporal ischemic lesion.

3.*12.2 Scores by Linguistic Skills and Levels* (see Tables 1 and 2). The number of correctly performed tasks was compared in the two languages by linguistic skills and levels using two one-way ANOVAs. There were no significant differences between the two languages either in linguistic skills [$F (1,6) = 2.8$, $p = .14$] or linguistic levels [$F(1,4) = 3.14$, $p < .15$].

3.12.3 Errors during spontaneous speech. Spontaneous speech was very slowed (L1= 75 words per minute). In the story description in Friulian the patient made a limited number of grammatical errors (see Appendices 1 and 2).

4. Discussion

As predicted by the corollary to "Murphy's law" applied to neurolinguistics (cf. Paradis 1988) grammatical errors made by Friulian aphasics depend on the language structure, which is highly rich in morphology. In the so-called agrammatic patients described here, almost all possible errors were observed, the most frequent of which were omissions of free-standing grammatical morphemes and substitutions of bound grammatical morphemes. There were also many substitutions of free-standing grammatical morphemes, while the least frequent errors were additions of free-standing grammatical morphemes. In particular, with the exclusion of perseverations, there were no additions of articles, conjunctions and auxiliary verbs in inappropriate grammatical contexts (Appendix 1). Patients made the same type of errors also in their L2. Italian is also a richly inflected language; errors in L2 were similar to those described by Miceli et al. (1989) and Miceli and Mazzucchi (1990). As predicted by Paradis (1988), there was no dissociation with regard to the type of grammatical errors made by agrammatic patients within a language. For example, none of the patients made only omissions of free-standing grammatical morphemes or only substitutions of bound grammatical morphemes (see Appendices 1 and 2). The percentage of morpho-syntactic errors in obligatory contexts shows that one patient did not make some types of errors (e.g. KB did not omit prepositions nor conjunctions in both languages), while the other three patients made all types of omissions (cf. Table 3). This feature has already been described by Miceli et al. (1989).

In the first 4 patients, the percentage of morphosyntactic errors in obligatory contexts in L1 and L2 was calculated over a 5-minute spontaneous speech sample (see Table 3). They all presented with aphasia with so-called agrammatism and with parallel recovery of the two languages. The analysis of morpho-syntactic errors made by the first four patients confirms the hypothesis that the so-called agrammatism is—as suggested by Miceli and Mazzucchi (1990)—a theoretical construct and not a natural category. In both languages these patients made omissions of free-standing grammatical morphemes and substitutions of bound grammatical morphemes (errors that are reported to be typical of agrammatism), but also a discrete percentage of errors came from substitutions and additions of free grammatical morphemes, which are considered specific to paragrammatism. A comparison of errors made by patients in the two languages revealed that the most significant difference was the percentage of omissions of obligatory pronouns in Friulian (38.25%) vs. Italian (1.25%). This reflects the peculiar grammatical structure of the two languages, as in Friulian all sentences, in addition to the subject noun, also require an obligatory pronoun (*Il frut al bef*–The boy drinks), whereas in Italian sentences include only one subject (Il bambino beve –The boy drinks) and in many cases if it is clear from the context, it can be even dropped (beve, he drinks). The peculiar morphosyntactic structure of Friulian vs. Italian and English makes even more evident the difficulty of so-called agrammatic patients with pronouns. For this reason, in the first four cases which were studied in more detail, more omissions of obligatory pronouns in Friulian vs. Italian were observed.

Another feature of Friulian is that many nouns in the masculine singular form are formed by combining the root of the word with a Ø affix (root + Ø), as are many verbs in different persons of the present tense (generally, the first and third persons). Friulian nonfluent aphasic patients can thus make errors in the conjugation of verbs producing the root of the verb with a Ø affix. These aspects which are also peculiar to English are not present either in Italian or Spanish (cf. Miceli et al. 1989; Miceli and Mazzucchi 1990; Benedet et al. 1998). KB (case 1) for example produced the following sentence "*Ti clamin a lavorà e _ viod cemût che tu vâs*", corrected sentence: *Ti calmin a lavorà e e viodin cemût che tu vâs* (they call you to work there and see (sees) how you cope with that). In this sentence, the patient did not produce the verb "viodi" (to see) in the first person singular (viodin), but the root of the verb "viod" + Ø, which corresponds to the first and the third persons singular of the present tense.

A type of error which is unusual for the Italian language was made by RT, who presented aphasia with a high percentage of mixing (see *Case* 7 and *Case 4*). In Italian RT produced many words omitting their obligatory final endings (e.g., *don -> donna, ram -> ramo, cad ->cade, anch -> anche*). So far, it was believed that this type of error was impossible, owing to the phonological structure of Italian which obligatorily requires that all words end with a vowel. In Friulan, by contrast, almost all words end with a consonant. This type of error probably depends on a sort of phonological mixing within a word. When the patient produced the word "ram" he used the root of an Italian word ("ramo" - branch) but, at the same time, he applied a phonological rule of Friulian to the word. This means that in a given language bilingual aphasics can produce a certain type of error while monolingual aphasics usually do not.

In conclusion, the most frequently made grammatical error in Friulian was omission of the second obligatory pronoun which must be present in practically all sentences in Friulian. It is thus evident that when the Friulian language system is placed under stress by an aphasic insult, above all its production system of obligatory pronouns breaks down.

Address correspondence to: Dr. Franco Fabbro, Istituto Scientifico "E.Medea", La Nostra Famiglia, Bosisio-Parini (Lecco), Italy. E-mail: fabbro@bp.lnf.it

References

Alajouanine, Th. (1963). *L'aphasie et le langage pathologique*. Paris: J.B. Baillère.

Albert, M.L., Goodglass, H., Helm, N.A., Rubens, A.B., & Alexander, M.P. (1981). *Clinical aspects of dysphasia*. Springer-Verlag, New York.

Aglioti, S., & Fabbro, F. (1993). Paradoxical selective recovery in a bilingual aphasic following subcortical lesions. *Neuroreport, 4,* 1359-1362.

Benedet, M.J., Christiansen, J.A., & Goodglass, H. (1998). A cross-linguistic study of grammatical morphology in Spanish– and English–speaking agrammatic patients. *Cortex, 34,* 309-336.

Brancherau, L. (1987). Analyse syntaxique et accès à la catégorie prép chez des patients agrammatiques. *Revue québécoise de linguistique théorique et appliquée, 6,* 27-244.

Briggs, G.C., & Nebes, R.D. (1975). Patterns of hand preference in a student population. *Cortex, 11,* 230-238.

Fabbro, F. (1999a). *The neurolinguistics of bilingualism. An introduction.* Hove: Psychology Press.

Fabbro, F. (1999b). Aphasia in multilinguals. In F. Fabbro (Ed.), *Concise encyclopedia of language pathology* (pp. 335-341). Oxford: Pergamon.

Fabbro, F., & Paradis, M. (1995a). Acquired aphasia in a bilingual child. In M. Paradis (Ed.), *Aspects of bilingual aphasia* (pp. 67-83). London: Pergamon.

Fabbro, F., & Paradis, M. (1995b). Differential impairments in four multilingual patients with subcortical lesions. In M. Paradis (Ed.), *Aspects of bilingual aphasia* (pp. 139-176). London: Pergamon.

Fabbro, F., Peru, A., & Skrap, M. (1997). Language disorders in bilingual patients after thalamic lesions. *Journal of Neurolinguistics, 10,* 347-367.

Francescato, G. (1967). *Dialettologia friulana.* Udine: Società Filologica Friulana.

Frau, G. (1985). *Friuli.* Pisa: Pacini.

Gregor, D.B. (1975). *Friulian language and literature.* New York: The Oleander Press.

Haiman, J., & Benincà P. (1992). *The rhaeto-romance languages.* London: Routledge.

Iliescu, M. (1972). *Le frioulan à partir des dialectes parlés en Roumanie.* The Hague: Mouton.

Luzzati, C., Willmes, K., & De Bleser, R. (1992). Aachener Aphasie-Test, Versione Italiana. Organizzazioni Speciali, Firenze.

Marchetti, G. (1985). *Lineamenti di grammatica friulana.* Udine: Società Filologica Friulana.

Miceli, G., & Mazzucchi, A. (1990). Agrammatism in Italian: Two case studies. In L. Menn and L.K. Obler (Eds.), *Agrammatic aphasia: A cross-language narrative sourcebook,* Amsterdam: John Benjamins.

Miceli, G., Silveri, C., Romani, C., & Caramazza, A. (1989). Variation in the pattern of omissions and substitutions of grammatical morphemes in the spontaneous speech of so-called agrammatic patients. *Brain and Language, 36,* 447-492.

Nazzi, Matalon Z. Marilenghe. (1977). *Gramatiche furlane.* Udin: Istitût di Studis Furlans.

Paradis, M. (1977). Bilingualism and aphasia. In H. Whitaker and H.A. Whitaker (Eds.), *Studies in neurolinguistics,* vol. 3, (pp. 65-121). New York: Academy Press.

Paradis, M. (1987). *The assessment of bilingual aphasia.* Hillsdale, NJ, Lawrence Erlbaum Associates.

Paradis, M. (1988). Recent developments in the study of agrammatism: The import for the assessment of bilingual aphasia. *Journal of Neurolinguistics, 3,* 127-160.

Paradis, M. (1998). Language and communication in multilinguals. In B. Stemmer and H. A. Whitaker (Eds.), *Handbook of neurolinguistics* (pp. 418-31). Academic Press: San Diego.

Paradis, M. (1999). *Valutazione dell'afasia bilingue.* Bologna: EMS.

Paradis, M. (in press). Bilingual and polyglot aphasia. In R.S. Berndt (Ed.), *Handbook of neuropsychology* (Second Edition). Oxford: Elsevier Science,

Paradis, M, & Canzanella, A. (1989). *Test per l'afasia in un bilingue.* Italian Version. Hillsdale, NJ: Lawrence Erlbaum Associates.

Paradis, M., & Fabbro, F. (1993). *Test pe afasie in tun bilengâl.* Friulian Version. Hillsdale, NJ: Lawrence Erlbaum Associates.

Rizzolatti, P. (1981). *Elementi di linguistica friulana.* Udine: Società Filologica Friulana.

Spinnler, H. & Tognoni, G. (1987). Standardizzazione e taratura italiana di test neuropsicologici. *The Italian Journal of Neurological Sciences*, Suppl. 8, 5-120.
Zannier, G. (1983). *El friulano*. Montevideo: Division Publicaciones y Editiones Universitad de la Republica.

Appendix 1.

GRAMMATICAL ERRORS IN FRIULIAN

1. OMISSIONS OF FREE GRAMMATICAL MORPHEMES

1.1 Omissions of articles

Case 3 (EM) "Gnò pari # faseve # muradôr"
Correct sentence (CS): Gnò pari *al* faseve il muradôr
Literal translation (LT): My father (he) was a (the) bricklayer.

Case 7 (RT) " A vevin # piçui"
Correct sentence (CS): A vevin i piçui
Literal translation (LT): They had (the) pets.

Case 9 (LT) "# # Rivade # autobulance"
CS: *A jè* rivade le autoambulance
LT: (It) The ambulance has arrived.

1.2 Omissions of prepositions

Case 1 (KB) " va a disi # cjase che ... "
CS: va a disi a cjase che ...
LT: go (to) home to tell that...

Case 4 (OR) "di lâ # scuela"
CS: di lâ a scuela
LT: we must go to school

Case 5 (LM) "Lui si è tornât # sposà"
CS: Lui si è tornât a sposà
LT: He (to) married again.

Case 9 (LT) "Al è lât # ospedâl"
CS: Al è lât in ospedâl
LT: He has gone to the hospital.

Case 11 (LV) "Al va # viodi ..."
CS: Al va a viodi ...
LT: He goes to see...

1.3 Omissions of conjunctions
Case 2 (CB) "O jerin in tre fantatis # # # ladis là"
CS: O jerin tre fantatis e *o sin* ladis là.
LT: There were three of us, all girls, and we (have) went there.

Case 4 (OR) "Ca al è colât ju # al **è** fàt mâl"
CS: Ca al è colât ju e al à fat mâl
LT: Here he has fallen down and he (**is**) injured himself.

Case 11 (LV) "Al è lât a viodi di chei ca # al è colât"
CS: Al è lât a viodi di chei ca e al è colât
LT: He has gone to see these and he has fallen.

1.4 Omissions of obligatory pronouns
Case 1 (KB) "e # netìn"
CS: e o netìn
LT: and we clean.

"Jê # gire e jo o salti"
CS: Jê e gire e jo o salti
LT: she (she) turns around and I (I) jump.

Case 2 (CB) "là # vin cjatât"
CS: là o vin cjatât
LT: there (we) have found.

Case 9 (LT) "Lui # # dite: a je rivade …"
CS: Lui al *à* dite: a je rivade …
LT: He (he) (has) said: she has arrived.

Case 11 (LV) "Che # menin a viodi"
CS: Che lu menin a viodi
LT: Here they take him to see.

1.5 Omissions of auxiliary verbs
Case 1 (KB) "Al # finît i ains"
CS: al a finît i ains.
LT: It is his birthday (He has completed his years).

"In talian # # cjapât sîs"
CS: In talian *o* ai cjapât sîs
LT: In Italian I (have) got D.

Case 2 (CB) "O jerin in tre fantatis # # # ladis là"
CS: O jerin tre fantatis *e o* sin ladis là
LT: There were three of us, all girls *and we* (have) went there.

Case 4 (OR) "Dopo # # # menât..."
CS: Dopo *o* soi stât menât …
LT: Then *I* was (been) taken...

"Jo # # voe di saltâ fûr"
CS: Jo *o* vevi voe di saltâ fûr
LT: I (*I*) (have) felt like going out.

Case 9 (LT) "# # rivade # autobulanze"
CS: A je rivade le autoambulance
LT: (It) The ambulance has arrived.

"Lui # # dite …"
CS: Lui *al* à dite …
LT: He (*he*) has said...

Case 11 (LV) "doi che si # fermât"
CS: doi che si son fermâts
LT: two (people) who have stopped.

1.6 Omissions of full verbs
Case 1 (KB) " E se o soi cun mes sûr # # a pallavolo"
CS: E se o soi cun me sûr *a* gjuiâ a pallavolo
LT: and I with my sister (*we*) play volleyball.

Case 3 (EM) "Dopo # sin # a Benevento"
CS: Dopo *o* sin lâs a Benevento
LT: Then *we* (have) went to Benevento.

---

2. VIOLATION OF WORD ORDER

Case 2 (CB) (E) "Ae vût fruts?" (T: Did you have any kids?)
(CB) "Si # ai vût doi **jò**"
CS: Si jò o ai vûs doi
LT: Yes, (*I*) have had two (kids) I.

Case 2 (CB) "Un biel apartament, # biele cjase, biele **dut**"
CS: Un biel apartament, une biele cjase, dut biel
LT: A nice flat, a nice house, beautiful (fem. sing.) all (masc.)

Case 3 (EM) "E dopo **jo** tre ains"
CS: E jo dopo tre ains
LT: and after (I) 3 years

3. SUBSTITUTIONS OF BOUND GRAMMATICAL MORPHEMES

3.1 Substitutions of verbs

Case 2 (CB) "E # uceluts **murì**"
CS: E i uceluts e son muarts
LT: and the birds (to) die.

Case 3 (EM) "E alore # **soi** lâts"
CS: E alore o sin lâts
LT: and then we are (am) gone.

"Al à **spand**"
CS: Al à spandût
LT: he has poured (pour)

Case 5 (LM) le femine e a dite "mi soi **sposât**"
CS: le femine e a dite: mi soi sposade
LT: the woman said: I got married (masc.)

Case 6 (PB) "A je une robe che al **van** e **vegnin**"
CS: A je une robe che e va e ven
LT: It is something that (she) come and (she) go

" e # omp # **disin** ..."
CS: e *l'*omp al dîs
LT: and the man (he) say.

Case 9 (LT) "# # **lade** tal ospedâl"
CS: Al è lât tal ospedâl
LT: he is gone (fem.) to the hospital.
Case 11 (LV) "I ucei **al è colât**"
CS: I ucei e son colâts
LT: the birds (he) is fallen.

"Al à spetât che **rive** une femine"
CS: Al a spetât che rivi une femine
LT: he has waited for a woman to come (fem. instead of masc.)

"Doi che si # **fermât**"
CS: doi che si son fermâts
LT: two (people) who have stopped (sing. instead of plural).

3.2 Substitutions of adjectives

Case 2 (CB) "**biele** dut"
CS: dut biel
LT: beautiful (fem. instead of masc.) all

3.3 Substitutions of nouns
Case 4 (OR) "Al ere un **nivei**"
CS: Al ere un nivel
LT: it was a levels.

Case 10 (VD) "Cul **assessôrs**"
CS: Cul assessôr
LT: with the local administrators (plural instead of sing.).

---

4. SUBSTITUTIONS OF FREE GRAMMATICAL MORPHEMES

4.1 Substitutions of articles
Case 3 (EM) "**Il** frute"
CS: Le frute
LT: the (masc. instead of fem.) child.

Cace 5 (LM) "**Une** biglietin"
CS: Un biglietin
LT: a (fem. instead of masc.) piece of paper

4.2 Substitutions of prepositions
Case 4 (OR) "... menât **sul** ospedâl"
CS: menât in ospedâl
LT: taken on the hospital.

4.3 Substitutions of conjunctions
Case 11 (LV) "*che lavora* **a** che al è malât"
CS: Ch'al lavore e che al è malât")
LT: that he works and (to) that he is ill.
4.4 Substitutions of obligatory pronouns
Case 6 (PB) "A je una roba che **al** va"
CS: A je une robe che e va
LT: It is something that (she) come

Case 8 (DC) "*Il signore* **e** viôt"
CS: Il siôr al viôt
LT: the man (she) sees

4.5 Substitutions of auxiliary verbs
Case 4 (OR) "Ca al è colât ju # al **è** fàt mâl"
CS: Ca al è colât ju e al à fat mâl
LT: Here he has fallen down *and* he (is) injured himself.

Case 5 (LM) "Cuant che jo mi **ai** sposad"
CS: Cuant che jo mi soi sposade
LT: When I got (was) married.

5. ADDITIONS OF GRAMMATICAL MORPHEMES IN INAPPROPRIATE CONTEXTS

5.1 Additions of prepositions
Case 4 (OR) "E à vût une volte **in** dopo tre ains"
CS: E à vût une volte dopo tre ains
LT: she has had one time in after three years.

Case 5 (LM) " Ca **a** la femina ..."
CS: Ca la femina ...
LT: here at the woman...

5.2 Additions of obligatory pronouns
Case 6 (PB) "A tu **capisitu**?"
CS: A tu capît?
LT: Have you understood (you)?

Appendix 2

GRAMMATICAL ERRORS IN ITALIAN

OMISSIONS OF FREE GRAMMATICAL MORPHMES

1.1 Omissions of articles
Case 1 (KB) "E # uccellini sono morti"
CS: E gli uccellini sono morti
LT: and (the) birds died.

Case 3 (EM) "dopo # malattia ..."
CS: dopo la malattia ...
LT: after (the) disease...

Case 4 (OR) "Ho fatto # muratore"
CS: Ho fatto il muratore
LT: I was (a) bricklayer.

Case 5 (LM) "Mi ha preso # tremore"
CS: (Mi ha preso un tremore)
LT: I have been taken by (a) tremor.

Case 6 (PB) "In # posto giusto"
CS: In un posto giusto
LT: in (the) right place

Case 7 (RT) "Allora # uomo ..."
CS: Allora l'uomo ...
LT: then (the) man...

1.2 Omissions of prepositions
Case 4 (OR) "Proprio # acciaieria ..."
CS: proprio in acciaieria
LT: Right there (at the) steel plant.

Case 5 (LM) "La moglie corre # chiamare aiuto"
CS: La moglie corre a chiamare aiuto
LT: the woman goes (to) ask for help.

Case 6 (PB) "# certi punti io non ci vedo"
CS: In certi punti io non ci vedo
LT: (at) certain times I cannot see

Case 8 (DC) "E # un certo punto..."
CS: E a un certo punto...
LT: and (at) some point in time...

1.3 Omissions of conjunctions
Case 8 (DC) "si **aprono** # guardano"
CS: Si apre **e** guardano
LT: they open (it opens) and they look

1.4 Omissions of obligatory pronouns
Case 2 (CB) "Come # dice"
CS: Come si dice
LT: as (they) say

1.5 Omissions of auxiliary verbs
Case 2 (CB) "E # trovato così ..."
CS: E ho trovato così
LT: and I (have) thus found

Case 4 (OR) "Sono stato in Svizzera e # lavorato là"
CS: Sono stato in Svizzera e ho lavorato là
LT: I have been to Switzerland and I (have) worked there

Case 3 (LM) "E # lavorato un anno solo"
CS: E ha lavorato un anno solo
LT: and he (has) worked only a year

"La moglie # vicino di lui"
CS: La moglie è vicino a lui
LT: the woman (is) next to him

Case 6 (PB) "Il senso della vita # che il leone mangia la gazzella"
CS: Il senso della vita **è** che il leone mangia la gazzella
LT: the meaning of life (is) that the leon eats the gazelle

1.6 Omissions of full verbs

Case 2 (CB) "E allora io # # la famiglia"
CS: E allora io *ho* lasciato la famiglia
LT: and so I (have) left my family

---

2. VIOLATION OF WORD ORDER

Case 7 (RT) "E gli uccelli piangono **anche**"
CS: E anche gli uccelli piangono
LT: and (also) the birds cry also

---

3. SUBSTITUTION OF BOUND GRAMMATICAL MORPHEMES

3.1 Substitution of verbs

Case 4 (OR) "**Lavorare** all'acciaieria"
CS: Ho lavorato in acciaieria
LT: To work in (I worked at the) steel plant

"Il vecchio **erano** italiano"
CS: Il vecchio era italiano
LT: the old man were (was) Italian

"Nessuno **buttare** via la sigaretta"
CS: Nessuno buttava via la sigaretta
LT: No one to throw (threw) away the cigarette

Case 7 (RT) "E gli uccelli **piangere** ..."
CS: E gli uccelli piangono ...
LT: and the birds (to) die

"La signora **chiamano** la gente"
CS: La signora chiama la gente
LT: the woman ask (asks) the people

3.2 Substitution of adjectives

Case 2 (CB) "**Mia** figlio"
CS: mio figlio
LT: my (fem. instead of masc.) son

Case 5 (LM) "Mia suocera è **morto** a novantadue anni"
CS: Mia suocera è morta a novantadue anni
LT: My mother-in-law (has) died (masc. instead of fem.) when she was 92

3.3 Substitution of nouns

Case 6 (PB) "Si ha fatto male a una **gambe**"
CS: Si è fatto male a una gamba
LT: He has (is) hurt himself in a legs

Case 7 (RT) "Allora due **uomo** ..."
CS: Allora due uomini ...
LT: then two man (men)

---

4. SUBSTITUTION OF FREE GRAMMATICAL MORPHEMES

4.1 Substitution of articles

Case 4 (OR) "**il** mattoni"
CS: i mattoni
LT: the (sing. instead of plural) bricks

Case 7 (RT) "Va a chiamare **le** gente"
CS: Va a chiamare la gente
LT: go and ask the (plural instead of sing.) people

"... **le** dito"
CS: il dito
LT: the (fem. plural instead of masc. sing.) finger

Case 9 (LT) "Va su **e** albero e prende **e** nido"
CS: Va sull'albero e prende il nido
LT: He climbs up and (the) tree and fetches and (the) nest

Case 10 (VD) "Si è rotto **la** ramo ..."
CS: Si è rotto il ramo...
LT: the (fem. instead of masc.) branch broke

4.2 Substitution of prepositions

Case 8 (DC) "si aprono gli occhi **a** vedere gli uccellini"
CS: aprono gli occhi per vedere gli uccellini
LT: they are opened (open) their eyes at seeing the birds

Case 9 (LT) "E' in ospedale **in** letto ammalato"
CS: E' in ospedale nel letto ammalato
LT: He is in hospital in (the) bed, he is ill

4.3 Substitution of obligatory pronouns
Case 6 (PB) "Cioè devo metter**ti** in un posto giusto"
CS: Cioè devo metter<u>mi</u> in un posto giusto
LT: that is, I have to find you (<u>myself</u>) in the right place.

4.4 Substitution of auxiliary verbs
Case 5 (LM) "Io **ho** stata ..."
CS: Io <u>sono</u> stata.
LT: I have (am) been

Case 6 (PB) "Si **ha** fatto male"
CS: Si <u>è</u> fatto male
LT: he has (<u>is</u>) hurt himself

---

5. ADDITION OF GRAMMATICAL MORPHEMES IN INAPPROPRIATE CONTEXTS

5.1 Additions of articles
Case 3 (EM) "A **l'**Udine"
CS: A Udine.
LT: at (the) Udine.

5.2 Additions of prepositions
Case 10 (VD) "Non andare via **tra** in mezzo..."
CS: Non andare via in mezzo ...
LT: Do not leave <u>between</u> in the middle of...

Table 1. LINGUISTIC LEVELS (percentage of correct answers)

Subjects	*S*	*A*	*YS*	*TL*	*Loc*	*Ass*	*Aphasia*	*Phonlogy* *L1*	*L2*	*Mrphlgy* *L1*	*L2*	*Syntax* *L1*	*L2*	*Lexicon* *L1*	*L2*	*Smantics* *L1*	*L2*	*Total* *L1*	*L2*
1 (KB)	F	15	8	I	FT	96	TM	95	95	65	69	88	93	91	95	93	87	86	88
2 (CB)	F	71	5	I	BG	4	B	81	76	52	43	51	55	61	66	42	55	57	59
3 (EM)	M	56	11	H	BG	28	B	79	82	13	69	50	56	65	68	47	42	51	63
4 (OR)	M	63	5	I	BG-I	3	W–B	75	78	43	43	53	50	63	68	50	71	57	62
5 (LM)	F	67	5	Tu	Th	1	TM	95	95	86	56	91	80	93	88	100	82	**93**	80*
6 (PB)	M	39	18	Tu	Th	3	A–B	96	95	91	78	75	77	90	92	82	92	87	86
7 (RT)	M	53	5	I	PT	24	TS	67	89	17	17	50	54	67	76	73	87	55	**64***
8 (DC)	M	50	13	H	BG	1	B	82	85	56	73	58	57	73	68	76	50	69	67
9 (LT)	F	54	5	I	BG	1	A	89	89	86	65	86	78	89	88	88	73	**88**	78*
10 (VD)	F	78	8	I	PT	1	W	59	62	30	60	60	56	68	72	65	77	56	**65***
11 (LV)	M	54	8	I	P	4	G	61	39	56	17	44	39	59	51	62	55	**56**	40**
12 (AT)	F	77	5	I	T	1	B	71	67	26	17	58	50	61	60	53	55	54	50

S= sex; A=age; YS= Years of schooling; TL= Type of Lesion (Tumor; Infarction; Hemorrhage); Loc= Localization of the Lesion (F: Frontal lobe; T: Temporal lobe; P: Parietal lobe; BG: Basal Ganglia; Th: Thalamus); Ass= Interval between the onset of the lesion and language assessment. Aphasia (B: Broca's Aphasia, W: Werniche's Aphasia, G: Global Aphasia, A: Anomic Aphasia; TM: Transcortical Motor Aphasia, TS : Transcortical Sensory Aphasia). * $p<.05$; ** $p<.01$

Table 2. LINGUISTIC SKILLS (percentage of correct answers)

Subjects	*Compreh*		*Repetit*		*Judgmnt*		*Lxcl Acc*		*Proposi*		*Reading*		*Writing*		*Total*	
	L1	*L2*	*L1*	*L2*	*L1*	*L2*	*L1*	*L2*	*L1*	*L2*	*L1*	*L2*	*L1*	*L2*	*L1*	*L2*
1 (KB)	91	91	91	100	94	96	82	86	80	86	91	94	100	100	89	93
2 (CB)	57	61	97	95	72	70	50	55	51	47	39	55	0	0	52	55
3 (EM)	62	65	83	82	86	76	38	54	24	44	51	75	25	25	53	60
4 (OR)	60	55	65	89	78	92	47	51	52	48	60	67	40	40	57	63
5 (LM)	93	81	94	97	92	96	94	83	88	74	92	82	N/A	45	92	85
6 (PB)	78	80	94	85	92	100	83	93	91	86	94	92	95	50	89	83
7 (RT)	63	62	35	82	66	80	55	66	52	52	75	82	60	35	58	65
8 (DC)	62	62	94	97	88	90	70	56	52	56	67	53	35	35	67	64
9 (LT)	88	79	97	100	92	90	87	74	84	62	89	94	60	80	85	82
10 (VD)	66	68	29	47	90	94	61	65	46	56	80	73	25	40	56	63
11 (LV)	53	50	53	8	98	96	61	44	56	22	19	35	20	15	51	39
12 (AT)	61	53	88	80	88	88	52	50	42	36	30	30	0	0	51	48

Table 3

PERCENTAGE OF MORPHOSYNTACTIC ERRORS IN OBLIGATORY CONTEXTS (in a 5-minute sample of spontaneous speech)

	1 (KB)		2 (CB)		3 (EM)		4 (OR)	
	L1	L2	L1	L2	L1	L2	L1	L2
OFGM								
Articles	8	4	7	15	80	29	–	1
Prepositions	–	–	5	3	16	27	5	5
Conjunctions	–	–	5	–	4	7	10	–
Obl. Pron.	38	–	43	3	42	–	30	2
Aux Verbs	15	–	18	10	40	100	26	24
Full Verbs	2	–	3	1	16	25	2	1
SBGM								
Verbs	3	1	5	3	–	–	3	11
Adjectives	–	1	7	2	–	–	–	–
Nouns	–	–	2	–	–	2	–	–
SFGM								
Articles	–	2	–	–	30	4	–	3
Prepositions	–	4	–	–	8	27	1	7
Conjunctions	–	–	–	–	–	–	–	–
Obl. Pron.	1	2	1	–	–	–	–	2
Aux Verbs	–	–	–	–	13	–	–	–
AGMIC								
Articles	–	2	3	–	–	–	3	2
Prepositions	–	–	–	6	–	–	3	2
Conjuctions	–	–	–	–	–	–	2	–
Obl. Pron.	–	5	–	–	–	–	–	–
Aux Verb	–	–	–	–	–	–	–	–

OFMG: *Omission of free grammatical morphemes*; SBGM: *Substitution of bound grammatical morphemes;* SFGM: *Substitution of free grammatical morphemes*; AGMIC: *Addition of grammatical morphemes in inappropriate contexts*.

Manifestations of morphological impairments in Greek aphasia: A case study

Kyrana Tsapkini*, Gonia Jarema*, Eva Kehayia°

*Université de Montréal, Montreal, Canada; and Centre de recherche, Institut universitaire de gériatrie de Montréal, Montreal, Canada, °McGill University, Montreal, Canada; and Jewish Rehabilitation Hospital, Laval, Canada

Abstract—The present study addresses the issue of morphological manifestations specific to non-fluent aphasia in Greek. The off-line performance of a Greek-speaking aphasic patient is investigated using Paradis'(1987) Bilingual Aphasia Test. His difficulties with inflectional morphology are further probed through a series of comprehension, production, repetition and reading tasks. Results obtained show a dissociation in the patient's processing of nouns and verbs related to language-specific morphological features of these grammatical categories. This study underscores the importance of taking the particularities of a given language into account when interpreting aphasic manifestations and sheds new light on the issue of syndrome variability.

Key words: aphasia, morphological impairment, grammatical categories, language-specific features, Greek.

Introduction

Inflectional errors are amongst the most prominent characteristics of aphasic non-fluent speech. They have been documented mainly in nouns and verbs. It has been found that non-fluent patients make more errors in inflection than in derivation and that they are more impaired in regular than irregular inflection (e.g., Miceli & Caramazza, 1988). Moreover, aphasic speech seems to be sensitive to the grammatical class of words, resulting in dissociations between nouns and verbs that have been interpreted in terms of their semantic (e.g., Gainotti, 1998), syntactic (e.g., Bastiaanse & Jonkers, 1998), morphological (e.g., Shapiro et al., in press) and neuronal (e.g., Ullman et al., 1997) representational differences. In the literature, the noun-verb distinction has been investigated mainly in terms of a categorial opposition. In most studies, it has been found that retrieving verbs is more difficult for aphasic patients than retrieving nouns in both sentence (Marshall et al., 1998) and single word (Berndt et al., 1997) elicitation tasks. However, the reverse dissociation has also been observed in patients impaired in naming, comprehension or retrieval of nouns (Danielle et al., 1994). These findings have been interpreted as evidence for differential processing of verbs and nouns, and in particular as an inability to access the phonological representations of verbs (Marshall et al., 1998). Another interpretation for the noun-verb distinction brings forth their morpho-syntactic differences (Bastiaanse & Jonkers, 1998). It has been shown that morphological processing of verbs can be impaired independently of that of nouns, resulting in grammatical class distinctions of morphological processing in aphasia (Shapiro et al., in press). Moreover, morphological impairment can be present without any syntactic impairment (Bates et al., 1991), and vice-versa, that is, grammatical class distinction may be manifested at the syntactic level (in sentences) but not at the single word level (Badecker, 1997). Furthermore, the particularities of each language stress the need to investigate aphasia in different languages (Jarema, 1998).

Modern Greek, a language where all stems need an inflection to surface to the word level, provides a case wherein both the verbal and nominal systems present a wide range of morphological and morpho-phonological operations, such as simple inflection, inflection involving stem allomorphy, and inflection with stem-final phonological change conditioned by the presence of the inflectional suffix. In this study, we investigate morphological impairment in verbs and nouns in Greek. The issue of rule application in aphasia has been investigated in verbs for the English past tense. It has been found that aphasic patients with frontal lesions, diagnosed as Broca's aphasics, are impaired in the application of the past-tense inflection but have no difficulty with irregular stored forms (Ullman et al., 1997). Given the particularities of the Greek language where both operations (rule application and stem allomorphy) can be at play in one and the same form, we investigate how this distinction manifests itself in the performance of Greek-speaking aphasics. The language also provides the opportunity to clarify whether the problems aphasics have with morphological structure are due to syntactic difficulties or morphological impairment *per se* and, more importantly, to reveal the effect of parametric variation in morphological impairments.

Description of the verbal and nominal systems in Modern Greek

In order to probe the effects of morphological and morphophonological operations in the processing of nouns and verbs, we adopted Ralli's (1988, 1997) linguistic analysis of the Greek verbal and nominal systems as a theoretical framework.

With respect to verbs, since all stems are bound in Greek, active verbs are formed by the addition of the inflectional suffix to the present tense stem, e.g., *pez-o* (I play). There are three different types of active past tense formation: 1) verbs with stem-internal change, e.g., *plen-o, e-plyn-a* (I wash, I washed), where the perfective stem *plyn-* is an allomorph of the imperfective stem *plen-,* 2) verbs with phonological change, e.g., *graf-o, e-grap-s-a* (I write, I wrote), and *lin-o, e-li-s-a* (I untie, I untied), where, in the presence of the perfective aspectual marker -s-, there is a phonological alternation and a stem-final consonant deletion, respectively, and 3) verbs with both a perfective allomorph and the addition of the aspectual marker *-s-*, e.g., *mil-o, mili-s-a* (I speak, I spoke), where *mili-* is the perfective allomorph of *mil-*. The second category can be seen as the equivalent of a rule-based paradigm, and the third category as the combination of rule-based (by virtue of the aspectual –s- marker) and stored-allomorph paradigms.

The nominal system in Greek also provides a range of morphological and morpho-phonological operations. Ralli (1988) describes Greek nominal forms in terms of feature representations and feature-passing operations. The main features characterizing Greek nouns are gender, case, number and inflectional class. There are three genders (masculine, feminine and neuter), four cases (nominative, genitive, accusative and vocative), and two numbers (singular and plural). The following three types of operations can be found in the formation of plural nouns: 1) allomorphic variation, *e.g., som-a, somat-a* (body, bodies), 2) stem-final phonological change conditioned by the presence of the plural marker, e.g., *pedi, pedi-a* (child, children) where the letter *i* in *pedia* is pronounced /j/, and 3) absence of any computation at the stem level, e.g., *vun-o, vun-a* (mountain, mountains), which can be considered the no-change condition.

In view of the particularities of both the verbal and nominal systems in Greek, we predict that Greek-speaking aphasics will exhibit morphological breakdown patterns that are language-specific, i.e., that reflect the degree of complexity of computations involved in the processing of morphological structures in Greek.

Previous findings on aphasic symptoms in Modern Greek

Previous neurolinguistic investigations of Greek addressed the issues of access and representation of inflected and lexical items as revealed by the performance of aphasic subjects in off-line and on-line experiments (Kehayia, 1988; Kehayia et al., 1990; Kehayia, 1997). The main finding of these studies was that morphology, i.e., rules of word-formation and underlying representations of morphemes, are not lost in aphasia. Rather, what is lost is access to morphemes and to the mechanisms that combine them. This, in turn, impairs the processing of morphologically complex words. Greek is an appropriate language to investigate this claim since all morphemes of major lexical categories are bound and must undergo inflectional affixation in order to surface to the level of the word.

In an off-line study (Kehayia et al., 1990), two Greek-speaking aphasics classified as non-fluent Broca's aphasics with agrammatism were tested using sentence repetition, comprehension and production tasks. These tasks investigated the morphological markers of number, case and gender. Moreover, they prompted the distinction of singular/plural for masculine, feminine and neuter nouns in the nominative and accusative cases that correspond to subject and object positions in the sentence. The repetition task involved 154 sentences probing the above distinction, and the same stimuli were used in a sentence-picture matching comprehension task. Each stimulus comprised two line drawings depicting the singular/plural contrast. The same pictures were used for the production tasks where patients had to provide the plurals. As is often found with patients with non-fluent aphasia, repetition and comprehension were less impaired than production. Nevertheless, in the repetition and comprehension tasks, the patients made more errors in the plural forms and these errors consisted of substitutions only. Omissions of suffixes were not observed, as is usually the case in languages with bound stems (Grodzinsky, 1986; Menn & Obler, 1990). The error rates were 14 and 17% for the two patients, respectively, in the repetition task, and 11 and 10% in the comprehension task. Given that these patients had mainly a production deficit, it is not surprising that the cumulative error rate in the production task was 36% for both patients. Again, errors involved substitutions of noun and verb plurals by their singular forms.

Kehayia (1988) postulated that for every Greek verb two stems are listed in the lexicon: the present stem (involved in the formation of the present and imperfect tenses) and the aorist stem (involved in the formation of all other tenses). She investigated four categories of verbs in the repetition, comprehension and production of two Greek-speaking patients: 1) category A verbs, i.e. active verbs forming the simple past (aorist) by affixation of the person/number/past tense inflection to the aorist stem, e.g. *pez-o, epex-**a***, (I play-I played), 2) category B verbs, i.e. active verbs in which the aorist stem is homophonous with the present stem and that form the simple past by affixing two suffixes to the aorist stem: the aspectual marker *-is-* and the person/number/past tense inflection, e.g. *metr-o*, *metr-**is**-**a***, (I count-I counted), 3) category C verbs, i.e.

passive/reflexive verbs that also feature two affixes: the passive/reflexive marker *–ik-* and the inflectional person/number/past-tense suffix, e.g. *hteniz-om-ai,htenis-**tik-a*** (I comb myself-I combed myself), and 4) irregular active verbs , e.g. *trog-o,efag-**a***, (I eat-I ate). Kehayia (1988) found a between-task deterioration progressing from comprehension, to repetition and production, as well as within-task variability depending on verb category. She concluded that the cumulative effects of double affixation increases processing load thus inhibiting performance, and that accessing the aorist stem with little morphological relatedness, as is the case with irregular verbs, results in impaired production. Kehayia (1988) thus proposed a differential storage for verbs of categories A, B and C, on the one hand, and verbs of category D, on the other. Throughout the verbal paradigm, the differentiating characteristic for the two types of storage is formal transparency. Thus, common storage is proposed for morphologically related verbs with formal transparency, while separate but linked stores are proposed for verbs with little or no transparency.

Experimental investigation

In this paper we investigate the performance of a Greek aphasic patient on several off-line tasks that targeted his processing of inflectional morphology. The tasks administered were the following: spontaneous speech, comprehension of complex morphological structures in sentence-picture matching, repetition of sentences, reading of sentences, cued elicitation of plural and past-tense forms in sentences, and verb and noun retrieval from pictures.

Subject

IS is a right-handed 59-year-old man who had suffered a left CVA 24 months prior to testing. His CT-scan revealed a hypodensity involving the basal ganglia and the neurological diagnosis was right hemiplegia with motor aphasia. At the time of testing his speech was moderately fluent and dysarthric, and he still had right upper-limb motor problems. Visual and auditory acuity, along with orientation in time and space were normal. He showed no signs of retrograde or anterograde amnesia, nor any signs of agnosia or apraxia. He had a short-term memory span of three digits. He had completed elementary school and, prior to his CVA, managed his own furniture factory.

BAT results

The patient was evaluated on the Greek adaptation (Paradis & Kehayia, 1987) of the BAT (Bilingual Aphasia Test, Paradis, 1987) for a general assessment of his off-line language deficits. The BAT examination revealed the following: In spontaneous production, his speech output was nearly normal, although effortful since he had articulatory problems. His grammar was at times incorrect, and he sometimes experienced word-finding difficulties when looking for specific words in his vocabulary (e.g., "angiogram"). He made no errors in the naming test, nor did he show any deficit following simple and complex commands. He performed at ceiling on the auditory differentiation task, and he did not exhibit any deficit in the syntactic comprehension task for either passive constructions or pronoun or genitive-possessive marker use in sentence-picture matching. However, he had difficulties deciding which item did not belong to a specific semantic category when he was asked to do a semantic categorization judgement (success rate: 3/5). He also missed 2/5 synonymy and 3/5 antonymy judgements in a task where he was given a word and was asked to choose the synonym or the antonym of a word among 4 orally presented choices. Moreover, he had great difficulty and exhibited great stress when he was asked to judge the antonym of a word among morphologically related items (e.g. *ikanos-anikanos*, capable-incapable). These problems, although pointing to a semantic deficit, could also stem from IS's short-term memory limitations as evidenced by his reduced digit-span. In the grammaticality judgement task, he did not make any errors, nor did he make any mistakes in judging the semantic correctness of sentences. He could also repeat nonwords without difficulty, although he was surprised by the task. He performed at ceiling in word-nonword judgments and he only made articulatory mistakes. He had no difficulties in repeating sentences. In the verbal fluency task, he produced in one minute 5 words that would start with the letter "P", a frequent word-initial letter in Greek, 2 words starting with the letter "F" which is rather infrequent word-initially, and 7 words starting with the letter "K", of which however 2/7 were proper names. In naming, he missed 3/20 words, but it must be noted that most of the items he had to name were common objects of daily use. When he had to construct sentences from a set of words, he performed correctly. However in the 2/5 cases where he was given 4 words, he omitted one of them, usually the second noun. When he had to provide antonyms he performed correctly 7/10 times and said he did not know the remaining items. However, when he was asked to produce an adjective from a given noun (abstract nouns such as beauty, honesty, etc.), he only produced 5/10 items. He performed even worse when he had to give the antonym of a word while keeping the same stem (3/10). In this task, he would provide a word with the opposite meaning but not with the same stem (an English equivalent would be to produce, e.g. 'open' instead of 'unlocked' when presented with the word 'locked'). It has to be noted, however, that these forms are much less frequent than their positive counterparts. When he had to produce a story describing a picture series, his speech output was satisfactory. He reached the end of the story and it made sense. In the mathematical calculations, he missed only 2/14 trials and commented, "I was even better before the CVA". He read 10/10 words and 7/10 sentences correctly. The errors he made in the sentences were in reading the verbs in the incorrect tense and voice. In oral comprehension of two small stories he missed 1/5 questions in the first and 1/6 in the second story because, as he said, "I did not pay attention to all the details". He was incapable of writing with his right hand because of his hemiplegia and he refused to write with his left hand; thus, he was not tested on any of the writing tasks. His written comprehension was tested with word-picture and sentence-picture-matching tasks where he scored 10/10 and 8/10 correct, respectively.

The patient's performance on the BAT revealed that he had problems mainly at the sentence level, and particularly with morphological relations. Since word-formation and derivation were tested in that assessment, we wanted to investigate whether inflectional relations were impaired and how.

Analysis of spontaneous speech

Since, during testing, the patient's speech revealed morphological errors, we further evaluated his spontaneous conversational and narrative capacities. The examiner prompted a conversation on issues that would both be interesting to him and induce him to narrate a story. Thus, he was asked to talk about his work, how he started his career, his daily life before and after the CVA and the history of his illness. We were interested in eliciting as many verbs and nouns as possible and in as many different contexts as possible. In general, he did not need much prompting and was very eager to collaborate and provide us with many details and information, despite his dysarthria and the required effort. His speech, although comprehensive, lacked subordinate clauses and other complex structures. He frequently interrupted his sentences when he could not retrieve a verb or a noun. Repeatedly, when he could not produce the appropriate form of a verb or a noun, e.g., a perfective past tense or a plural form, he would resort to less complex forms, e.g., he would use the historical present. His nouns would lack the article even when obligatory, and although the production was prolific, it sounded chopped and elliptical. Below we provide examples of the types of errors he made to illustrate his performance in conversational and narrative speech.

Target: vazame rafia ystera,
Gloss: we were putting up (2nd pers. plur. imperf. past) shelves (plur.) afterwards
Target English equivalent: we were putting up shelves afterwards
Defective sentence: vazame rafi ystera
Gloss: we were putting up shelf (sing.) afterwards

Target: to proi ksipnisa, pira ta hapia, ystera ipia ena boukali gala
Gloss: in the morning I woke up, I took the pills, then I drank (1st pers. sing. perf. past) a bottle (noun, neut. sing. accusative with indefinite article) of milk
Target English equivalent: in the morning, I woke up, I took the pills, then I drank a bottle of milk
Defective sentence: to proi ksipnisa, pira ta hapia, ystera pino boukali gala
Gloss: in the morning I woke up, I took the pills, then I drink (1st pers. sing. present) bottle (noun neut. sing. accusative without indefinite or any other article) of milk

Target: apo 6:30 i ora ksypnousa ke eperna to aftokinito
Gloss: I would wake up at 6:30 and take (1st pers. sing. imperf. past) the car (noun, neut. sing accusative with definite article)
Target English equivalent: I would wake up at 6:30 and take the car
Defective sentence: apo 6:30 i ora ksypnousa ke aftokinito
Gloss: I would wake up at 6:30 and (omission of verb and definite article) car

Target: kathisa epano sto krevati
Gloss: I sat on the bed (noun, neut. sing. accusative)
Target English equivalent: I sat on the bed
Defective sentence: kathisa pano sto...
Gloss: I sat on the.... (omission of noun)

Target: to heri kai to podi mou itan ola akinita
Gloss: my hand and my foot were both immobile (adjective, neut., plur. nominative)
Target English equivalent: my hand and my foot were both immobile
Defective sentence: to heri kai to podi mou itan ola ...
Gloss: my hand and my foot were both .... (omission of adjective)

Target: mou elegan pia ine, i Anna, i Vaso, de mporousa na po to onoma
Gloss: they were telling me who they were, Anna, Vaso, I could (1st pers. sing. imperf. past) not say their name

Target English equivalent: they were telling me who they were, Anna, Vaso, I could not say their name
Defective sentence: mou elegan pia ine, i Anna, i Vaso, de mporo na po to onoma
Gloss: they were telling me who they were, Anna, Vaso, I can (1st pers. sing. present) not say their name

Target: ego, 15 meres kathisa, de mprousa katholou, sikothika, ekatsa, de mporousa, eipa tha figo
Gloss: I stayed (1st pers, sing, past) 15 days, I couldn't stand it at all, I got up, I sat down, I couldn't (1st pers, sing, imperf. past), I said (1st pers, sing, perf. past) I will leave
Target English equivalent: I stayed 15 days, I couldn't stand it at all, I got up, I sat down, I couldn't, I said I will leave
Defective sentence: ego, 15 meres kathome, de mporousa katholou, sikothika, ekatsa, de mporo tha figo
Gloss: I stay (1st pers, sing, present) 15 days, I couldn't stand it at all, I got up, I sat down, I can't (1st pers. sing. present) ....(omission of verb) I will leave

Target: ystera me pirane me ena karotsi
Gloss: then they transferred me with (preposition) a (article, neut. sing. indefinite) wheelchair
Target English equivalent: then they transferred me with a wheelchair
Defective sentence: ystera me pirane karotsi
Gloss: then they transferred me (omission of preposition, omission of indefinite article) wheelchair

Target: nomize oti ego imouna nekros
Gloss: he thought (3rd pers. sing. imperf. past) that I (pronoun, 1st person sing) was dead
Target English equivalent: he thought that I was dead
Defective sentence: ego nomize oti imouna nekros
Gloss: I (pronoun, 1st pers. sing., correct form but illegally topicalised outside the embedded clause) he thought that was dead

Verbal morphology

Comprehension of past tense forms
Since the BAT examination did not suggest that the patient had a comprehension deficit, we wanted to investigate whether he had any specific problems comprehending morphological relations. We administered a modified version of a sentence-picture matching test used to probe Greek aphasic patients' comprehension skills (Kehayia, 1988). Thus, the patient was confronted with two pictures presented on the same page and depicting the same action, but one action could only be occurring in the present, whereas the other could only be completed. For example, for the verb 'to cut' there was a picture with a girl cutting a bunch of flowers with a pair of scissors and another picture of the same girl holding the cut flowers. Then the examiner would say a sentence describing the picture in either the present or the perfective past tense. For example, "the girl cuts the flowers", or, "the girl cut the flowers". The task the patient had to perform

was to point to the picture that corresponded to the sentence given by the examiner. The position of the present and past tense pictures (top or bottom of the page) was randomized in order to exclude the possibility that the patient would develop a spatial strategy to facilitate his performance. We used 18 verbs, 6 from each verb category, presented both in present and perfective past tense form. Thus, there were 6 verbs that form the perfective past tense by attaching the rule-based aspectual marker to their perfective stem-allomorphs, 6 verbs that form the perfective past tense by attaching the rule-based aspectual marker to their imperfective stem (i.e., there is no allomorphy involved), and 6 verbs that form the perfective past tense on their perfective stem-allomorphs bearing a stem-internal vowel change. The order of tense was randomized. Each verb was presented only once in either the past or the present form in each session, and the entire test was completed in two sessions. The patient's performance was at ceiling (36/36) for the present and the past tense sentences grouped together.

Cued elicitation of past tense forms

In this task, the patient was shown a picture of someone performing an action, and was also cucd with the sentence describing the picture, e.g., "the man is stealing the silverware". Then he was asked to produce the same sentence in the past tense with the probe: "what did he do yesterday?" Thus he had to produce the perfective past tense form of the verb in the picture. (Note that, although the example of the present form in English is given in the present continuous, in Greek there is no such distinction between present continuous and simple present. However, as described above, for the past tense there are perfective and imperfective forms that differ in the presence or absence of an aspectual marker. In some cases where the perfective was not the only plausible form for a given situation (i.e., the action could also be performed continuously, thus triggering the imperfective form), the patient was prompted additionally with "what did the person do only once?". The patient was tested on a total of 43 sentences with the accompanying pictures. The verbs used in these sentences belonged to the three morphological categories described above, i.e. (1) the category where the perfective past tense is formed with the addition of the rule-based aspectual marker to the perfective stem-allomorph, (2) the category where the rule-based aspectual marker is affixed to the imperfective present-tense stem and further induces a phonological change, and (3) the category where there is no rule-based aspectual marker involved, but where the perfective past tense is formed with the stem-allomorph resulting from an internal stem-vowel change of the imperfective present-tense stem. It should be noted that the first category where both a stem-allomorph and a rule-based aspectual marker are needed to form the perfective past tense form is specific to the language and thus of particular interest in this investigation.

The percentage of verbs belonging to each category represented roughly their percentage in the language. Thus, there were 11, 24 and 8 verbs in each of the three categories, respectively. The percentages of errors the patient made were 9/11, 9/24 and 0/8 for each category. We counted as errors all responses where IS either did not produce any response (in most cases he expressed his frustration for this difficulty), or he would produce the incorrect present or past imperfective form even when he knew it was inappropriate. There were only 2 instances of omissions in the data since he would resort to the imperfective past and present forms almost immediately after being confronted with a "difficult" form. His performance across the three categories was significantly different (Pearson x^2 (2)=13.16, $p < .005$). However, the basic question we wanted to address was which of the two perfective features, i.e., stem-allomorphy or the rule-based aspectual marker was problematic for IS. We thus analysed two more comparisons by isolating two verb categories at each time. In order to compensate for the additional statistics we decided to lower the acceptable level of significance from .05 to .01. Thus, we compared the categories that shared a common feature, i.e., the presence of a rule-based aspectual marker or the presence of a stem-allomorph. To answer the first question, i.e. whether the two categories with the rule-based aspectual marker elicit the same performance, we compared the first category featuring the stem-allomorph and the aspectual marker with the second category featuring the same stem and the rule-based aspectual marker. The data revealed that the patient made significantly more errors with the verbs of the first category where he had to compute both features (Pearson x^2 (1)=5.9, $p < .01$). To answer the second question, i.e. whether the two categories which both entailed the processing of a stem-allomorph in the past differed from each other, we compared the first category featuring both the stem-allomorph and the rule-based aspectual marker, with the third category featuring only a stem-allomorph to signify the perfective past-tense form. The comparison showed that IS was significantly more impaired for the category with both the stem-allomorph and the aspectual marker than for the stem-allomorph-only category (Pearson x^2 (1)=12.43, $p < .0005$, Fisher's two-tail exact test $p < .001$).

The last two comparisons showed that it is neither the mere presence of stem-allomorphy that creates difficulties for the patient (in fact, he showed a 100% success rate for the category of stem-allomorph-only past tense forms), nor just the computation of the rule-based aspectual marker. We can postulate that the difficulties in production of past tense forms for the category that requires both the stem-allomorph and the rule-based aspectual marker arise from the cumulative processing load of the combined computations that are required for those verbs in order to correctly produce the perfective past tense form. This finding sheds new light on the debate of whether aphasics have problems with regular (rule-based) or irregular (stored allomorph-based) past tense formation (e.g., Ullman et al, 1995; Kehayia, 1988). The particular case of Greek shows that the regularity-irregularity distinction is not a clear-cut, all-or-nothing and mutually exclusive way to describe linguistic reality and pathological performance. The Greek-speaking patient described in the present study conforms, on the one hand, with the universally claimed processing load difficulty of aphasic patients but, on the other, does not fall into previous categorizations proposed for his type of problem, namely the rule-based vs. stem-allomorph distinction in past tense formation.

Repetition of present and past-tense forms

It could be argued that results from the cued elicitation task may simply be a manifestation of a production deficit, e.g. with the phonological realization of the rule-based aspectual marker *-s-*. If those representations are impaired or unavailable for production, then the difficulties observed would be arising from a different level of processing than the one postulated and therefore would be manifested in other tasks that require the production of the phonological form of past tense, such as in repetition. We investigated this possibility by administering a repetition task to the patient using the same materials as the ones in the elicitation task. The order of the sentences was identical in both tasks.

The patient performed at ceiling level for all sentences in the present tense (43/43) and made only one error in the repetition of the past tense sentences (42/43). The error consisted of a substitution with the imperfective past tense of a verb featuring the rule-based aspectual marker *-s-*, but no stem-allomorphy, although bearing a phonological change at the stem-boundary triggered by the aspectual marker. Thus, in that category he scored 23/24 correct. The repetition task showed that the phonological representations of verbs are not impaired in this patient. Thus any difficulties observed in cued elicitation with particular verb categories are related to the cognitive demands of the task. Therefore, his problems were at the level of accessing and computing the perfective past-tense morphology, rather than at the phonological output level of these forms.

Reading of present and past-tense forms in sentences

Since IS's phonological representations of past-tense forms were not impaired, as evidenced in his performance on the repetition task, we investigated whether the computation of these forms would be more impaired when accessed through their graphemic representations. A reading task was thus administered using the 43 sentences from the previous tasks. Prior testing of the patient had shown that the same verbs in isolation did not pose any difficulty and that the patient's performance was almost at ceiling (97% correct utterances). The sentences in both the present and the perfective past-tense form were written in large-size letters (SuperGreek font for Macintosh, size 24) and randomized so that IS would not know what tense to anticipate. He was instructed to read them as accurately and as clearly as possible. All responses were recorded.

With respect to the present tense, the patient made 3/43 errors, overall. Two of those errors occurred in the second category with the single-stem and the rule-based aspectual marker in the past (2/24). In one case the patient read incorrectly the imperfective past-tense form instead of the present, and in the other the perfective past-tense form instead of the present. The third error was in the stem-allomorph category where the patient produced the imperfective past-tense form. However, these errors did not reach statistical significance (Pearson x^2 (2)= 1.27, $p = .53$). With respect to the past tense, the patient made 9/43 errors overall, that were distributed as follows: 2/11 in the stem-allomorph plus rule-based aspectual marker category where he produced imperfective past-tense forms, 7/24 in the single-stem plus rule-based aspectual marker category where he produced the present-tense form, and, 0/8 in the stem-allomorph category. However, the percentage of errors in the three categories did not differ significantly (Pearson x^2 (2)= 3.16, $p = .2$), even when compared in pairs (first and second: Fisher's two-tail exact test $p = .68$; second and third: Fisher's two-tail exact test $p = .15$; first and third: Fisher's two-tail exact test $p = .48$). Therefore, although IS showed a tendency to make more errors in reading, we cannot conclude from these data that he had any specific problem accessing phonological representations from the graphemic ones. Since it has been shown that representations in the two modalities can be independently impaired (Rapp & Caramazza, 1994), we wanted to further investigate the graphemic output representations by eliciting written verb forms However, the patient refused to perform the task due to his right hemiplegia and complete inability to write with his left hand.

Nominal morphology

Comprehension of singular and plural forms

As with verbs, we first tested the patient's comprehension of plural forms for different morphological categories of nouns. We confined our investigation to neutral nominal forms in order not to introduce additional features such as gender and case that would confound his performance, thus obscuring the locus of his impairment. Neutral nouns in Greek preserve the same form in both the nominative and accusative cases; thus, the case variable would not influence IS's performance. For the purpose of this investigation, we therefore tested whether morphological structure at the stem level plays a role in plural formation. The task included three types of variation in plural formation. In the first category, there were 14 nouns that form their plurals by adding the plural suffix to a stem-allomorph. In the second category, there were 26 nouns that form their plurals on the same stem which however undergoes a phonological change in the presence of the inflectional suffix. In the third category that consisted of 18 nouns, the stem is the same for both singular and plural forms and there is no phonological change. All 58 nouns were depicted in both the singular and the plural (2 or 3 exemplars of the same item) on the same page. However, the location of the plural was varied randomly (top or bottom of the page). 95% of the pictures were enlarged reproductions of stimuli from the Snodgrass (1991) standardized stimuli and the remaining 5% were taken from the BAT neurolinguistic testing battery (Paradis, 1988). All nouns were imageable line drawings and they were matched as well as possible for visual complexity. The instruction given to the patient was to point at the picture that corresponded best to the sentence provided by the examiner. The sentences were simple constructions of the type: "this is a ...." or "these are ....". The test was administered in two sessions and each sentence was shown only once per session to elicit comprehension of either the plural or the singular form of the noun. IS had no problems comprehending any of the items and performed at ceiling level (correct responses: 58/58). We thus established a basis for the lexical semantics of plural forms for all three morphological types of neutral nouns tested.

Cued elicitation of plural forms

In this task the patient was shown the same pictures as in the previous task, but this time he was given the singular form and was asked to produce the plural form, e.g., "this is a nail", "and here?". He saw all pictures in one testing session. He made only 3 mistakes in retrieving the plural form of three nouns (2/26 errors in the second and 1/18 errors in the third category) which consisted of producing the singular instead of the plural form. However, these errors did not reach significance (Pearson x^2 (2)= 1.11, p = .57). Therefore, we conclude that, unlike in the case of verbs, he seemed to have no marked problems with nominal morphology, at least with respect to the feature of plurality. In Greek, morphology is overall simpler in nouns than in verbs. There is no need for complex computations at the level of the stem. That is, the only operation the patient had to perform was accessing the stem-allomorph and, as was the case for verbs, stem-allomorphy alone did not seem to increase processing load, and therefore errors.

Repetition of singular and plural forms

A repetition task was also administered to IS. Specifically, he was asked to repeat all forms in the singular and in the plural, balanced and randomized, as in the previous task. He repeated all 58/58 nouns despite his articulatory difficulties and scored 100% correct. The fact that he did not have problems with the category of nouns that require a phonological change in the plural showed that his difficulty was not at the phonological level. Thus, the finding that he could not retrieve the plural form of a noun in spontaneous speech cannot be attributed to the fact that its phonological representation was impaired or lost.

Reading of singular and plural forms

A reading task was administered to IS in order to investigate the access of plural forms through their graphemic representations. Each noun was presented one at a time and the patient was instructed to read it as accurately and clearly as possible.

With regard to the singular forms, the patient made 3/58 errors overall, producing the diminutive forms of the nouns instead. All these nouns belonged to the second category featuring phonological change at the stem level. However, these errors did not reach statistical significance (Pearson x^2 (2)= 1.11, p = .57). As for the plural forms, the patient made 6/58 errors overall, which were distributed among the three categories as follows: 2/14 in the stem-allomorph category, 4/26 in the single-stem plus phonological change category, and, 0/14 in the stem-allomorph category. Again, the categories were not significantly different from each other (Pearson x^2 (2)= 3.02, p = .22), even when compared in pairs (first and second: Fisher's two-tail exact test p = 1; second and third: Fisher's two-tail exact test p = .13; first and third: Fisher's two-tail exact test p = .18). Therefore, although IS showed a tendency to make more errors in reading than in repetition, we cannot conclude from these data that he had any specific problem in accessing plural forms through their graphemic representations.

General Discussion

Morphological impairments in aphasia have already been documented in different languages (Menn & Obler, 1990). The purpose of this study was to explore morphological breakdown in an as yet scarcely documented language, Greek, and to account for morphological problems in two major grammatical categories, verbs and nouns, through a series of different tasks. In our results, we did not obtain a notable breakdown in the case of nouns in contrast to a significant morphological deficit in verbs. This suggests that morphological impairment in nouns and verbs may follow different patterns across languages, and that aphasic symptoms may be differentially manifested for these two categories depending on the particular characteristics of the language involved. A dissociation in the morphological processing of nouns and verbs has also been reported earlier, although in the opposite direction (see Shapiro et al., in press). The authors present a case of an English-speaking patient who exhibited a deficit in producing the nominal plural marker -s but had no problems producing the phonologically identical third-person singular marker of verbs. Thus, it is shown that morphological processing is a dimension that can be selectively impaired within each grammatical class after language breakdown in aphasia. Our results further underscore that the language-specific morphology of grammatical classes can be reflected in the breakdown patterns of aphasic performance. The fact that we obtained diverse patterns of performance between our patient and previously studied patients in different languages, coupled with the fact that this can occur even within a single grammatical category (in our case verbs), suggests that aphasic symptoms in each language can fall into more generally claimed trends *and* also reveal strictly language-specific patterns.

In addition to contributing to the search for universal patterns, the study of morphological impairments in Greek presents interesting new dimensions because morphological breakdown in Greek is not an "all-or-nothing" phenomenon, given the morphological richness of the language and the fact that all words need an inflectional affix to surface to the word level. More specifically, verbal inflection in Greek encompasses a range of interesting phenomena from phonological change during the application of the regular past-tense rule to the combination of allomorphic stem retrieval with the regular past-tense rule. Thus, in the case of verbs, the Greek language provided the opportunity to take some distance from dichotomies commonly found in the literature such as rule-based vs. stored-allomorph mechanisms because of the presence, in Greek, of a category that combines both of these mechanisms. The issue of morphological breakdown in Greek aphasia appears even more intriguing with the investigation of aphasics' performance with respect to nominal inflection. Greek nominal inflection provides instances where the straight-forward rule-based vs. storage-based distinction can be further explored with the existence, in the language, of allomorphic plural stems that include the singular form (e.g., stoma-stomata), regular plural-rule application with phonological but not stem-final orthographic change (e.g., pedi-ped/j/a) , and single-stem inflection without any change at the level of the stem (e.g., vuno-vuna). Given the particularities of the language, the scope of this study is thus not restricted to confirming universal patterns in the breakdown of rule-based or stored representations, but extends to the investigation of the role that grammatical category plays in this distinction.

Neurolinguistic investigation of morphological impairments in verbs has shown regular/irregular dissociations in Italian (Cappa & Ullman, 1998). Patients performed worse at producing irregular present tense and past participle forms than regular ones. However, the opposite pattern has also been documented (Ullman et al.,1997), i.e., patients produced irregular verbs more accurately than regular ones. Moreover, Ullman et al. (1997) claimed that the regularity-irregularity distinction is the manifestation of different brain mechanisms dedicated to these functions: the "procedural" and the "declarative" systems served by anterior and posterior brain areas, respectively. A possible artifact in English is that regular past-tense forms are usually more phonologically similar to their base forms (e.g., mark-marked) than irregular forms (e.g., teach-taught), so that regular forms are more sensitive to phonological similarity effects. This may, however, be irrelevant to the issue of morphological regularity.

Verbal inflection also seems to cause problems in off-line tasks in Greek, especially in production, but the pattern of errors is a function of the regularity of the stem and the number of affixes involved in past tense forms (Kehayia, 1988). In our patient, we observed that rule-based access is more impaired than access through the stem-allomorph. Whenever the rule needed to be computed, IS's performance slowed down, especially when processing load was increased by the additional operation of stored-allomorph retrieval. With regard to nouns, Kehayia et al. (1990) observed that aphasic patients tend to show impairment in plural production, indicating that plural inflection implies computational difficulties. However, in these cases patients also had to compute features other than number, e.g., gender and case. In the present investigation, we tested only number by selecting neuter nouns in which the feature of case can be held constant. Since our patient had no significant problems with nominal number, one can conclude that the processing of this one feature by itself did not impose any extra computational demands that would have resulted in impaired performance. Thus, taken together, our results for nouns and verbs allow us to propose a unified account of IS's performance in terms of a computational load deficit.

Our claim that the patient did not just exhibit problems with retrieving the allomorphs is supported by the fact that he did not show any impairment in the stem-allomorphic verb category, nor did he have any difficulties with the noun category that requires retrieval of the stem-allomorph. Thus, his problem seems to be manifested only when the computational demands exceed his capacities. A computational load deficit in aphasia, although documented previously in the aphasic literature, takes a different shape in this Greek patient because of the specificities of the morphological system of the language. Taking together the results of previously documented Greek patients (Kehayia et al., 1990; Kehayia, 1988) and those of the present patient, one may further claim a dissociation between the two types of deficits manifested: a deficit in accessing the allomorphic stems in the previously studied patients and a computational deficit in processing the perfective rule together with the allomorphic stem in our patient. The patients documented so far show a differential morphological impairment, as is usually the case in aphasia where variability is the norm, but more importantly, they show how the language determines the way in which these impairments are realized in language breakdown. In English and German (see Clahsen, 1999, for a review) it has been found that it is usually the regular rule-based forms that show an impairment in aphasia, but this does not seem to be the case in a highly inflected language such as Greek. Thus, in Greek, problems can arise not just when having to compute an extra suffix (e.g., the rule-base aspectual marker alone) but rather in accessing the allomorphic forms (Kehayia, 1988) or in carrying out more more complex computations (e.g., both accessing the allomorphic form *and* computing the rule-based aspectual marker as is the case in our patient).

In conclusion, in this paper we have discussed manifestations of morphological deficits in Greek aphasia. We investigated verbal and nominal inflection and accounted for morphological impairments that are manifested in non-fluent aphasics' performance precisely because of the particularities of the language. Further research needs to be conducted in order to fully investigate breakdown patterns particular to Greek in other areas, e.g. syntax.

Acknowledgements

The research reported here was supported by an MCRI grant from the Social Sciences and Humanities Research Council of Canada (#412-95-0006) awarded to Gonia Jarema (Université de Montréal), director and co-principal investigator; Eva Kehayia (McGill University), co-principal investigator, and Gary Libben (University of Alberta), co-principal investigator. We are grateful to patient IS for his participation and his patience throughout the testing period. We are indebted to Dr Nikos Artemis, Dr Rania Argyropoulou-Raka, and Dr Magda Tsolaki for making the AHEPA and Papanicolaou General Hospitals' archives available for us and for their help in recruiting patients. We would also wish to thank Helene Kaufman and Lara Riente for their help in proofreading this paper.

Address correspondence to: Kyrana Tsapkini, Centre de recherche. Institut de gériatrie de Montréal, 4565 Chemin Queen-Mary, Montéal H3W 1W5, Canada.
E-mail: tsapkink@magellan.umontreal.ca

References

Baayen, H., & Schreuder, R. (1997). Morphology: why, how, when, when not, and why not. In G. Booij & J. v. Marle (Eds.), *Yearbook of morphology 1996,* (pp. 1-7). Dordrecht: Kluwer Academic Publishers.

Baayen, H., & Schreuder, R. (1999). War and peace: Morphemes and full forms in a noninteractive activation parallel dual-route model. *Brain and Language, 68*, 27-32.

Badecker, W. (1997). Levels of morphological deficit: indications from inflectional regularity. *Brain and Language, 60*, 360-380.

Bastiaanse, R., & Jonkers, R. (1998). Verb retrieval in action naming and spontaneous speech in agrammatic and anomic aphasia. *Aphasiology, 12*, 951-969.

Bates, E., Chen, S., Tzeng, O., Li, P., & Opie, M. (1991). The noun-verb problem in Chinese aphasia. *Brain and Language, 41*, 203-233.

Berndt, R. S., Mitchum, C.C., Haendinges, A.N., & Sandson, J. (1997). Verb retrieval in aphasia. 1. Characterizing single word impairments. *Brain and Language, 56*, 68-106.

Cappa, S., Ullman, M. (1998). A neural dissociation in Italian verbal morphology. Paper presented at the 5th Annual Meeting of the Cognitive Neuroscience Society, San Francisco, CA.

Caramazza, A., Laudanna, A., & Romani, C. (1988). Lexical access and inflectional morphology. *Cognition, 28*, 297-332.

Clahsen, H. (1999). Lexical entries and rules of language: a multidisciplinary study of German inflection. *Behavioral and Brain Sciences, 22*, 991-1060.

Daniele, A., Giustolisi, L., Silveri, M.C., Colosimo, C., & Gainotti, G. (1994). Evidence for a possible neuroanatomical basis for lexical processing of nouns and verbs. *Neuropsychologia, 32*, 1325-1341.

Gainotti, G. (1998). Category-specific disorders for nouns and verbs: A very old and very new problem. In B. Stemmer and H. A. Whitaker (Eds.), *Handbook of neurolinguistics* (pp. 3-11). San Diego, CA: Academic Press.

Grodzinsky, Y. (1986). Language deficits and the theory of syntax. *Brain and Language, 37*, 480-499.

Jarema, G. (1998). The breakdown of morphology in aphasia. In B. Stemmer and H. A. Whitaker (Eds.), *Handbook of Neurolinguistics*. San Diego, CA: Academic Press.

Joanisse, M., Seidenberg, M.S. (1999). Impairments in verb morphology after brain injury: A connectionist model. *Proc. Natl. Acad. Sci. USA, 96*, 7592-7597.

Kehayia, E., Jarema, G.,, & Kadzielawa, D. (1990). Cross-linguistic study of morphological errors in aphasia: Evidence from English, Greek, and Polish. In J.-L. Nespoulous and P. Villiard (Eds.), *Morphology, phonology and aphasia* (pp. 140-155).

Kehayia E. Morphological representation of inflected and derived words in Greek speaking individuals. Proceedings from the Second International Conference on Greek linguistics, October 1997.

Kehayia, E. (1988). Morphological impairments in agrammatic aphasia: A comparative Study. Unpublished Ph.D. Dissertation, McGill University, Montreal, Canada.

Marshal, J., Pring, T., & Chiat, S. (1998). Verb retrieval and sentence production in aphasia. *Brain and Language, 63*(2), 159-183.

Menn L., & Obler, L.K. (Ed.). (1990). *Agrammatic aphasia: A cross-language narrative sourcebook*. Philadelphia: John Benjamins.

Miceli, G., & Caramazza, A. (1988). Dissociation of inflectional and derivational morphology. *Brain and Language* 35, 24-65.

Nadeau, S. E., & Rothi, I. J. (1992). Morphologic agrammatism folowing a right hemisphere stroke in a dextral patient. *Brain and Language, 43*, 642-667.

Paradis, M. (1987). The assessment of bilingual aphasia. Hillsdale, NJ, LEA.

Pinker, S. (1999). *Words and rules: the ingredients of language*. Basic Books: New York.

Prather, P., Zurif, E., Stern, C., & Rosen, T. J. (1992). Slowed lexical access in nonfluent aphasia: a case study. *Brain and Language, 43*, 336-348.

Prather, P. A., Zurif, E., Love, T., & Brownell, H. (1997). Speed of lexical activation in nonfluent Broca's aphasia and fluent Wernicke's aphasia. *Brain and Language, 59*, 391-411.

Ralli, A. (1988). *Eléments de la morphologie du Grec Moderne: La structure du verbe.* Unpublished Ph.D. Dissertation, Université de Montréal, Montreal, Canada.

Ralli, A. (1997). Inflectional features and the morphological component hypothesis. Paper presented at 20th GLOW. Rabat, Marocco: March 19-21, 1997.

Schreuder, R., Baayen, R.H. (1995). Modeling morphological processing. In L. B. Feldman (Ed.), *Morphological aspects of language processing* (pp. 131-154). Hillsdale, NJ: LEA.

Shapiro, K., Shelton, J., & Caramazza, A. (in press). Grammatical class in lexical production and morphological processing: evidence from a case of fluent aphasia. *Cognitive Neuropsychology*.

Ullman, M. T., Corkin, S., Coppola, M., Hickok, G., Growdon, J. H., Koroshetz, W. J., & Pinker, S. (1997). A neural dissociation within language: Evidence that the mental dictionary is part of declarative memory, and that grammatical rules are processed by the procedural system. *Journal of Cognitive Neuroscience, 9*, 266-276.

Aphasia in Hebrew Speakers

Mira Goral

The Graduate Center of The City University of New York

Abstract – This paper presents a review of studies reporting aphasia and related language deficits in Hebrew speakers. First, a brief introduction to the main characteristics of Hebrew is provided. Then, studies that address Hebrew features are described, presented based on the language deficits at their focus. The contribution of each study is reviewed, specific participant and lesion information is included when available, as are specific examples of the impaired language skills. A summary of the characteristics of aphasia in Hebrew is then provided.

Key words: aphasia; Hebrew; morphology; reading

Introduction

The manifestation of language breakdown in aphasia is influenced by the nature of the lesion causing the language deficit and by language-specific features. To introduce some language-specific features pertaining to Hebrew, I begin with a very brief overview of Hebrew grammar. (For a detailed account of modern Hebrew see, for example, Berman, 1978; Rosen, 1966). Modern Hebrew, spoken in Israel today, is a product of its ancient relatives (e.g., Biblical Hebrew, Mishnaic Hebrew) and a revival process that began at the end of the 18th century and continued into the beginning of the 20th century (see, for example, Ravid, 1995; Sivan, 1976).

In Hebrew, as in other Semitic languages, most words are constructed of a root morpheme and a morphological pattern (*binyan*). The root is an abstract, unpronounceable morpheme, usually consisting of three consonants (e.g., *LMD*, *KTB*). The morphological patterns, also bound morphemes, consist of vowel or vowel-and-consonant templates (e.g., CaCaC, miCCaC). These two morphemes, a root and a pattern, combine non-linearly to form words (see Table 1). Roots are usually associated with a general meaning (e.g., the root *LMD* is associated with the meaning "learn"), which may be modified, depending on the specific pattern (e.g., the root *LMD* forms the words "learn," "be learned," "teach," "pupil"). Patterns may be associated with a general meaning (such as profession, action, reciprocal) but their form-meaning relationship is not consistent.

The root-pattern derivational system for verbs is highly regular, with only seven possible verbal patterns and mostly productive roots (i.e., roots that appear in various words, all related in their meaning). The nominal system is less regular, with numerous patterns and with productive roots as well as roots that exist in one or a few words only. Borrowed words usually assume a native pattern when incorporated into the language and can be conjugated accordingly, even though they do not contain a native root.

Root	Pattern	Word	Meaning	Category
LMD "learn"	CaCaC	lamad	learned (3rd pers. sing. masc., past)	verb
LMD "learn"	CiCeC	limed	taught (3rd pers. sing. masc., past)	verb
LMD "learn"	tCCiC	talmid	pupil (sing. masc.)	noun
KTB "write"	CaCaC	katav	wrote (3rd pers. sing. masc., past)	verb
			reporter (sing. masc.)	noun
KTB "write"	hitCaCeC	hitkatev	corresponded (3rd pers. sing. masc., past)	verb
KTB "write"	miCCaC	mixtav	letter (sing. masc.)	noun

Table 1. Examples of Hebrew words and their morphological structure

Hebrew has a relatively rich inflectional system. Verbs are inflected for person, gender, number, and tense (see Table 2). The inflectional markers (suffixes and prefixes) vary in the different verb patterns and in the different tenses. There are three tenses: one past tense, one present tense, and one future tense, as well as an imperative form (derived from the future tense form).

Verb	Meaning
lamadti	learned (1st pers. sing. masc.+fem.)
lamadta	learned (2nd pers. sing. masc.)
lamadet	learned (2nd pers. sing. fem.)
lamad	learned (3rd pers. sing. masc.)
lamda	learned (3rd pers. sing. fem.)
lamadnu	learned (1st pers. plur. masc.+fem.)
lamadtem	learned (2nd pers. plur. masc.)
lamadten	learned (2nd pers. plur. fem.)
lamdu	learned (3rd pers. plur. masc.+fem.)

Table 2. An example of verb conjugation in the past tense. Root: LMD. Pattern: CaCac

Nouns are inflected for number and gender and must agree with their adjectives, which also mark number and gender (see Table 3). Some prepositions may be conjugated according to person, gender, and number (e.g., *be* "in", *bi* "in me" 1st pers. sing.; *baxem* "in you" 2nd pers. plur. masc.). Several prepositions are bound morphemes and are added as prefixes to the word that follows them (e.g., *mi* "from," *misavta* "from grandmother"). When the identified article *ha* follows a bound preposition, the consonant of the definite article is deleted and the vowel is transferred to the preposition. For example, *bayit* "a house," *bebayit* "in a house," *habayit* "the house," *babayit* "in the house."

In terms of word order, Hebrew has a predominant SVO order with several structures that require or allow VSO order. Adjectives follow the nouns they modify.

Noun	Meaning	Adjective	Meaning
talmid	pupil (sing. masc.)	tov	good (sing. masc.)
talmida	pupil (sing. fem.)	tova	good (sing. fem.)
talmidim	pupils (plur. masc.)	tovim	good (plur. masc.)
talmidot	pupils (plur. fem.)	tovot	good (plur. fem.)

Table 3. Examples of gender and number agreement in nouns and adjectives

The Hebrew phonetic inventory contains 19 consonants and five vowels. Various morpho-phonological changes occur within both the verb and the noun systems (e.g., in compounds that contain female or plural nouns as their left constituent). One such alternation is referred to as spirantization: Three stop consonants alternate, in certain word contexts, with their corresponding fricatives (p-f, b-v, k-x). Thus, a root consonant may be realized in the words derived from that root as the stop or the corresponding fricative (e.g., see above, from the root *KTB* ***k**atav* vs. *mi**x**tav*).

Hebrew is written from right to left. Primarily the consonants (though sometimes certain vowels) are represented by letters; the vowels are usually not represented in writing. There is a vowelization system (*nikud*), consisting of dots and lines that are inserted above and below the letters, but this system is used only for written material related to religious scripts, poetry, and beginning readers. Because most vowels are missing in the unvoweled written representation, there are many homographs in Hebrew. For example, the consonant string *ktb* (which theoretically can be read with any vowel combination: katav, kitiv, kitav, kativ, ktav, etc.) can denote the past tense verb *katav* "he wrote" or the noun *ktav* "orthography". During reading, potential ambiguity resulting from homographs is often resolved based on the regularity of the morphological patterns and the use of contextual cues.

Aphasia in Hebrew Speakers

I turn now to a review of studies reporting language deficits in Hebrew speakers. Several studies clearly address Hebrew-specific phenomena; they will be introduced based on the main deficits they address. I begin with studies on syntactic and morphological deficits. These focus on Hebrew morpho-syntactic features, including verb-agreement and tense inflections, root morphology, and morpho-phonological alternations. I proceed with two studies of reading deficits, which incorporate various features of Hebrew orthography, including the right-to-left writing direction and the lack of graphemic vowel representation. Additional studies that deal with aphasia more generally (studies that focus on phonological deficits, pragmatic deficits, and rehabilitation issues in Hebrew speakers and polyglots) will only be mentioned below.

I. Morphological Deficits

A. The morpho-syntax of agrammatism

Addressing a commonly described characteristic of agrammatism in the literature published prior to his paper, Grodzinsky (1984) demonstrated that "omissions of inflectional morphemes" may apply only to agrammatism in some languages but not in others. For languages such as English, with minimal inflectional morphology and verb stems that are free morphemes, omissions of inflections may seem a sufficient description of the output of agrammatic patients. But in some languages in which bare stems are not necessarily free morphemes, omission of inflectional morphology will leave the aphasic speaker with an unpronounceable verb stem. Deficits in inflectional morphology in such languages are then expected to be realized in morpheme substitutions, not omissions.

The Hebrew examples Grodzinsky provided included person substitutions and verb pattern (*binyan*) substitutions as in (1) and (2).

(#1)	Target:	nasanu
	Gloss:	went (1st pers. plur., past)
	English equivalent:	We went
	Aphasic production:	nas'u
	Gloss:	went (3rd pers. plur., past)

(#2)	Target:	hifsaqti
	Gloss:	stop (1st pers. sing., past, *binyan hif'il*)
	English equivalent:	I stopped
	Aphasic production:	nifsaqti
	Gloss:	was stopped (1st pers. sing., past, *binyan nif'al*) [a passive form, not used in 1st pers.]

Grodzinsky's observation changed the standard description of agrammatism in the literature. Comparing data from various languages with varying morphological makeups (e.g., Hebrew, Italian, Russian, English) can demonstrate that the manifestation of agrammatic language deficit is language dependent, constrained by the type of language spoken and its morphological (or other) grammatical characteristics.

In a later study, Friedmann & Grodzinsky (1997) provided a syntactic account for the pattern of inflectional deficits demonstrated by a Hebrew-speaking agrammatic aphasic. Their account, based on Chomsky's linguistic theory the Minimalist Program (Chomsky, 1992) and Pollock's hypothesis regarding split inflection (Pollock, 1989), can explain the dissociation between the impaired production of tense markers and the spared production of agreement markers demonstrated by the reported case, as well as predict other agrammatic deficits according to severity of impairment.

Participant

The participant (RS) was a Hebrew-speaking 70-year-old right-handed woman with 14 years of education who was diagnosed with Broca's aphasia four years prior to the reported study. A CT scan revealed low density in the left anterior-inferior temporal lobe and asymmetry between larger left frontal horn and smaller right. Her speech output was characterized by short phrases, non-fluent production, and phonemic paraphasias. Her comprehension was judged to be intact as were her naming and reading skills.

Task and Procedure

Extensive lists of words and sentences were used in a repetition task and a sentence-completion task, administered to elicit production of inflectional morphemes. Correct and incorrect use of tense and agreement markers in verb and copula structures were recorded and evaluated. Comprehension of grammatical morphemes was evaluated using grammaticality judgment tests (free judgment, contrastive judgment, and forced-choice judgment) and a tense-comprehension test. Production of Wh-questions was also tested using various elicitation tasks.

Results and Conclusion

While single-word repetition yielded a low error rate (3 out of 43), sentence repetition yielded 37% errors and sentence completion yielded more than 50% errors in both oral and written production. Strikingly, all errors (including morpheme substitution and copula omission) were tense errors, while production of agreement markers was near normal (see Table 4 for error distribution; no specific examples are provided in the paper). Performance on the comprehension tests revealed intact grammatical comprehension. Performance on the Wh-question elicitation tasks was poor.

	Sentence Repetition	Sentence Production	
		Oral	Written
Tense	37	50	82.1
Agreement	0	2	6.9

Table 4. RS's percent error in sentence repetition and sentence completion tasks (based on Friedmann & Grodzinsky, 1997)

The account given by the authors for the clear dissociation of grammatical markers, namely, spared agreement marking and impaired tense marking, is based on the syntactic theory and the representation of inflection (INFL) in the underlying structure of sentences. Specifically, tense and agreement are represented as separate inflectional processes and can be selectively impaired. Moreover, tense marking is "higher up" in the tree representation of the sentence structure and thus (assuming bottom-up processes of inflectional markers' specification) may be impaired with no effect on agreement marking (represented lower in the tree structure). Friedmann & Grodzinsky further postulate that an underspecified part of the syntactic (tree) structure will cause agrammatic production and will affect other structures higher up in the tree. In contrast, there will be no effect on structures below the impaired one. Thus, while tense errors may be seen without the existence of any agreement errors, agreement errors are not expected to be found without any tense errors. In cases of severe agrammatism, hypothesized by the authors as deficits further down in the tree structure, both tense and agreement errors are expected.

These predictions can certainly be tested, particularly in languages in which tense and agreement markers can be readily dissociated. Indeed, two cases of Hebrew agrammatism with comprehensive descriptions of deficits are available (Baharav, 1990). In both cases, inflectional errors are evident, though with different distributions, as described below.

As part of a large cross-linguistic study of agrammatism (Menn & Obler, 1990), Baharav provided data from two agrammatic speakers and two control speakers. The data included production of conversational speech and narrative. The analysis focused on syntactic and morphological aspects of the agrammatic language production.

Participants
Two non-fluent aphasic speakers and two neurologically intact speakers were included in the study. They were all right-handed men. Their ages at the time of the study ranged from 65 to 76. One patient (MS) had suffered an ischemic infarction resulting in lesions in the left fronto-parito-temporal region extending into the periventricular white matter. He was diagnosed with severe Broca's aphasia with agrammatism and severe anomia. MS was tested ten years after the onset of his aphasia. The other patient (MD) had suffered a CVA resulting in damage to the left fronto-temporal and parietal areas. He was diagnosed with mild Broca's aphasia with agrammatism. MD was tested seven years post the onset of his aphasia.

Task and Procedure
Speech production was collected during conversation (history of illness), story-telling (Little Red Riding Hood), and picture description (the Cookie Theft; the Wechsler-Bellevue Picture-Sequence). Production was analyzed for distribution and type of errors made with morphemes, grammatical categories, syntactic structures, use of tenses and for fluency, using measures of rate of production and phrase length.

Results and Conclusion
MS demonstrated impaired morphological performance. He correctly produced 30% of all required (free and bound) morphemes. He omitted 42% and made substitution errors in 28% of the morphemes he produced. Omissions included prepositions, definite articles and pronouns. Substitution errors included substitution of both gender and tense markers of adjectives, verbs, and copula. In addition, MS overused conjunctions, adverbs, fillers, negatives and exclamations in his speech, as compared to his neurologically intact control.

MD correctly produced 50% of all required morphemes. He omitted 24% and substituted 26% of the morphemes. When morphological errors in all other categories but verbs were considered, MD omitted 25% of the morphemes (as compared to 59% for MS) and substituted 21% (as compared to 11% for MS). Omitted morphemes included definite markers, object marker, copula, and relative markers. Substitutions included use of demonstrative *ze* (impersonal deictic) instead of personal pronouns and gender errors. Tense substitutions were rare (there were a few instances of production of present tense where past tense was judged to be more appropriate and a few infinitive forms substituting finite forms). As found for MS, MD overused conjunctions, adverbs, fillers, negatives and exclamations. Examples of morphological errors produced by MS and MD are provided in Table 5.

Baharav's analysis of the distribution of grammatical classes revealed great inter-subject variability and no consistent differences between the output of the patients and their controls. Nor were consistent differences found between the type of sentences used by the patients and those of their controls. The author summarized the analyses pointing out that the two agrammatic patients demonstrated several shared production characteristics but also differed from each other on a number of grammatical measures. Both patients showed deficits in inflectional morphology but not derivational morphology. They both made gender substitution errors and tense errors including substitution of infinite forms for finite verbs. They generally used a variety of verbs, and the same distribution of word type and sentence type as their controls, although both patients showed a tendency to omit verbs, producing incomplete sentences. They differed in their rate of omission and substitution errors and in the type of grammatical morphemes that were found to be more or less impaired.

Patient, Error Type	MS, Gender Substitution
Target	kipa aduma holexet (or: halxa)
Gloss	LRRH* (sing. fem.) go (3rd pers. sing. fem., present) (or past)
English Equivalent	LRRH is going
Aphasic Production	kipa aduma holex
Gloss	LRRH (sing. fem.) go (3rd pers. sing. masc., present)
Patient, Error Type	MS, Gender Substitution
Target	mashehu axer
Gloss	something (sing. masc.) else (sing. masc.)
English Equivalent	something else, another thing
Aphasic Production	mashehu axeret
Gloss	something (sing. masc.) else (sing. fem.)
Patient, Error Type	MD, Gender Substitution
Target	savta amra
Gloss	grandmother (sing. fem.) say (3rd pers. sing. fem., past)
English Equivalent	Grandmother said
Aphasic Production	savta amar
Gloss	grandmother (sing. fem.) say (3rd pers. sing. masc., past)
Patient, Error Type	MD, Pronoun Omission
Target	ani medaber lo kol kax tov
Gloss	I speak (sing. masc., present) no so good
English Equivalent	I speak (or I am speaking) not so good
Aphasic Production	medaber lo kol kax tov
Gloss	speak (sing. masc., present) no so good

LRRH = Little Red Riding Hood

Table 5. Examples of morphological errors (based on Baharav, 1990)

Baharav concluded that a strict syntactic theory cannot account for the differences found between the two patients and for the lack of differences between the syntactic characterization of the patients and their controls and proposed a more cognitive-based theory of deficits at the language planning stages of speech production.

The patterns of inflectional errors demonstrated by the two patients in Baharav (1990) are not both consistent with the hypotheses put forward by Friedmann & Grodzinsky (1997). Recall that according to their hypotheses, while tense errors are expected to be found without agreement errors, agreement errors are not expected without tense errors. Furthermore, only in cases of severe aphasia, both types of errors are expected. In accordance with the latter, MS, the patient with the more severe agrammatism, demonstrated both tense and agreement errors. However, in contrast to the former hypothesis, MD, the patient with the milder agrammatism, demonstrated agreement errors but few frank tense errors.

It should be noted that results from spontaneous production (used in Baharav, 1990) may differ from results obtained using various elicitation tasks (Freidmann & Grodzinsky, 1997). Dissociation patterns of these two types of inflectional markers, agreement and tense, could be further investigated with agrammatic speakers of languages with rich morphological systems. Moreover, dissociations in the breakdown of specific morphological markers can be studied. For example, dissociation of gender and number agreement, gender and person agreement, or number and person agreement can be explored with speakers of languages that mark these features with distinctive markers.

In both studies, inflectional morphology was found to be impaired while derivational morphology appeared intact. Dissociation of inflectional and derivational morphology has been described in the aphasia literature, with most studies documenting intact derivational morphology (e.g., Miceli & Caramazza, 1988). Several studies, however, demonstrated that derivational morphology may also be impaired (Mathews & Obler, 1997; Barkai, 1980).

B. The morpho-phonology of an aphasic

Barkai (1980) provided a comprehensive description of a case of a man who suffered a TBI resulting in language disturbances including dysgraphia and speech errors such as deviant verb forms and paraphasias. Errors associated with the root-based structure of verbs as well as phoneme spirantization were analyzed with respect to phonological and morphological approaches.

Participant

A 33-year-old right-handed man suffered a TBI caused by shrapnel resulting in damage to the anterior and superior parts of the left parietal lobe and probably to the superior part of the frontal lobe with right hemiplegia as well as hearing loss. (No further information is provided.)

Task and Procedure

Spoken and written production were recorded and analyzed early in the course of recovery, particularly in the third and fourth months post-onset. The data were collected during free conversation and writing to dictation.

Results and Conclusion

In writing to dictation, most words were correctly written. Errors did occur on most verbs that involved metathesis, namely, verbs in the verb pattern *hitpa'el* made of roots that begin with a sibilant (e.g., *SPR histaper vs. BGR hitbager*). For example, given the word *hizdaqeq* "was in need for" from the root *ZQQ*, the patient failed to switch the order between the pattern-consonant /t/ and the root-consonant /z/ (and to adjust the voicing of the /t/) as in (3).

(#3) Target (written): hzdqq
Gloss: [hizdaqeq] need (3rd pers. sing. masc., past, *binyan hitpa'el*)
English equivalent: He was in need of
Aphasic production: htzqq
Gloss: [hitzaqeq] need (3rd pers. sing. masc., past, *binyan hitpa'el*) without the required morpho-phonological changes

A second type of error found in the patient's writing was his failure to contract bound prepositions and the definite article as in (4).

(#4)	Target (written):	bgn
	Gloss:	[bagan] in (+identified article) garden
	English equivalent:	In the garden
	Aphasic production:	bhgn
	Gloss:	[behagan] in the garden (uncontracted)

In spontaneous speech, the patient made errors that were characterized by production of verbs constructed of the intended root but the wrong verb class (*binyan*) as in (5). Additional examples are presented in Table 6. The patient was rarely aware of his mistakes.

(#5)	Target:	levate
	Gloss:	pronounce (infinitive of the root *BTA* in *binyan pi'el*)
	English equivalent:	To pronounce
	Aphasic production:	livto
	Gloss:	infinitive of the root *BTA* in *binyan pa'al* (non-existent)

Target Verb	nivhelet
Gloss	get scared (3rd pers. sing. fem., present; root: BHL, binyan: nif'al)
English Equivalent	She is getting scared
Aphasic Production	mitnavhelet
Gloss	3rd pers. sing. fem., present, root: BHL, binyan: hitpa'el
Target Verb	kibsa
Gloss	launder (3rd pers. sing. fem., past; root: KBS, binyan: pi'el)
English Equivalent	She laundered
Aphasic Production	hixvisa
Gloss	3rd pers. sing. fem., past; root: KBS, binyan: hif'il
Target Verb	higdilu
Gloss	enlarge (3rd pers. plur., past; root: GDL, binyan: hif'il)
English Equivalent	They enlarged
Aphasic Production	gadlu
Gloss	enlarge (3rd pers. plur., past; root: GDL, binyan: pa'al)

Table 6. Examples of errors resulting from root-pattern non-existent combinations (based on Barkal, 1980)

In addition to these morphological errors, spontaneous speech during the early period post-onset revealed errors in spirantization as in (6) and (7).

(#6)	Target:	xoshvim
	Gloss:	think (plur. masc., present)
	English equivalent:	We/you/they think
	Aphasic production:	koshvim
		/k/ substituting /x/

(#7)	Target:	kovesh
	Gloss:	conquer (sing. masc., present)
	English equivalent:	I/you/he conquer(s)
	Aphasic production:	kobesh
		/b/ substituting /v/

The author took the type of errors the patient made as support for morphological theories that are based on the notion that the Hebrew root is conceptualized as a morpheme, despite its abstract representation. The errors made by the patient were not random, but rather substitutions of the target *binyan* with another *binyan* as he formed non-existent words from existing morphemes, suggesting on-line morphological composition rather than lexical access of fully composed forms.

The spirantization errors produced by the patient can be identified as phonologically based (i.e., phonemic paraphasias) or morphologically based errors. In light of the specific distributions of his patient's spirantization errors, Barkai argued that the theory best accounting for these errors is morphological rather than phonological.

While most studies of morphological deficits in aphasia report inflectional deficits (e.g., Tyler & Cobb, 1987 for English; Miceli & Caramazza, 1988 for Italian), Barkai's patient demonstrated derivational errors in speech production. The root-and-pattern derivational processes of most words in Hebrew can be used to explore derivational processes in aphasia. Other derivational processes should be studied in various languages with various derivational systems (Mathews & Obler, 1997).

In sum, this section presented some characteristics of morphological (including morpho-syntax and morpho-phonology) deficits in aphasia. Omission and substitution patterns of inflectional deficits were discussed (Grodzinsky, 1984; Baharav, 1990). While omissions and substitutions of free morphemes can be estimated based on obligatory context, the use of bound morphemes is more strictly determined by language-specific constraints. The overall use of bound inflectional morphemes was analyzed (Baharav, 1990) as well as dissociations of specific inflectional markers (Friedmann & Grodzinsky, 1997). Further studies can explore patterns of impairment and sparing of specific inflectional markers in Hebrew as well as in other languages. In addition to inflectional deficits, derivational errors in aphasia were demonstrated (Barkai, 1980), suggesting on-line derivational processes in Hebrew verb production. Further investigation of linear and non-linear derivational processes in aphasia is warranted. Systematic assessments of the use of derivational and inflectional morphology in the output of aphasic speakers of languages with rich morphological systems will add to our understanding of morphological deficits in aphasia.

II. Reading Deficits

Recovering alexia

Sroka, Solsi, & Bornstein (1973) reported a case of pure word blindness following a small CVA in the left occipital lobe. The main deficit found in the patient was alexia without agraphia. The alexia was temporary and after several months seemed to have resolved.

<u>Participant</u>

The patient was a 40-year-old woman with a high-school education who suffered a small CVA. Cerebral angiography revealed vascular malformation in the left posterior cerebral artery. Brain scans performed on admission showed a lesion in the temporo-occipital region. In a similar scan performed two months post-onset those findings were no longer evident.

Task and Procedure

A variety of cognitive and language tasks were administered upon admission, during the two and a half months of her hospitalization, and in the first few weeks after discharge. Reading and writing were reportedly assessed, but no detailed information about specific tasks and procedure was provided.

Results and Conclusion

Upon admission, the patient was found to be oriented and to suffer no object agnosia, prosopagnosia, aphasia or verbal memory deficit. She demonstrated right homonymous hemianopsia and color agnosia. In addition, she was unable to read (in any of her three languages: Hebrew, Slovakian, and German) although her writing, in both writing directions (from right to left in Hebrew and from left to right in German and Slovakian), was intact.

With time, both the color agnosia and the alexia receded. Her reading difficulty receded simultaneously in Hebrew (learned in adulthood) and in Slovakian (her mother tongue) and she was gradually able to recognize letters and words, until she completely regained her reading ability. At first, she regained ability to recognize some letters but there were fluctuations in her performance (for same letters on different tasks or different days). Short words were read correctly more often than long words (in both languages). At initial stages of her reading recovery (specific MPO was not reported), the patient drew the letters on the palm of her hand or later in the air in order to be able to read them. Her reading was usually accompanied by lip movement and once she finally pronounced a word, she often repeated it several times.

Sroka et al. concluded that their patient suffered from agnostic alexia, manifested in both reading directions and for all the languages the patient knew. They noted the unusual complete recovery (consistent, however, with the patient's brain-scan data) of the alexia in all three languages.

Interestingly, both the nature of the patient's reading difficulty and the course of recovery appeared parallel in both Hebrew and Slovakian despite the fact that the two languages use different orthographies and opposite writing directions.

A partial recovery of reading skills is reported by Birnboim & Share (1995). They described a case of acquired surface dyslexia, with relatively preserved writing skills, who gradually reacquired reading ability.

Participant

The case (JV) reported in Birnboim & Share was of a 19-year-old patient with a high-school education who suffered a TBI followed by a coma lasting two months. She suffered a left temporo-occipital fracture and right hemiparesis. In the first year post-onset, the patient had poor orientation and severe amnesia. Her speech was characterized by short sentences, perseverations, and incoherence. Five years post-onset her language and cognition skills were still severely impaired. Following JV's enrollment in a rehabilitation program and a change in her motivation to learn and communicate, she began demonstrating improvement in her cognitive ability and reading skills. Verbal and visual memory skills were still impaired. Her reading age was assessed to be 7.

Task and Procedure

With the goal of understanding the patient's reading difficulty, JV was comprehensively assessed using various lists of words in isolation and in context. Various parameters that might influence her reading were incorporated into the word lists, including word type, frequency, length, regularity of spelling, and existence of homographs. Specific characteristics of Hebrew orthography, namely, the existence of homographs that share all graphemes but represent different words as well as the existence of two graphemes representing the same phoneme were used to dissociate lexical processes and grapheme-to-phoneme decoding processes of reading.

Results and Conclusion

Overall, JV's reading was slow and effortful. She made 28% errors in reading unvoweled single words and 46% errors reading the same words voweled. This difference was not statistically significant. The errors included a high proportion of vowel errors, often creating neologisms (e.g., *eifo* "where" read as *eifa*). Inflected or long words were more difficult than uninflected short words. When word length was tested separately, there was no difference between 3-4-letter words and 5-7-letter words. In context, JV demonstrated similar distribution of errors found in single word reading and did not appear to benefit from contextual cues. Comprehension of the material read was impaired.

Regular nonwords were read relatively well but "strange" nonwords, that is, foreign words that did not follow Hebrew patterns, resulted in errors. In addition, JV was not sensitive to spelling errors of the type that substituted between two graphemes representing the same phoneme (an English example would be "kat" for "cat"). In contrast to her impaired reading, JV's spelling skill appeared to be intact.

The authors took JV's performance to be relying on phonological, non-lexical decoding. Her visual representation of words appeared to be impaired. Context, which is crucially used in Hebrew to distinguish between homographs (a by-product of Hebrew unvoweled orthography) did not help JV choose the intended word when encountering homographs. Reading comprehension was also impaired, possibly due to erroneous word reading that did not benefit from contextual cues.

While JV was able to reacquire some reading skills, her reading remained the laborious grapheme-phoneme decoding process characterizing beginning readers' performance and lack of lexical access during reading.

In sum, Hebrew orthography offers a unique opportunity to study phonological processes during reading and to distinguish them from processes of direct lexical access. In the unvoweled version of Hebrew script, it is mainly consonants that are represented by the graphemes while vowels have to be determined by lexical and morphological constraints. In contrast, when the vowelized script is used, the orthography represents virtually one-to-one grapheme-to-phoneme correspondence. Reading performance and the use of morphological information in the absence of specific phonological information can be studied with Hebrew readers. Several researchers have addressed these issues with neurologically intact readers (e.g., Shimron, 1993; Ben-Dror, Frost, & Bentin, 1995; Frost, 1998). The aphasic presented in Birnboim & Share (1995) demonstrated phonological errors in reading and did not benefit from lexical and contextual constraints. Her performance can thus be attributed to breakdown of direct lexical access in reading as a result of brain damage. Additional studies of Hebrew reading deficits following aphasia could contribute to our understanding of intact and impaired reading processes.

Summary

An extensive search for studies that report cases of aphasia in Hebrew speakers yielded two types of studies: those that address a specific attribute of Hebrew and investigate the acquired language deficits vis-à-vis that aspect of the language and those that address general issues in aphasia, applicable to all languages.

Among the Hebrew-specific features, two aspects of Hebrew morphology are of interest: the systematic derivation of words from two bound morphemes (roots and morphological patterns) and the relatively rich inflection paradigm.

Barkai's patient produced non-existent combinations of existing roots and existing patterns (Barkai, 1980). Such errors suggest that these two abstract morphemes have a psychological reality for Hebrew speakers and may play a role during word production. Indeed, if Hebrew verbs were represented and accessed as whole-word units, errors of the type demonstrated by Barkai's patients would be highly unlikely. This is particularly interesting given the non-linear nature of Hebrew verb formation. The presence of derivational errors in the absence of inflectional errors demonstrates that derivational processes of word production can be selectively impaired.

Inflectional morphemes in Hebrew mark gender, person, number, and tense. While impaired inflectional morphology has been reported in the literature, it would be useful to address morpho-syntactic processes and systematically study the impairment of the various inflectional markers. Based on an existent syntactic theory, Friedmann & Grodzinsky (1997) predicted the possibility of a dissociation in the breakdown of gender agreement and tense marking. They demonstrated that the predicted dissociation was found in at least one agrammatic aphasic, who produced tense errors but virtually no agreement errors. But the opposite pattern, unexpected according to their theory, was evident in one of Baharav's (1990) patients, demonstrating agreement errors with virtually no tense errors. Further evidence for specific impairment patterns can be sought in additional aphasic speakers of Hebrew or any language with a rich morphological system.

In addition to the morphology-syntax interface, the interaction between morphology and phonology can be investigated using certain aspects of Hebrew grammar. Barkai (1980) interpreted the spirantization errors produced by his patient on the basis of the systematicity of phonological alternation according to morphological constraints.

Another characteristic of Hebrew that can interact with the manifestation of language deficits concerns Hebrew orthography. The underspecified phonology in the more common (unvoweled) Hebrew writing system suggests that during reading, grapheme-to-phoneme decoding and lexical access processes interact. Birnboim & Share (1995) used some of the characteristics of Hebrew orthography (e.g., frequent homographs and homophones that are spelled differently) to investigate the reading deficits of a case of acquired dyslexia. Further studies of reading deficits as well as of normal reading can employ the unique characteristics of Hebrew to explore the interaction between phonological and lexical processes in reading and to identify specific manifestations of breakdown of these processes in the various forms of alexia. For example, if lexical and contextual constraints are assumed to be crucial for reading unvoweled Hebrew, skilled Hebrew readers may be expected to be more likely to preserve these processes. At least in one Hebrew case of acquired dyslexia these very lexical aspects of reading appeared to be impaired (Birnboim & Share, 1995).

Other studies with Hebrew-speaking aphasics explored general aspects of aphasia such as pragmatic skills (Kasher et al., 1999), the distribution of paraphasias (Ani, 1996), phonological perception (Eviatar et al., 1999), and processes associated with aphasia rehabilitation (Gil et al., 1996; Rappaport et al., 1999; Fredman, 1975; Lapidot, 1995; Albert & Obler, 1978). In the studies of Kasher et al., Ani, and Gil and her colleagues, the lack of specific examples did not enable the addressing of language-specific issues. Similarly, the examples provided in Eviatar et al. from the performance of a Russian-Hebrew bilingual (1999) did not speak to the issue of the role of language specifics in the manifestation of the deficit. However, such studies that describe selective impairment in aphasics who speak more than one language can potentially address language-specific issues by way of comparing patterns of deficits in two (or more) languages.

The relation between the two (or more) languages of aphasic speakers had been the focus of early reports of polyglot aphasia (e.g., Halpern, 1949). The focus of those studies was comparing the order and degree of the recovery of the various languages of polyglot speakers. Even though these reports focus on patients with more than one language, unfortunately, they lack (as do the more recent reports of polyglot aphasia) systematic evaluation of various attributes of the languages under investigation or systematic comparisons of patterns of language deficits according to the different and similar characteristics of the languages.

Further studies exploring the manifestation of specific features of Hebrew syntax, morphology, phonology, and pragmatics in aphasia, as well as studies comparing these characteristics across languages within and across individuals, would contribute to our understanding of acquired language deficits specifically and the mechanisms of language generally.

Acknowledgments

I would to like to thank Loraine Obler for her helpful comments on earlier drafts of this paper and for the continuous advice, insight, and encouragement she has offered me and many other students.

Address correspondence to: Mira Goral, The Graduate Center of the City University of New York, 365 Fifth Avenue, New York NY 10016, U.S.A. E-mail: mgoral@gc.cuny.edu

References

Albert, M.L., & Obler, L.K. 1978. *The bilingual brain: Neuropsychological and neurolinguistic aspects of bilingualism*. New York: Academic Press.

Ani, B. 1996. Phonology as human behavior: Aphasia. *Journal of the Israeli Speech Language and Hearing Association,* 18: 105-128.

Baharav, E. 1990. Agrammatism in Hebrew: Two case studies. In L. Menn & L.K. Obler (Eds.), *Agrammatic Aphasia: A Cross-Language Narrative Sourcebook* (pp. 1087-1190). Amsterdam/Philadelphia: John Benjamins Publishing Company.

Barkai, M. 1980. Aphasic evidence for lexical and morphological representations. *Afroasiatic Linguistics*, 7: 163-187.

Ben-Dror, I., Frost, R., & Bentin, S. 1995. Orthographic representation and phonemic segmentation in skilled readers: A cross-language comparison. *Psychological Science*, 6: 176-181.

Berman, R.1978. *Modern Hebrew Structure*. Tel Aviv: University Publishing.

Birnboim, S., & Share, D. 1995. Surface dyslexia in Hebrew: A case study. *Cognitive Neuropsychology*, 12: 825-846.

Chomsky, N. 1992. A minimalist program for linguistic theory. *MIT Occasional Papers in Linguistics*. Cambridge, MA: MIT.

Eviatar, Z., Leikin, M, & Ibrahim, R. 1999. Phonological processing of second language phonemes: A selective deficit in a bilingual aphasic. *Language Learning*, 49: 121-141.

Fredman, M. 1975. The effect of therapy given in Hebrew on the home language of bilingual or polyglot adult aphasics in Israel. *British Journal of Disorders of Communication*, 10: 61-69.

Friedmann, N. & Grodzinsky, Y. 1997. Tense and agreement in agrammatic production: Pruning the syntactic tree. *Brain and Language*, 56: 397-425.

Frost, R. 1998. Toward a phonological theory of visual word recognition: True and false trails. *Psychological Bulletin*, 123: 71-99.

Gil, M., Cohen, M., Korn, C., & Groswasser, Z. 1996. Vocational outcome of aphasic patients following severe traumatic brain injury. *Brain Injury*, 10: 39-45.

Grodzinsky, Y. 1986. Language deficit and the theory of syntax. *Brain and Language*, 27: 135-159.

Halpern, L. 1949. Hebrew in recovery from sensory aphasia in polyglots. Translated in: M. Paradis (Ed.), 1983. *Readings on Aphasia in Bilinguals and Polyglots*. Montreal: Marcel Didier.

Kasher, A., Batori, G., Soroker, N., Graves, D., & Zaidel, E. 1999. Effects of right- and left-hemisphere damage on understanding conversational implicatures. *Brain and Language*, 68: 566-590.

Khamis, R., Venkert-Olenik, D., & Gil, M. 1995. Bilingualism in aphasia: The effect of L2 treatment on language performance of L1. *Proceedings of The International Symposium on Communication Disorders in Bilingual Populations*, 73-82.

Menn, L., & Obler, L.K. (Eds.) 1990. *Agrammatic aphasia: A cross-language narrative sourcebook*. Amsterdam/Philadelphia: John Benjamins Publishing Company.

Miceli, G., & Caramazza, A. 1988. Dissociation of inflectional and derivational morphology. *Brain and Language*, 35: 24-65.

Mathews, P. , & Obler, L.K. 1997. Processing derivationally suffixed words in agrammatism: Stress-change and length effects. Paper presented at the Academy of Aphasia, Philadelphia.

Paradis, M. 1983. *Readings on aphasia in bilinguals and polyglots*. Montreal: Marcel Didier.

Paradis, M. 1995. *Aspects of bilingual aphasia*. Oxford: Pergamon.

Pollock, J.Y. 1989. Verb agreement, universal grammar, and the structure of IP. *Linguistic Inquiry*, 20: 365-424.

Rappaport, Z., Gil, M., Ring, H., & Schechter, I. 1999. Isolation of speech area syndrome (ISAS): A follow-up study -- a rehabilitative approach. *Disability and Rehabilitation*, 21: 181-186.

Ravid, D. 1995. *Language change in child and adult Hebrew: A Psycholinguistic Perspective*. New York/Oxford: Oxford University Press.

Rosen, H. 1966. *A textbook of Israeli Hebrew*. Chicago: University of Chicago Press.

Shimron, J. 1993. The role of vowels in reading: A review of studies of English and Hebrew. *Psychological Bulletin*, 114: 52-67.

Sroka, H., Solsi, P., & Bornstein, B. 1973. Alexia without agraphia with complete recovery: Functional disconnection syndrome. *Confinia Neurologica*, 35: 167-176.

Tyler, L.K., & Cobb, H. 1987. Processing bound grammatical morphemes in context: The case of an aphasic patient. *Language and Cognitive Processes*, 2: 245-262.

Manifestations of aphasic symptoms in Hungarian

Andrew Kertesz* and Judit Osmán-Sagi°

*Department of Clinical Neurological Sciences, University of Western Ontario, St. Joseph's Hospital. London, Ont. Canada; °Institute for Psychology of Hungarian Academy of Sciences, Budapest, Hungary

Abstract—The characteristics of Hungarian aphasics reflect the difference in the features of Hungarian as a Finnish-Ugric language. These features are the highly complex use of inflectional morphemes, which are concatenated, providing markers for several functions in one word. Hungarian aphasics were systematically studied for features of agrammatism in language output, as well as in comprehension. The results of these studies suggest that in Hungarian there is a direct mapping of inflectional markings to semantics. The competition between definite and conditional conjugation is a major source of error just like in French, as well as competition between first and third persons. Omission errors occurred frequently, especially among Broca's aphasics omitting the indirect objects and Wernicke's aphasics the direct objects. Broca's aphasics also showed a lower level of pronoun use and article omission. Omissions and substitutions amounted to telegraphic speech in some patients, although this is not as marked as in English because of the high rate of omission in normal Hungarian. Wernicke's aphasics tended to produce paraphasic nouns and pronouns with some errors in inflection. Vowel harmony in the inflections was particularly resistant to deficit. Studies of sentence comprehension revealed that subject-verb agreement cues were most affected in Wernicke's aphasics and animacy cues were the weakest in Broca's aphasics. Although word order is rather free in Hungarian, canonical word orders were used for interpretation by all aphasics.

Systematic studies of comprehension in Hungarian aphasics show that phonemic contrasts in words are more sensitive than sound discrimination tasks. Higher levels of sentence processing are influenced by the availability of case marking suffixes, which are numerous in Hungarian.

Key words: Hungarian aphasia, agrammatism, case markings, inflection, thematic roles, phonemic contrast, aphasia types

Introduction

Hungarian is a Finnish-Ugric language with a unique phonology, grammar and lexicon. Very few lexical items of body parts, hunting or fishing are in common with Finnish, indicating their early separation at a period of hunting-gathering.

Hungarian is a highly inflected language, in contrast to English which is a mainly monomorphemic system. In Hungarian several inflections can be attached to a single stem which results in a concatenation of inflectional morphemes (with strict rules of vowel harmony). Some words can contain even four suffixes at a time, similar to

Turkish. Compare, for instance, the six common inflectional markings in English: past, third singular, plural, progressive, adverbial, and possessive (three of which are homophonous) to the 70 inflectional suffixes in Hungarian. None of the six markings in English can be combined with any other. No wonder Arnold Pick (1913) referred to English as "an essentially formless language of high standing." The distinction between English as an isolating language and Hungarian as agglutinating language results in different aphasic manifestations of agrammatism.

Definition of agrammatism as telegraphic speech had its origins in the study of languages, such as English, French, and German with many free standing, grammatical morphemes. Pick (postulated the cause of "telegraph style" aphasic speech was an economy of effort of impaired output processes in his 1913 article on "agrammatism." The agrammatism model of Kean (1979) emphasizes the omission of morphological markings on a phonological basis. Pick (1913), originally, felt that speakers of inflectional languages should produce paragrammatical errors rather than omissions. The nature and the regulation of the substitutions remain obscure. The model of competition has been postulated to explain some of the phenomena observed (Bates & Wulfeck, 1989; MacWhinney & Bates, 1989). According to this model, errors are expected where cues to marker selection strongly conflict. If there is a large set of possible markings then there would be a lot of substitutions.

In German and Italian, article selection depends on gender and number, and in German it also depends on case. The more options in the German system would lead to more errors in aphasic speakers, according to the competition model. However, Bates et al. (1987) found errors were restricted in scope and tended to occur in only one of the three dimensions. Omission errors in German were more frequent in Broca's aphasics. The tendency in general was to avoid difficult case forms by substituting a simpler, morphosyntactic frame. This has also been explained on the basis of complex computational paradigms, a recent extension of the "economy of effort" model of Pick (1913).

Certain features of Hungarian account for some of the errors made by Hungarian aphasics. Hungarian seems to have a closer relation between meaning and morphological markers. Because there is no gender in Hungarian, there is no need to record or retrieve formal class information about the noun. Most of the important markings are suffixes and they can be prepared without the exact semantic specification of the noun. Plurality is also marked independently of the case so there can be a fairly direct mapping back to semantics. Case, on the other hand, is marked quite clearly and regularly and based on cognitive distinctions or the meaning of the sentence rather than arbitrary syntactic subcategorization such as gender. Therefore, the problems in suffix selection in Hungarian can be attributed to the process that maps directly from semantics to lexical items (MacWhinney, 1976).

Nevertheless, Hungarian has extremely complex inflectional case forms. For instance, there are nine locative cases and several have semantically complex mapping between particular case markings and particular verbs. On the phonological level, the inflectional paradigms are quite irregular and the suffixes need to be adjusted to the stem in a fashion that is most frustrating for a foreigner to learn. Interestingly some of the phonological adjustments seem to be spared in Broca's aphasics, which contradict the phonological model of agrammatism.

Agrammatism and Sentence Production

MacWhinney and Osmán-Sagi (1991) studied the production system of Hungarian aphasic patients with special attention to competing case markings. The central case markings, those which are most tightly specified by the case frame of the verb, were:
1. Nominative, which is the uninflected and unmarked form of the noun. 2. Accusative, case suffix has the form "- t," which competes rather directly with the instrumental as well as often with the locative case (Zsilka, 1967). This seems to be a strong source of competition. 3. Dative "- nak, nek," which has an originally directional meaning like the English dative marker "to" but it also competes with the accusative pairs such as giving something to somebody. This kind of competition is similar but appears stronger than in English. 4. Instrumental or comitative suffix "- vel" corresponds to the English word "with" and it competes tightly with the accusative and dative in many semantic frames. Locatives suffixes and postpositions are numerous including a full set of 9 case suffixes and a set of 12 locative postpositions competing to produce a set of contrasts that mark position and directional movement. The ones that were involved in aphasic substitutions are: a. sublative (ra) corresponds to the English "onto," b. superessive (on) corresponds to the English preposition "on," c. inessive (ban, ben) corresponds to the English preposition "in," d. ablative (tól) corresponds to the English preposition "from," and e. The postposition under "alatt."

Verb markings are dozens in number but the main ones that had aphasic substitutions were the following: 1. infinitive suffix "ni." 2. 1st singular indefinite "ok." 3. 1st singular definite "om," used in the first person singular and the object is definite. 4. 3 singular definite "ja". It is used in the present declarative when the subject is the third person singular and the direct object is definite. 5. Conditional suffix is "na" corresponding to the English word "could." 6. 3 plural indefinite is "nak" which is a difficult one. It is used in the third person plural and when a direct object is indefinite or when the verb is intransitive.

The competition between definite and conditional conjugation in Hungarian is similar to French and it is a source of speakers error both in normal and aphasic patients. There was also a competition between definite and indefinite conjugation and between the first and third persons.

In the picture description task of MacWhinney and Bates (1978) in nine Broca's and five Wernicke's aphasics in Hungary, both groups had much higher rate of omission of inflectional markings of all argument types (MacWhinney & Osmán-Sagi, 1991). Subject ellipsis was particularly strong. There was a tendency to for Broca's aphasics to omit the indirect object and for Wernicke's aphasics to omit the direct object. Across argument types, Wernicke's had a much higher level of pronoun usage than did Broca's. Broca's also showed a very high level of article omission. Hungarian aphasics showed an elevated omission of case markings, and there were 14 substitutions of one case marking for another. These errors all involved the substitution of some close semantic competitor. Neither the view of Broca's as agrammatic nor the view of Wernicke's as paragrammatic was strongly supported.

Lexical omissions were difficult to interpret because subject omission is common in normal Hungarian. Verb omission, which is more definitely pathological, occurred in 11% of Broca's and 8% of Wernicke's cases. Substitution was severe in a few patients. Altogether there was a higher amount of case omission compared to Turkish and these aphasics came closer to producing what is usually thought of as telegraphic speech. Article omission is often sanctioned in normal speech and this was not a significant feature of Hungarian agrammatism. Broca's aphasics tended to omit nouns but Wernicke's aphasics, when confronted with word finding difficulty, tended to produce paraphasic nouns and pronouns. Some of these included errors inflection as well. The investigators expected violations of morphophonological rules mentioned above. However, these seemed resistant to impairment in this group of aphasics.

In summary, despite the inflectional complexity of Hungarian language, basic inflectional markings were less severely affected than in German and agrammatism is not as definite as it is in English with the omission of closed class words. Turkish has more regular inflectional rules and may be less affected. Inflectional markings in Hungarian have a more direct semantic relationship to words and tend to be better preserved. The hypothesis of the authors was that the results matched best with the competition model of agrammatism, manifesting only in areas where cues to marker selection strongly conflict such as confusing locatives with other locatives or similarly marked sentence elements.

Sentence comprehension Hungarian Aphasics

Hungarian is also different from other languages because the markers fully distinguish all persons, in all numbers, and all tenses. These markers not only indicate the person and number of the subject, but also the definiteness of the object. In other words, a single suffix in a Hungarian verb is used to marked both subjects - verb agreement and object - verb agreement. Unlike in other languages, the Hungarian article is not marked for case number nor gender, and it plays a fairly minimal role in sentence interpretation.

Experiments of sentence comprehension were carried out where case marking, subject-verb agreement, animacy and word order were varied, to detect the most important cues allowing sentence comprehension in aphasics (MacWhinney, Osmán-Sagi, & Slobin, 1991;MacWhinney & Osmán-Sagi, 1997). The results indicate the use of case marking cues was diminished in Wernicke's aphasics, but subject verb agreement cues were the most severely impaired. Animacy cues were weakest in Broca's and word order, a false friend in this instance, was used by all, especially conduction aphasics. Canonical word orders were overused in interpretations.

Thematic role interpretation in Hungarian Aphasics

Thematic role interpretation in aphasic patients was studied in enactment task (MacWhinney, Osmán-Sagi, & Slobin, 1991). In sentences with subject, direct object and verb, word order, place of case marking suffix, animacy of nouns, and detectability of direct object case marking connected to the wordstem were the variables. According to results in this task, Wernicke's patients utilized the main and unambiguous cue for thematic role interpretation - case marking suffix - less than Broca's aphasic patients. This result was replicated later (MacWhinney & Osmán-Sagi, 1997). A defect at the morphological level of speech processing, participating in detection of case marking suffix was hypothesized as an explanation for this phenomenon.

Hungarian hierarchies of comprehension

A systematic assessment of comprehension processes level by level was carried out by Osmán-Sagi (unpublished material, in preparation). Twenty aphasic patients participated in this study. All of them were of vascular origin in a chronic stage. They were capable to move, some of them with hemiparesis or hemiplegia. Fluent patients were significantly older than nonfluent and anomic patients. No significant differences were found in education and aphasia onset time. Fluent patients had somewhat milder aphasia than nonfluent ones, because of global and severe Broca's aphasics were included in the latter group. Not every task was applied to every patient and statistical analysis was done task by task. The results are summarized according to the tasks:

Global Comprehension

On the comprehension tasks of the Western Aphasia Battery (WAB) (Kertesz, 1982) (translation by Judit Osmán-Sagi) no significant differences were found between nonfluent and fluent groups. This is related to the milder Wernicke's and conduction patients compared with more severe global and Broca's patients. The group of anomic patients in all three tasks differ from the other two groups significantly.

Speech sound discrimination

In 210 pairs of CV nonword syllables the patients had to decide are the two syllables different or are they the same. The consonants of the syllable could differ in one phonemic feature: in voicing or in the place of articulation, or in vowel pairs. In 132 meaningful word pairs, half of them differed in one consonant. **Results**: no significant differences between nonfluent and fluent groups. (from the anomic group only two patients participated in this task). There are tendencies of higher performance of fluent group at pairs differing in voicing, while nonfluent groups performed better at pairs differing in place of articulation.

Spoken word/pictures matching

Fifty spoken nouns were given one by one to match to four pictures. In 20 items the target word has a distractor picture differing in one phonemic feature from the target word (target word: toboz (pinecone), distractor picture: doboz (box). One of the distractors are from the same semantic category, and one picture is neutral. Forty spoken verbs were given without phonemic contrasts.

Results: Nonfluent group and anomics matched nouns to pictures significantly better than fluent patients. In verbs differences are lower. This feature could be explained with the presence of phonemic contrast in noun matching. Comparing items without and with phonemic contrast distractor the combined aphasic groups' scores are higher in the part without phonemic contrast than with it. Performance of nonfluent group does not differ significantly in these two parts, while fluent and anomic patients were better at matching items without phonemic contrast. Error analysis revealed that without phonemic contrast no significant differences were found between phonological, semantic and visual errors with phonemic contrast significantly more phonological than semantic errors were produced ones. Differences in error types between nonfluent and fluent groups occurred only in phonological errors: nonfluent patients made highly significantly ($p < 0.00004$) more phonological errors with phonemic contrast. In fluent patients this difference is less significant ($p < 0.05$). Semantic errors in nonfluent patient are higher in part with phonemic contrast ($p < 0.1$) in fluent patients this difference is not significant.

Sentence comprehension

This task matches a spoken sentence to a choice of two pictures. Sentences types: Active SVO; OVS (no passives in Hungarian), CO: conjoined subject [The mother and the father look at the boy (A mama es a papa nezik a fiut)], CS: conjoined object [The boy looks at the mother and the father (A fiu nezi a mamat es a papat)], R1: subject relative clause [The boy who is behind the tree looks at the girl (A fiu, aki a fa mogott all, nezi a lanyt)], R2: object relative clause [The boy looks at the girl, who is behind the tree (A fiu nezi a lanyt, aki a fa mogott all)]. No differences were found in the overall performances of nonfluent and fluent groups, anomic patients performed significantly better.

Semantic discrimination of word pairs
Patients were given 132 word pairs for decision: do they mean the same or do they have a different meaning? Word pairs were from different word classes, and non-homonyms differ in meaning distance. Results: global performance of nonfluent group was significantly lower than that of the other two groups. Results by word classes significantly differ at nouns and at adjectives, not at the verbs. Meaning distance: best performance with the homonyms: fluent patients' performance is the worst at the words with close meanings ($p < 0.03$). The performance of nonfluent group is very low at the pairs with common semantic features. The word pair results correlate well with Raven scores.

Discussion

Results of speech sound discrimination tasks do not back up the hypothesis about basic difficulties in perceptual processing of grammatical morphemes in earlier works (Luria, 1966). These tasks assess lower level processing of speech sounds and defects in detection. Interpretation of the results suggest a higher level of interaction with the lexicon or semantic representation of words. English speaking aphasics also preserve phonological discrimination according to studies of Blumstein et al. (1977) and Boller (1978).

In word level speech comprehension matching tasks were used. According to overall results nonfluent patients performed better at noun matching then fluent patients. This is attributable to the presence of phonemic contrast distractors for nouns.

Phonemic contrast distractors appeared to elicit more phonological errors in nonfluent patients. Performance of the semantic task is more sensitive to produce an aphasic deficit than the sound discrimination task in this patient population. We hypothesize that the matching task needs more working memory capacity than the discrimination task. This could be limited in all of the patients (except anomic ones) as evidenced from the Token test. Next phase of this study will assess working memory capacity and the effect of perceptual difficulties of grammatic morphemes.

Several interactions of the various hierarchies of processing were detected by this series of studies. The influence of phonology in the sentence comprehension task supports the utilization of phonemic cues by speech therapists. The interaction of phonology with semantics is evident from the positive results of word discrimination tasks and no correlation with nonword discrimination. Higher level of sentence processing such as thematic interpretation are clearly influenced by the availability of case markings suffixes, which are numerous in Hungarian.

Acknowledgments

Grant Support for J. Osmán-Sagi: Hungarian State Research Fund OTKA N/2-600-2881-585; 2604; T-018391; T-030114.

Address correspondence to: Dr. Andrew Kertesz, Department of Clinical Neurological Sciences, St. Joseph's Health Center, 268 Grosvenor Street, London, Ontario, N6A 4V2.
E-mail: kertesz@lri.stjosephs.london.on.ca

References

Bates, E., Friederici, A., & Wulfeck, B. (1987). Grammatical morphology in aphasia: evidence from three languages. *Cortex, 23,* 545-574.

Bates, E., & Wulfeck, B. (1989). Crosslinguistic studies of aphasia. In B. MacWhinney & E. Bates (Eds.), *The crosslinguistic study of sentence processing* (pp. 328-371). New York: Cambridge University Press.

Blumstein, S.E., Cooper, W.E., Zurif, E., & Caramazza, A. (1977). The perception and production of voice-onset time in aphasia. *Neuropsychologia, 15,* 371-383.

Boller, F. (1978). Comprehension disorders in aphasia: A historical review. *Brain and Language, 5,* 149-165.

Kean, M.-L. (1979). Agrammatism: a phonological deficit? *Cognition, 5,* 69-83.

Luria, A.R. (1966). *Higher cortical functions in man.* London: Tavistock.

MacWhinney, B. (1976). Hungarian research on the acquisition of morphology and syntax. *Journal of Child Language, 3,* 397-410.

MacWhinney, B., & Bates, E. (1978). Sentential devices for conveying givenness and newness: a cross-cultural developmental study. *Journal of Verbal Learning and Verbal Behavior, 17,* 539-558.

MacWhinney, B., & Bates, E. (1989). The crosslinguistic study of sentence processing. New York: Cambridge University Press.

MacWhinney, B., & Osmán-Sagi, J. (1991). Inflectional marking in Hungarian aphasics. *Brain and Language, 41,* 165-183.

MacWhinney, B., & Osmán-Sagi, J. (1997). Agreement processing in Hungarian aphasics. *Acata Linguistica Hungarica, 44,* 73-86.

MacWhinney, B., Osmán-Sagi, J., & Slobin, D.I. (1991). Sentence comprehension in aphasia in two clear case-marking languages. *Brain and Language, 41,* 234-249.

Pick, A. (1913). *Die agrammatischen Sprachstörungen. Studien zur psychologischen Grundlegung der Aphasielehre.* Berlin: J. Springer.

Zsilka, J. (1967). *The system of the Hungarian sentence patterns.* Bloomington, IN: Research Center for Languages and Semiotics.

A longitudinal study of agrammatism in Polish: A case study

Hanna K. Ulatowska*, Maria Sadowska°, Danuta Kądzielawa‡

**University of Texas at Dallas, °Polish Academy of Sciences ‡University of Warsaw*

Abstract—Grammatical disturbances characteristic of the Polish language are illustrated in a longitudinal study of a patient with aphasia. Disturbances of the inflectional system of nouns and verbs consisted of substitution errors on inflectional suffixes and verb prefixes. Errors also occurred in stem alternations in both nouns and verbs. Forms which were more complex and less frequent were more disturbed. There was also extensive use of high-frequency diminutive forms. Errors decreased over time with no change in the basic patterns of disturbance. Preservations of specific structures in the language were also noted.

Key words: Polish, aphasia, agrammatism, longitudinal

Introduction

Cross-linguistic studies in aphasia have shown that language-specific features determine the patterns of omissions and substitutions in agrammatism (Menn and Obler, 1990). By suggesting additional explanations of error patterns derived from specific languages, these studies can contribute significantly to the understanding of the nature of agrammatism in general. Polish exhibits many grammatical categories, extensive inflectional and derivational systems, and morphophonemic phenomena. For these reasons it allows us to observe a great variety of language changes in aphasia.

The person with aphasia presented here is especially interesting for the following reasons: (1) A well-defined clinical picture associated with a focal brain lesion of a particular location; (2) preservation of language characteristics of specific aphasia type and characteristics of the personality of this person as shown by her rich linguistic repertoire; (3) preservation of the ability to communicate despite her linguistic deficits; and (4) availability of extensive data compiled systematically over four years of rehabilitation and observational data collected over 12 subsequent years of continuous contacts during which this subject returned to work and an active life. The above factors create an ideal opportunity to observe what is preserved and what is disturbed in the language of the aphasic subject, as well as, how these symptoms change over time. More importantly, the factors reveal features characteristic of aphasic disturbances in Polish.

Review of the Literature on Agrammatism in Polish

The investigation of agrammatic disturbances of language in aphasia in Polish was conducted concomitant with the general development of aphasia studies in Poland. It included descriptions and experimental studies of disturbances in inflectional forms, syntactic structures and lexical formations. The purpose of these studies was to explain the factors, which formed the general picture of the disturbances, and also to compare the phenomena in various types of aphasia. Additionally, there were investigations which were based on the comparative analyses of agrammatism, derived from the materials of aphasic speakers using their native language, aphasic speakers using different languages, and also on the persons learning Polish as a foreign language. The experimental investigations, which were focused on describing the character of aphasic disturbances of grammatical forms, syntactic disturbances in sentences and the description of differences between Broca's aphasia and Wernicke's aphasia, were presented in the work of Tomaszewska-Volovici (1976). The author pointed to the co-existence of two factors contributing to the picture of grammatical disturbances in aphasia, namely disturbances in the inflectional system and the phonetic alterations of inflectional forms. Furthermore, Tomaszewska-Volovici (1976) has described the area of disturbances of sentential structure and deletion of various syntactic structures, which were not considered as a manifestation of agrammatism strictly speaking, but as a result of the difficulties in the word finding. The observed phenomenon showed a similarity in the basic disturbances of grammatical forms in these two different types of aphasia without a particular predisposing factor. Another study of the Polish language, by Mierzejewska (1977), focused on the aphasic disintegration of the sound form of words and on the influence of the phonetic factor on the formation of secondary alterations of grammatic forms. Furthermore, Zarębina (1973) illustrated the repertoire of inflectional forms and syntactic structures in various individuals with aphasia. Strachalska (1978) described additional studies focusing on the aphasic disturbances in lexical forms, which fueled other studies done on the Polish language and its grammatical forms. She recognized the influence of the two factors contributing to the picture of the disturbances: the phonetic factor and the morphological factor. It appeared that the high frequency of use of a given form in the language deters its disintegration. However, the type of aphasia did not influence the quality of the disturbances when we compared Broca's aphasia and Wernicke's aphasia (since one can observe the same manifestations in the functioning of these two factors). The differences consisted only in the quantity of the individual type of disturbances, as well as the dynamics and the ease of word finding.

The view that the language structure and its characteristic features influence the symptoms of aphasic disturbances inspired the initiation of collaborative studies of aphasic dissolution in different languages, where the morphology of the Polish language was the primary framework (Mierzejewska, 1982). Sadowska (1991) described the role that the characteristic features of the Polish language played in the difficulties seen in native speakers with Wernicke's aphasia as compared to persons who used Polish as a foreign language. Despite the differences in the mechanism causing these difficulties, there appeared many similarities in the character of the disturbances of inflectional forms: in the use of suffixes, in morphophonological alternations, difficulties in coordination of inflectional forms, in agreement relations, in prepositional constructions, and also in the use of aspect in verbs. Kądzielawa (1978) investigated the evaluation of grammatical correctness in the sentences of brain-damaged individuals. This investigation, which was conducted on the Polish language, allowed the author to formulate conclusions pertaining to rules in Polish and in natural language in general. It appeared that grammatical rules function in a form of internal models, which condition the correct understanding of the meaning of the expression and the construction of the language. The language disturbances in aphasia do not destroy these models. Instead, they only modify them. These modifications of grammatical structures are produced because of a tendency to observe the primacy of the sentence's meaning over the principle of formal correctness of the sentence.

Jarema and Kądzielawa (1990) conducted a single case study of a patient with aphasia secondary to a fronto-temporal lesion of the left hemisphere. This study was based on the narrative discourse from the fable, Little Red Riding Hood, in the context of comparative studies of agrammatism on different languages. It showed a difference in the type of disturbance to morphology and syntax. The dissolution of the morphological system was manifested primarily by deletion and wrong distribution of grammatical morphemes. Deletion mainly affected pronouns, while the substitution remained in the same grammatical categories and involved both free and bound morphemes. Mainly reduction and simplification of syntactical structures characterized the disturbances in syntax. These features are integral to the Polish language and are elucidated in the case study presented here. This case study of agrammatism involves an individual with aphasia followed over many years and has been presented previously in several other works (Ulatowska and Sadowska 1988, 1989a, 1989b, 1992a, 1992b, 1992c).

Description of Grammatical Features of the Polish Language

The Polish language is a good representative of a language of an inflectional type. In its historical evolution, it has undergone many changes, which have affected all levels of the language (Doroszewski, 1963; Grzegorczykowa, Laskowski, & Wróbel, 1999). Some of these changes have increased the degree of its complexity. For example, many morphological alternations in inflectional and derivational forms occurred as a result of the phonetic changes in palatalization and depalatalization of consonants and vocalic changes. In noun inflections, changes involved shifts, which led to the occurrence of variants and polymorphism of many inflectional suffixes. These shift changes often led to the lack of uniformity in distributional criteria of those suffixes. For example, genetive singular of masculine gender has two suffixes *–a* or *-u*, which are semantically conditioned, and genitive plural has three suffixes, *-ów*, *-i*, and *–y*, which are phonologically conditioned.

In verb conjugation, there was a reduction to three basic tenses and also a shift of function expressing tense, perfective aspect and imperfective aspect to lexical and derivational categories. Thus, the category of aspect ceased to be a strictly grammatical category. The factor, which additionally increases complexity of verbs, is the system of prefixation. A verb prefix can be a marker of perfective aspect, as well as a marker of both aspect and semantic meaning or only semantic meaning. For example, in *z-robił*, *z-* indicates perfective aspect of the verb *robi*; in *za-robił*, *za-* indicates perfective aspect and a change in the semantic meaning of the verb; and in *za-miatał*, *za-* only modifies the semantic meaning of the verb stem.

During the evolution of verb conjugation, another change occurred. Namely there emerged two alternative forms of periphrastic future tense in imperfective aspect, which can be formed by finite verb form of auxiliary *być* plus infinitive, or finite verb form of that auxiliary plus preterite, for example, *będę pić* or *będę pił* (masculine gender) or *będę piła* (feminine gender).

Both semantic and syntactic criteria exist, which serve to differentiate the following grammatical categories in the Polish language: nouns, adjectives, pronouns, numerals, verbs, prepositions, conjunctions, interjections and particles. They reflect either inflectional or non-inflectional categories.

Inflection

Inflection includes: declension of nouns, adjectives, pronouns, numerals, and conjugation, which includes verbs. The basic categories of the contemporary system of declension consist of case, number, and gender; while conjugation consists of person, number, gender, mood and voice. The category of number, both in declension and conjugation, consists of the singular and the plural. The category of case includes seven forms: nominative, genetive, dative, accusative, instrumental, locative and vocative. The existence of these forms, both in the singular and the plural numbers, create a potential possibility of the occurrence of 14 paradigmatic forms of each inflected word. However, this potential number is counteracted by the syncretism of forms, which reduces the total number of possible inflectional forms.

Genetive has the highest frequency (33.97%), with the other cases having the following frequencies: Nominative- 28.03%, Accusative- 15.33%, Locative- 13.52%, Instrumental- 6.52%, Dative- 1.47%, and Vocative- 1.16% (Szpiczakowska, 1992).

The category of gender in declension consists of masculine, feminine and neuter. There are also two sub-genders of the masculine: animate and inanimate in the singular, and personal and non-personal in the plural. The category of gender in conjugation is marked in the preterite and consists of masculine, feminine and neuter. On the other hand, in the singular, neuter is marked only in the third form. In the plural, there is a differentiation of masculine personal and non-masculine personal. The analogical distinction occurs in the periphrastic future tense, which consists of auxiliary verb and preterite.

The category of tense consists of present, future and preterite. As mentioned before, the shifts of marking of tense and aspect by lexical means result in the three tenses that occur only in imperfective verbs, whereas perfective verbs exhibit only the preterite and future tense. The category of person has three forms in the singular and three forms in the plural. The category of mood consists of indicative, conditional and imperative. There are two forms of voice, active and passive.

Syntax

Sentence relations

Agreement:

This relation occurs in various elements of the sentence and consists of form agreement between subject and predicate according to number and gender, and between noun and modifiers according to number, gender and case. It is a very important feature of sentence structure in Polish (Buttler, 1973).

Government:
This relation occurs between the verb and object, or preposition and its object where the verb or preposition requires its object to be in a given case.

Word order in sentences
The canonical word order in a simple sentence in the Polish language consists of the subject group followed by the predicative group. However, because of the inflectional character of the Polish language this order is changeable. Thus, the order of the whole groups or the order of their elements can be altered. These order changes can cause various semantic modifications as they are utilized to change the distribution of information in the sentence. The order of elements indicates the distribution of the new and old information, and it also identifies the information, which has to be emphasized. In written texts, where there is no possibility of using intonation and stress, the order of the elements in the sentence is the only means of expressing topic and comment. In complex or compound sentences the freedom of word order is similar to that of simple sentences. Thus, the word order in sentences in the Polish language is flexible but not completely free.

Derivation

Word formation in the Polish language is produced through affixal or non-affixal, so-called regressive, derivation, and through compounding of two free stems (Grzegorczykowa & Puzynina, 1999). In the contemporary Polish language derivational processes are still very active although their dynamics and productivity have been undergoing various evolutions. Nouns exhibit the richest derivation, and its range increases all the time. It is especially evident in the following semantic classes: the names of tools, the names of performers of actions, abstract names referring to actions and states, nouns of places, and feminine nouns (Waszakowa, 1994).

Another characteristic feature of the derivational processes is the great productivity of diminutive formations. The diminutive forms occur in the series of several degrees of intensity and are very frequent in the language, especially in its colloquial variety.

The Patient

Clinical information

The patient in this study was a 39-year-old, right-handed female, with a degree in psychology. For a number of years, she suffered from untreated high blood pressure. On January 30, 1983, she experienced an acute headache and lost consciousness. The angiogram revealed an aneurysm in the left middle cerebral artery located just before trifurcation. It was narrow and 8 mm in length. There was a slight shrinkage of the artery. The patient underwent surgery and the aneurysm was clipped. Postoperatively, she incurred severe fluent aphasia. The patient was sent to a rehabilitation institute where she received speech therapy. After a year and a half, the patient took a job as a salesperson and continued her speech therapy. Four years after the surgery, a CT scan showed a hypodensive focus of irregular shape. It was 46 x 28 mm in size, located at the base of the left temporal lobe and corresponded to softening tissue of the original lesion.

Language profile

In the first period after the stroke, the patient presented with acoustic-mnestic aphasia according to Luria's classification or Wernicke-type aphasia with severity level 3, according to BDAE scale of 0 - 5.

The majority of errors in the patient's language were caused by inhibition of sensory-verbal traces characteristic of acoustic-mnestic aphasia and consistent with the site of the brain lesion. The patient exhibited difficulties in producing multi-syllabic words, words with complex phonological structure, series of words not related semantically, and also long complex phrases and sentences. Finding words in appropriate forms was also problematic. Phonological and semantic paraphasias and other word form disturbances appeared as well. These difficulties occurred in all modalities (i.e., speech, reading, writing, and also in repetition). However, reading and writing were more preserved than speech or repetition. There were also some difficulties in comprehension of structurally complex sentences. There were no difficulties with differentiation of sounds, phonologically similar words, or in comprehension of simple grammatical constructions.

The patient was administered standardized language tests, which included the Polish version of the Boston Diagnostic Aphasia Examination (BDAE), the Boston Naming Test (BNT), and the Token Test. The tests were administered at four different points in time: shortly after her stroke, four years post-stroke while she was in therapy, 13 years post-stroke as part of the investigation of metaphorical language in aphasia and lastly, at 16 years post-stroke to collect the additional comparative data for the present study. The comparison of the results of these tests is included in the table below.

		Time of Examination			
	Test	Initial	After 4 years	After 13 years	After 16 years
Severity of aphasia:	BDAE	3	4	4.5	4.5
Naming:	BDAE	97/114	102/114	114/114	114/114
	BNT	20/80	29/80	22/30	20/30
Comprehension:	BDAE	98/119	118/119	117/119	119/119
	Token Test	6/16	13/16	DNT	12/16

Table 1. Scores on language tests over time

The results of the tests indicate some improvements between the first two testings when the patient was undergoing therapy. However, stabilization of language function occurred during the later testings when the patient returned to active life and no longer worked systematically on her language.

Cognitive profile

Cognitive tests were administered in the later period of the investigation, namely 13 and 16 years after the stroke. The tests included subtests of Wechsler's Intelligence Test (stories, block design and similarities), Raven's Progressive Matrices (part A and B) and Choynowski's Memory Scale (version A—immediate and delayed recall). The following table shows the comparison of raw scores on the tests obtained at the time of the assessments.

Test	Time of Examination	
	13 years after stroke	16 years after stroke
Wechsler Intelligence Scale		
Stories	11	11
Block Design	25	17
Similarities	15	17
Raven's Progressive Matrices	24	22
Choynowski's Memory Scale		
Immediate Recall	7	4
Delayed Recall	2	6

Table 2. Scores on cognitive tests over time

The results show that the patient performed at approximately the same level over time and the differences represent acceptable variations.

Findings

Inflection

Declension of nouns

The category of case was tested in paradigms where verbs were given which govern a particular case together with nouns in masculine, feminine and neuter in nominative case. There were 18 stimuli. The testing was done two and four years after the stroke. The best-preserved cases, at both points of time, were genitive and instrumental; the most disturbed were dative and locative. The errors were substitutions of the required suffixes, by suffixes of the wrong case but most often of the same number. The substitution of accusative case by nominative case, also occurred, for example *widzę karp* (nominative) instead of *widzę karpia* (I see a carp). In that case, the error occurs in the syncretism of accusative and genitive of the masculine animate gender. The aforementioned relative preservation of the form of genitive and instrumental may be conditioned by the high frequency of genitive in the language and a small number of specialized suffixes in instrumental.

The investigation of inflectional forms in agreement relations in sentence context did not show any errors. There were occasional errors of agreement relations found in the texts. Interestingly, these errors occurred only in more complex forms, for example:

Target form: *opowiadał o chłopcu czternastoletnim*
Gloss: He talked about boy (loc., sing., masc.) fourteen-year (loc., sing., masc.)
Target English equivalent: He talked about a fourteen-year-old boy.
Defective production: *opowiadał o chłopce czternastoletniego*
Gloss: He talked about boy (loc., sing., fem.) fourteen-year (gen., sing., masc.)

The disturbances of agreement relations were much less frequent than the government relations, which indicate that the former may be more resistant to the damage in aphasia. The investigation of cases in the context of texts consisted of inserting the appropriate noun suffixes. In the tests given three years after the stroke, no errors were found. In the tests repeated 16 years after the stroke, there was only one isolated error, i.e. *miała sześć młodych kotek* (gen., pl., fem.) instead of *kotków* (gen., pl., masc.) (she had six young kittens). Also, the errors in inflections of nouns occurred in the tests of government relations with verbs and prepositions. They occurred at various points in time and consisted of combinations of verbs with nouns in dative case. For example, *dziwię się myślami* (I am puzzled about the thoughts), the patient used instrumental case instead of dative case. This type of error was not noticed in the test of judgment of grammaticality of inflection in sentences, such as *dużo ludzi dziwi się stosunkami w kraju* instead of *stosunkom* (many people are surprised at the relations in the country). Inflectional errors in government relations with prepositions in the context of sentences showed difficulties in producing the right forms, for example:

Target form: *polityk głosi o kryzysie*
Gloss: Politician talks about crisis (loc., sing., masc.)
Target English equivalent: The politician talks about the crisis.
Defective production: *polityk głosi o kryzysu*
Gloss: Politician talks about crisis (loc., sing., fem.)

In the above sentence, the locative suffix *–ie* was replaced by another locative suffix, which does not require stem alternation involving palatalization. Thus, the substitution can be interpreted as a strategy of avoidance of stem alternation, which may be considered one of the possible explanations of disturbances in suffix distribution. At the present time, the patient still makes many errors in noun inflection, especially in cases, which require stem alternation.

Conjugation of verbs

Aspect:

In verbs, aspect was the category which was studied the most. It was studied without context, where the forms were elicited with 20 stimuli for each aspect and the instruction, "Jan performed many activities. How do we say it, assuming that he did not complete them, (imperfective aspect) or that he completed them (perfective aspect)?". Aspect was also studied in sentence context with 10 stimuli.

The testing done two and 16 years after the stroke showed improvement in producing the forms of both imperfective and perfective aspect. The errors or inability to produce these forms in the earlier testing occurred primarily with verbs, which undergo stem alternation or suppletion of form in the perfective versus imperfective forms, for example, *wziął - brał* (took), or *znalazł - znajdował* (found). Another error was forming the perfective form from *zamiatał - zamiatł* (was sweeping) instead of *zamiótł* (swept). Also, there occurred errors of adding a wrong prefix in perfective aspect, such as *zasiwiał* (turned gray) instead of *osiwiał* (turned gray). This error re-occurred in the second testing, where the same prefix was added, whereas all other forms of both aspects were correct.

Four years after the stroke, aspect was also tested in the sentence context where the number of errors decreased presumably because the context facilitated the selection of the appropriate form. The example of the incorrect selection from the perfective/imperfective pair (*pisać - napisać*) was *Miałam trudności z pisaniem, więc list ten napisałam przez długi czas* (I had difficulties with writing so I wrote this letter for a long time). The testing of aspect 12 years later, showed that the same type of errors still occurred but their numbers decreased. No difference was found in the number of perfective, as compared with imperfective aspect. In the earlier testings of judgment of grammaticality of aspect, no errors were found at two and four years post-stroke. This may be due to the fact that the sentence context strongly favored the use of imperfective aspect by the presence of temporal adverbs expressing durative feature of action, for example *całymi godzinami* (hour by hour) or *wieczorami* (...all evenings).

Tense:

The formation of future tense was examined by giving the context of *jutro* (tomorrow) followed by an infinitive. The patient used a finite verb form instead of an infinitive. She did not use it in the preterite as is appropriate, but instead used it in the present, for example *będę piję* instead of *będę pić* (I will drink); or *będziemy cierpimy* instead of *będziemy cierpieli* or *cierpiały* (we will suffer).

In the preterite where there is a distinction in the suffix of masculine personal gender *-li* and non-masculine *-ły*, there were many errors consisting of substitution of the non-masculine suffix by the masculine personal gender. This error occurred both in the initial and the most recent testing and was evident in both sentence and text context.

Summary of inflectional system

On the basis of the above findings, it can be concluded that the disturbances occur in the inflectional system of both nouns and verbs across different categories such as case and gender in nouns, aspect, and tense, as well as person in verbs and gender in the preterite. In the disturbances of the case system, there is a tendency towards better preservation of the more frequent cases such as genitive or the cases which are formed by a smaller set of suffixes, such as instrumental. On the other hand, the cases which are less frequent in the language, such as dative, are more likely to be disturbed.

In the inflectional form of both nouns and verbs, those which undergo morpho-phonemic alternations are especially vulnerable. The prefixal system in verb forms, particularly in the perfective aspect, is also frequently disturbed. The errors consist of substitutions of prefixes in the verb forms. The errors in the suffixes of finite verbs in the preterite are also substitutions of the two possible forms, where the most frequent form of masculine personal forms substitute for the less frequent non-masculine forms.

Despite the quantitative changes in the investigations conducted over time, which consisted of a decrease in the number of errors, the type of disturbance remains the same. There are definitely fewer errors in writing than in speech. Completion of most of the tasks demands a considerable amount of time and concentration from the patient. The tasks of judgment of grammaticality were much easier and required less time.

At the present time, one notices much more frequent self-correction and monitoring of errors by the patient, even in the cases where the self-correction is not achieved.

Syntax

Syntax was examined primarily in the context of texts, both in the initial period after the stroke and also at later points of time. The texts were retold by the subject from the stories given to her, but they were also produced spontaneously. Most of them were narrative, but some were expository texts and letters written by the subject to the authors over a period of 15 years. The main feature of the sentences in the texts was preservation or preference for the order of subject, verb, object (SVO). Sentences were relatively short (about eight words) and the majority of them were simple sentences. Subordinate clauses consisted primarily of relative, noun, and temporal clauses. In the letters, a clear tendency to use a telegraphic style with a large number of clause equivalents was observed. These clauses often caused problems with clarity and interpretation of meaning. The telegraphic style seemed to be a strategy used purposely by the subject in order to avoid difficulties arising in more complex sentence structures. It is important to note that agrammatism, exhibited in inflectional forms and also in syntactic relations, did not affect the comprehensibility of the texts. Both four years after the stroke and recently, on examination of the function of noun cases in the sentence structure which did not have canonical order (SVO), the subject did not make any errors. However, the subject herself admitted that even now she has difficulties in understanding texts consisting of more complex structures and longer sentences. Thus, it seems that the syntax of the sentences of this subject is characterized primarily by the reduction of more complex syntactic structures with preservation of the canonical word order in sentences.

Derivation

The findings reported concern four types of constructions: agentive nouns, locative nouns, feminine nouns, and diminutives.

Agentive nouns

Agentive nouns elicited with probe questions such as, "What do you call someone who makes furniture?" were tested at four points in time: one year, two years, three years and 16 years after the stroke. There were four different stimuli. Even during the first testing, most of the answers were correct. The difficulty which arose was not caused by the derivational processes, but by problems with producing the words as lexical items.

In the earlier testing, there were disturbances in producing morphophonemic alternation of the stems with correct use of the suffix, for example, *windarz* (*windziarz*) (lift operator) and *gazetarz* (*gazeciarz*) (newspaper boy). In the last testing, there appeared a form *wspinacz na górach* (*ten kto wspina się po górach*) (he who climbs the mountains) (mountain climber). This form is a neologism, which was produced through the addition of the suffix *-acz* to the verb stem, which is productive with verb stems. The comparison of the test results at different points in time did not reveal any significant changes, and the ability to produce these forms was relatively well preserved.

Locative names

The formations were elicited with the probe question, "What do you call a place ... e.g. where planes land?". This formation was tested one year post-stroke and then again 16 years later, with 10 stimuli. During the first testing, all answers were correct. During the second time, the patient could not give two forms, presumably because of the difficulties of finding a given lexical item. Thus, the results showed the preservation of this type of derivation. There was no latency in producing the responses.

Feminine names

The formations were created from the given masculine forms. They were elicited with 21 stimuli by using the following probe question, "Please form a feminine name from the following nouns, for example *dentysta* (a male dentist)". The task required adding one of five different suffixes expressing that function and was performed correctly at both times of testing, i.e., two years and 16 years after the stroke.

Diminutives

The formations were elicited with a probe question, "What do you call a little ... for example, flower?" The testing was done 2 years, 4 years and 16 years after the stroke. In this task, there were 33 words, which required addition of various suffixes and produced alternations in the stems. During the first two testings, there were some errors which did not occur during the last testing. The errors consisted of replacing the required suffix with a wrong one, specifically the more productive suffix *–ek*, for example, *talerzek* instead of *talerzyk* (little plate), or *serduszek* instead of *serduszko* (little heart). The other type of error was the absence of alternation in the stem and adding a wrong suffix, for example *kapeluszek* instead of *kapelusik* (little hat) or *krawatek* instead of *krawacik* (little tie). During the last testing, the patient self-corrected errors of this type, although there still occurred some errors in more complex forms, for example *poleczko* instead of *pólko* (little field). Also during the last testing, a tendency to produce double diminutives was noticed, which did not occur during the earlier testing. Double diminutives consist of a sequence of two diminutive morphemes, and function as intensifiers of single diminutives, for example *główeczka, główka* (little head), *dzwoneczek*, *dzwonek* (little bell), *koteczek*, *kotek* (little cat). Moreover, the double diminutives were given as the first possibility. The tendency to use many diminutives was characteristic of the patient's speech. Several people who had frequent social contacts with the patient noticed that the tendency to use diminutives increased over time. The patient herself stated that she was aware of the highly frequent use of diminutives in her speech and that she was annoyed by it because she could not control it. She also confirmed that this tendency (to use diminutives) was characteristic of her premorbid speech.

Summary of derivational system
The results of the investigation of the patient's derivational system showed that, in general, there were no changes in derivational processes. The occasional errors consisted of substitution of the appropriate suffix with a wrong one which belonged to the same category. For example, the diminutive suffixes were replaced by other diminutive suffixes of the same derivational category. The phenomenon, which was an evident disturbance, was a frequent absence of alternation in the stems. This disturbance, which persisted over time and covered all language areas, was also present in the inflectional system.

Discussion

The findings of our investigation of agrammatism include phenomena which can be considered as language-general, i.e., documented in the previous studies of typologically different languages, and those which are considered as specific to this study. Those belonging to the first category will be only briefly mentioned, whereas the specific ones will be discussed in more detail since they are the main focus of the case presented here.

Language-general features

The language-general features, which were confirmed in our investigation, are summarized according to the level of the language structure they represent.

In inflection and derivation:
- the inflectional system is impaired more than the derivational system;
- disturbances of the morphophonological type occur both in inflection and derivation;
- agrammatism in the inflectional system in an inflectional language such as Polish consists of substitution of inflectional morphemes and not their deletion;
- there is no crossover in substitution of suffixes between inflectional and derivational systems;
- verb inflection is the most disturbed; and
- deletion of the functors occurs, especially those with a low semantic load, e.g., the particle *się* in reflexive verbs.

In syntax:
- canonical word order in clauses is preserved;
- grammatical complexity in clauses is reduced;
- phrase and clause length are reduced; and
- a tendency to use telegraphic style occurs.

Additionally,
- agramatism occurs in different modalities, i.e., in speech and in writing; and
- comprehension and judgement of grammaticality are better than the ability to produce forms.

Language-specific features

Phenomena related to the features inherent in the Polish language are influenced by two factors, the structural factor connected to the structure of individual forms and the frequency factor connected to frequency of occurrence of forms in the language.

Structural factor
Explanation of the functioning of the structural factor is based on an assumption that the processing load is connected directly to the degree of complexity of a given structure, which in turn leads to frequent disturbances of more complex structures. In the Polish language, the complexity of structures can be related to the functioning of different language components, i.e., phonological, morphological, syntactic, semantic or a combination of these in the formation of a given inflectional or derivational structure. For example, we observed the functioning of the phonological and the morpho-phonological component in the formation of a form with wrong alternation of the type such as *windarz* instead of *windziarz,* derived from the noun *winda* or the inflectional form *o kryzysu* (sing., gen.) instead of *o kryzysie* (sing., loc.). Functioning of the morphological component is especially evident in disturbances of noun inflections, which exhibit polymorphism of suffixes, for example, with locative case. There are disturbances of gender marking in verbs, which can be seen in the differentiation between *czytali* (masc.) and *czytały* (non-masc.) in the preterite. Other instances of disturbances occur in the periphrastic future tense, where there are two possible forms of infinitive or preterite after an auxiliary form, in the frequent use of multiple diminutives, and in the deletion of the reflexive particle.

The morphological-semantic component influences disturbances in verb prefixation, which has two functions: marking the grammatical aspect and modifying the meaning of the verb, such as, *zasiwiał* instead of *osiwiał.* Finally, the morphological-syntactic component is evident in disturbances of agreement relations between noun inflections governed by verbs or prepositions, for example with, *dziwię się myślami* (instr., pl.) instead of *dziwię się myślom* (dat., pl.).

Frequency factor
Explanations of the frequency factor can be derived from the principle that more frequent forms are more resistant to disturbance. This explains why the genetive case is relatively well preserved in the Polish language. Also, the overuse of the suffix *-ek* in diminutive forms, for example, *talerzek* instead of *talerzyk* can be explained by the frequency of that suffix. It is highly probable that the high frequency of the diminutive form in the Polish language explains the very high occurrence of these forms in the language of the patient.

Characteristics of the patient

Finally, it is also important to mention how some characteristics of the patient's communicative style and personality may be reflected in her agrammatism and her language. It is possible that the excessive use of diminutives and consequently, errors in diminutives are not only related to their frequency and their complexity in the Polish language, but also to the patient's idiolect and her personality. Since diminutives are often exponents of emotional load, they can be related to the patient's high emotionality and gregarious social nature. Thus, the features of premorbid idiolect and personality may produce additional sources of change to some forms, such as diminutives in this case. On the other hand, a premorbid tendency of this patient to use informal style often associated with telegraphic style, allowed her to use this style as an adaptive strategy. This in turn, may have contributed to the avoidance of using more complex structures, especially verbs and in this way, camouflaged the extent of her agrammatism in certain communicative contexts. It was the longitudinal nature of this investigation that allowed us to observe, over time, many fascinating accomodations of this patient to her deficits. However, the most important observation, which we gained from the longitudinal nature of the study, is that although there was an improvement in the patient's overall linguistic functioning, the *nature* of the language impairment did not change. Extensive use of diminutives and telegraphic style remained pervasive across time.

Concluding Remarks

This study has greatly improved our knowledge of the ways in which the symptoms of aphasia interact with the intricacies of the Polish language. First, the qualitative nature of the study showed us areas of particular vulnerability, reflected in errors on structures of high complexity, such as stem alternations and prefixal and suffixal verb systems. Second, the longitudinal nature of the study revealed structures which are relatively resistent to improvement over time, such as gender distinctions in preterite verb forms, in contrast with structures such as certain noun suffixes which do improve. Finally, the study showed us some compensatory strategies, such as telegraphic style, which emerged over time thanks to one specific feature of the Polish language, i.e., a high tolerance for elliptical structures due to the highly inflectional nature of the language.

Address correspondence to: Hanna K. Ulatowska, Ph.D., University of Texas at Dallas, Callier Center for Communication Disorders, 1966 Inwood Rd., Dallas, Texas 75235, U.S.A.
E-mail: hanna@utdallas.edu

References

Buttler, D. (1973). Składnia [Syntax]. In D. Buttler, H. Kurkowska, H. Satkiewicz (Eds.), *Kultura języka polskiego* (pp. 301-448). Warszawa: PWN.

Choynowski, M. (1962). *Skala pamięci* [Memory Scale]. Warszawa: Pracownia Psychometryczna PAN.

De Renzi, E. & Vignolo, L. (1962). The token test: A sensitive test to detect receptive disturbances in aphasics. *Brain, 85*, 665-678.

Doroszewski, W. (1963). *Podstawy gramatyki polskiej* [Foundations of Polish grammar]. Warszawa: PWN.

Goodglass, H., & Kaplan, E. (1983). *Assessment of aphasia and related disorders.* Philadelphia, PA: Lea & Febiger.

Grzegorczykowa, R., Laskowski, R., & Wróbel, H. (Eds.) (1999). *Gramatyka współczesnego języka polskiego. Morfologia* [Grammar of contemporary Polish. Morphology]. Warszawa: PWN.

Grzegorczykowa, R., & Puzynina, J. (1999) Słowotwórstwo rzeczowników [Derivation of nouns]. In R. Grzegorczykowa, R. Laskowski, H. Wróbel (Eds.), *Gramatyka współczesnego języka polskiego. Morfologia* (pp. 389-468). Warszawa: PWN.

Jarema, G. & Kądzielawa, D. (1990). Agrammatism in Polish: A case study. In L. Menn & L. Obler (Eds.), *Agrammatic aphasia: A cross-language narrative sourcebook* (pp. 817-893). Philadelphia, PA: J. Benjamins.

Kaplan, E., Goodglass, H. & Weintraub, S. (1983). *Boston Naming Test.* Philadelphia, PA: Lea & Febiger.

Kądzielawa, D. (1978). Ocena poprawności gramatycznej zdań przez chorych z ogniskowymi uszkodzeniami mózgu [Judgement of grammaticality of sentences in patients with focal brain injuries]. In S. Urbańczyk, J. Basara, & K. Rymut (Eds.), *Badania lingwistyczne nad afazją* (pp.75-81). Wrocław: Ossolineum.

Menn, L. & Obler, L. (Eds.), (1990). *Agrammatic aphasia: A cross-language narrative sourcebook.* Philadelphia, PA: J. Benjamins.

Mierzejewska, H. (1977). *Afatyczna dezintegracja fonetycznej postaci wyrazów* [Aphasic disintegration of phonetic form of words]. Wrocław: Ossolineum.

Mierzejewska, H. (1982). Zagadnienia teoretyczne badań porównawczych nad afazją [Theoretical problems in comparative studies in aphasia]. In S. Urbańczyk, J. Basara, & K. Rymut (Eds.), *Badania lingwistyczne nad afazją* (pp. 9-30).Wrocław: Ossolineum.

Raven, J. C., Court, J. H. & Raven, J (1978). *Coloured Progressive Matrices – Revised.* London: H. K. Lewis & Co.

Sadowska, M. (1991). Neurolingwistyka i glottodydaktyka [Neurolinguistics and glottodidactics]. *Poradnik Językowy, 9-10,* 390-398.

Strachalska, B. (1978). Zaburzenia formacji słowotwórczych języka polskiego w afazji akustyczno-mnestycznej i ruchowej [Disturbances of derivational forms in aphasia in the Polish language]. In S. Urbańczyk, J. Basara, & K. Rymut (Eds.), *Badania lingwistyczne nad afazją* (pp. 203-210). Wrocław: Ossolineum

Szpiczakowska, M. (1992) Charakterystyka ilościowa kategorii gramatycznych rzeczownika [Quantitative description of grammatical category of nouns]. In W. Miodunka (Ed.), *Język polski jako obcy. Programy nauczania na tle badań współczesnej polszczyzny* (pp. 185-189). Kraków: Uniwersytet Jagielloński.

Tomaszewska-Volovici, H. (1976). *Agrammatyzm w afazji* [Agrammatism in aphasia]. Wrocław: Ossolineum.

Ulatowska, H. K. & Sadowska, M. (1988). Features of agrammatism in Polish: A case study. *Journal of Neurolinguistics, 3*(1), 77-88.

Ulatowska, H. K. & Sadowska, M. (1989a). Discourse and agrammatism. *Polish Psychological Bulletin, 20*(2), 127-138.

Ulatowska, H. K. & Sadowska, M. (1989b). Cechy agramatyzmu u osoby z uszkodzeniem lewego płata skroniowego [Agrammatism in a patient with left temporal lesion]. *Neurologia i Neurochirurgia Polska, 22*(3), 243-245.

Ulatowska, H. K. & Sadowska, M. (1992a). Some observations on aphasic texts. In S. J. Hwang & W. R. Merrifield (Eds.), *Language in context: Essays for Robert Longacre* (pp. 51-66). Arlington, TX: Summer Institute of Linguistics and the University of Texas at Arlington.

Ulatowska, H. K. & Sadowska, M. (1992b). Przetwarzanie tekstu w afazji [Transformation of texts in aphasia]. *Poradnik Językowy, 6,* 432-446.

Ulatowska, H. K. & Sadowska, M. (1992c). Tekst w afazji [Texts in aphasia]. In T. Dobrzyńska (Ed.), *Typy tekstów* (pp. 47-58).Warszawa: IBL.

Waszakowa, K. (1994). Tendencje rozwojowe w słowotwórstwie polszczyzny końca XX wieku. [Developmental tendencies in lexical formations in Polish of the end of the twentieth century]. In S. Gajda & Z. Adamiszyn (Eds.), *Przemiany współczesnej polszczyzny końca XX wieku.* (pp. 53-60). Opole: Wyższa Szkoła Pedagogiczna..

Wechsler, D. (1981). *Wechsler Adult Intelligence Scale – Revised.* San Antonio, Texas: The Psychological Corporation.

Zaręba, M. (1973). *Rozbicie systemu językowego w afazji.* [Disintegration of language system in aphasia]. Wrocław: Ossolineum.

The Manifestation of Aphasic Symptoms in Spanish

Alfredo Ardila

Memorial Regional Hospital, Hollywood, Florida

Abstract—Few systematic descriptions of aphasia characteristics are available about the Spanish language. Three different language aspects are examined in this paper: phonology, aphasic substitutions (paraphasias), and morphosyntax. It has been observed that phonological errors in Spanish speaking aphasics more frequently involve vowels than consonants. It is proposed that this is related to the salience of vowels observed in Spanish. Phonological paraphasias are about 10 times more frequent than verbal paraphasias in conduction aphasia. In Broca's aphasia, they are only five times more frequent, whereas in Wernicke's aphasia the number of phonemic and verbal paraphasias is roughly the same. It is difficult to know how well this distribution fits in other languages, due to the absence of cross-linguistic comparisons. Agrammatism in Spanish has certain distinguishing characteristics, particularly due to the significant flexibility of the word order in the sentence and the use of some preposition to distinguish the object from the subject. Certain aspects of Spanish grammar are relatively resistant in cases of brain pathology, such as the subject-verb concordance. Some relatively unusual types of sentences, such as passive sentences, are significantly impaired in cases of agrammatism. Obviously, those grammatical aspects that are stronger (i.e., more crucial to distinguish the agent and the patient, such as the use of the preposition "a") are also better preserved in cases of Broca's aphasia associated with agrammatism. It is concluded that, despite similarities with aphasia described in other Indo-European languages, certain aphasia features can be considered characteristic of the Spanish language.

Key Words: Spanish, aphasia, paraphasias, agrammatism

Acquired language disturbances correlate with specific language idiosyncrasies. Spanish, as any other language, possesses phonological, lexical, grammatical, and semantic peculiarities. Comparing aphasia symptomatology across different languages, some common characteristics, but also specificities, are expected. As an example, the article omissions represent the most evident sign of agrammatism in Spanish. Such sign is simply nonexistent in some other languages, such as Russian, simply because articles are nonexistent in Russian.

Unfortunately, few systematic descriptions of aphasia characteristics are available about the Spanish language. Even though the interest in aphasic disturbances is quite strong in the Spanish-speaking world, only a few aphasia analyses have been published. Departing from those few reports, in this paper an analysis of aphasias in Spanish speaking individuals will be presented. Three different language aspects will be examined: phonology, aphasic substitutions (paraphasias), and morphosyntax.

Phonology

A few published journal articles have analyzed the phonological disorders in Spanish. Ardila, Montañes, Caro, Delgado, and Buckingham (1989) reported the phonological changes observed in a group of 37 Spanish-speaking aphasics (Table 1). Patients were divided into four groups: those with Broca's aphasia, conduction aphasia, Wernicke's aphasia, and anomia. It was found that vocalic changes are particularly infrequent in Spanish. In the motor types of aphasia (Broca's and conduction aphasia—conduction aphasia can be interpreted as a motor type of aphasia; Luria, 1976) vocalic changes represented less than 10% of the total number of substitutions. In Wernicke's aphasia and anomia they represented about 25%. Voiced/ voiceless changes in stop consonants were also rather infrequent. They represented less than 5% of the total number of changes in the motor types of aphasia and about 10% in Wernicke's aphasia and anomia. Most of the phonological or literal paraphasias were due to errors in the place of articulation, manner of articulation, or both. In motor aphasias, phonological paraphasias are due in about one-quater of the cases to phoneme omissions. Phoneme metatheses (e.g., mano → namo) are particularly unusual in Spanish. In anomic aphasia they represent barely 5% of the aphasic phonemic substitutions.

Table 1. Characteristics of 744 phonological paraphasias in 37 Spanish-speaking aphasics. Different types of errors and mechanisms utilized are presented (Adapted from Ardila et al.1989)

	Broca (n=10)	Conduction (n=9)	Wernicke (n=8)	Anomia (n=10)
TYPE OF ERROR				
Manner of articulation	46	57	35	32
Place of articulation	13	11	9	22
Place and manner of articulation	28	23	19	16
Voiced/voiceless (oral stops)	4	4	8	8
Vocalic errors	9	5	29	22
MECHANISMS UTILIZED				
Substitution	62	52	72	78
Omission	20	25	12	2
Reduplicative substitution	8	15	8	10
Addition	5	4	6	5
Reduplicative addition	2	3	1	0
Exchange	1	1	1	5

It is interesting to emphasize the very low frequency of vocalic changes observed in Spanish-speaking aphasics. It may be assumed that they are due to the vocalic characteristics of Spanish. As a mater of fact, the vocalic system in Spanish is extremely simple and includes only five vowels. Syllables are formed around the vowels. Usually, vowels are not reduced in spontaneous language and vowels have a significant salience. That is, they are very clearly produced and easily heard. Furthermore, when learning to write, children present usually errors in consonants, not in vowels (Ardila, Rosselli & Ostrosky, 1996; Bravo-Valdivieso, 1982, 1988). In other words, vocalic errors are unusual not only in cases of acquired language disturbances, but also in other conditions.

Ardila and Rosselli (1992) analyzed language repetition errors in a group of 41 Spanish-speaking aphasics. The three repetition subtests from the Boston Diagnostic Aphasia Examination—Spanish version (Goodglass & Kaplan, 1979) were used (words, high probability and low probability sentences) (Table 2). Aphasic patients were divided into five groups: extrasylvian motor aphasia (i.e., transcortical motor aphasia or dynamic aphasia), Broca's aphasia, conduction aphasia, Wernicke's aphasia, and anomia. It was found that repetition errors were unusual in extrasylvian motor aphasia.

Some errors were recorded only in low probability sentences. Errors were due to word omissions and changes in word order. It should be noted that Spanish presents a significant flexibility in sentence word order. In their repetitions, extrasylvian motor aphasia patients tended to make sentences more usual and probable. In Broca's aphasia, errors were mainly due to phonological paraphasias (phoneme omissions, phoneme substitutions, and phoneme anticipations). Repetition of sentences was agrammatical with evident omission of grammatical connectors. Percentage of errors was similar under the three conditions (words, high probability sentences and low probability sentences). In conduction aphasia, phonemic errors, self-corrections and successive approaches to the target word were observed. A significant difference was observed between the high and low probability sentences. Repetition of high probability sentences (as well as simple spontaneous speech) can be relatively correct. Conversely, production of unusual phoneme sequences and unusual word sequences was abnormal. Phonological paraphasias were particularly evident. In Wernicke's aphasia phonological paraphasias were observed in word and in sentence repetition. Sentence repetition was notoriously harder than word repetition, probably due to limitations in verbal memory. In anomic aphasia, errors were found in sentence repetition, particularly in repetition of long sentences. Word omissions and semantic paraphasias were observed.

It was concluded that repetition errors are associated with perisylvian aphasias (Broca, conduction and Wernicke), but, all the aphasia groups, including extrasylvian (transcortical) motor aphasia, present some errors in language repetition tasks. Repetition errors, however, are not only quantitatively but also qualitatively different. Depending upon the repetition test, errors can be very evident or minimal and even absent in a particular group of aphasic patients. Different mechanisms can underlie errors in aphasia.

Table 2. Percentage of correct repetition in different types of aphasia in the three repetition subsets (words, high probability and low probability sentences) of the Boston Diagnostic Aphasic Examination (Adapted from Ardila& Rosseli, 1992).

	Extrasylvian motor (n=6)	Broca (n=5)	Conduction (n=6)	Wernicke (n=13)	Anomia (n=4)
Words	98	46	63	74	100
High probability sentences	95	50	53.7	45	71.2
Low probability sentences	67.5	45	21.2	22.5	52.5

Paraphasias

In the aphasia domain, a significant effort has been devoted to the analysis of paraphasias. Jakobson (1964) interpreted paraphasias as paradigmatic errors in the phoneme or word selection process. Lecours and Lhermitte (1969) illustrated the existence of different types of errors in aphasics' language deviations and proposed to distinguish different types of paraphasias. Blumstein (1973) observed that substitutions represented the most common type of error found in phonological paraphasias, followed by simplification errors (omissions) and additions.

Lecours (1975) proposed the concepts of paradigmatic distance (formal similarity between the substituting and substituted units) and index of formal similarity (number of common phonemes between the substituting and substituted words). Several authors have introduced a difference between phonetic and phonemic changes (Blumstein, 1973; Lecours & Caplan, 1975; Lecours & Lhermitte,1969; Ryalls et al, 1988). Phonetic (example., [t] → [t']) are not designated as "phonetic paraphasias" but as "phonetic deviations " (Ryalls et al., 1988). The name paraphasia is not used because they do not represent errors at a linguistic level. As a matter of fact, they result from an inappropriate realization of the phonemes. As a general rule, in motor aphasias, an abundant number of phonetic deviations are found. Some phonemic errors found in motor aphasias, however, could be the result of such significant phonetic deviations that are erroneously perceived as phonemic changes (Buckingham, 1989; Lecours & Caplan, 1975). In this regard, they represent phonemic changes for the listener, but phonetic distortions for the speaker (Buckingham & Yule, 1987). For the aphasic patient they represent a motor articulatory defect; for the listener they are phonemic paraphasias. Luria (1976) emphasized that the literal (i.e., phonemic) paraphasias observed in afferent motor aphasia (conduction aphasia), even though perceived as phonemic substitutions, are indeed articulatory substitutions.

Table 3 presents some examples in Spanish of the different types of deviations observed in aphasics' language.

Table 3. Examples of aphasic deviations in Spanish.

Type of deviation	example
Phonemic or literal paraphasias	
Omission	perder -> peder
Addition	camino -> carmino
Displacement	tortuga -> toturga
Substitution	mesa -> tesa
Verbal paraphasias	
Formal	cajetilla -> carretilla
Morphologic	nochemente
Semantic	
same semantic field	nariz -> oreja
antonymous	salir -> entrar
superordinate	caballo -> animal
proximity	papel -> lápiz
Unrelated	casa -> nariz
Sintagmatic paraphasias	el acuario del pez -> la jaula del león
Circumlocutions	
Description	moneda -> redonda, pequeña
Instrumental function	reloj -> para la hora
Neologisms	camisa -> surinjor

Ardila and Rosselli (1993) analyzed the frequency of different types of paraphasias in 30 Spanish-speaking aphasics. The sample was divided into five different groups: extrasylvian (transcortical) motor aphasia, Broca's aphasia, conduction aphasia, Wernicke's aphasia, and anomia. Three subtests from the Boston Diagnostic Aphasia Examination, Spanish version (Goodglass & Kaplan, 1979) were used: Oral description of Plate #1 (The Cookie Theft), repetition, and naming. A total of 833 errors were analyzed.

Table 4. Mean frequency of different types of paraphasias found in different aphasia types (standard deviations in parentheses). A total of 833 errors were analyzed (Adapted from Ardila & Rosselli, 1993).

	Extrasilvian Motor (n=5)	Broca (n=5)	Conduction (n=6)	Wernicke (n=11)	Anomia (n=3)
Phonemic paraphasias					
Omissions	-	8.4 (5.6)	3.0(2.3)	4.5(4.3)	-
Additions	-	1.8 (1.2)	1.3 (1.1)	1.4(1.2)	-
Dispacements	-	1.0 (1.2)	1.7(0.9)	1.0(1.2)	-
Substitutions	-	7.4(6.2)	9.5(8.4)	9.6(5.4)	0.6(0.4)
Verbal paraphasias					
Formal	0.6(0.8)	1.0(1.0)	1.5(0.9)	4.6(4.5)	1.0(0.8)
Morphologic	-	0.8(0.4)	-	2.4(1.5)	-
Semantic					
semantic field	0.2(0.4)	2.2(1.7)	0.8(0.8)	5.1(2.4)	7.0(0.8)
antonyms	-	-	0.2(0.3)	0.5(0.9)	-
superordinate	-	-	-	1.5(1.9)	1.0(1.4)
proximity	-	-	-	0.2(0.3)	0.5(0.4)
Unrelated	-	-	0.2(0.3)	4.5(6.0)	3.7(5.1)
Syntagmatic	0.2(0.4)	-	-	0.5(0.8)	-
Circumlocutions					
Description	-	-	0.2(0.3)	1.2(2.0)	0.6(0.4)
Function	-	-	-	1.5(1.9)	0.6(0.9)
Neologisms	-	1.0(0.9)	2.3(3.5)	10.9(13.8)	-

Phonemic paraphasias were significantly associated with perisylvian aphasias (Broca, conduction and Wernicke). In extrasylvian (transcortical) motor aphasia, just a few verbal paraphasias were noted. In Broca's aphasia, the number of paraphasias was particularly high, as a result of phoneme omissions and substitutions. Sporadically, other types of paraphasias are also observed. Phonemic paraphasias were quite frequent in conduction aphasia, as a result of phoneme substitutions, but also phoneme omissions and displacements. Wernicke's aphasia patients present all the types of paraphasias mentioned above. The amount of literal and verbal paraphasias was roughly equivalent. Anomic patients present especially semantic verbal paraphasias due to substitutions within the same semantic field. Occasionally, superordinate words and circumlocutions are also found. Table 4 summarizes the frequency of paraphasias found in this group of Spanish-speaking aphasics. It is difficult to know how this frequency compares with the frequency found in other languages.

The ratio "phonemic paraphasia/verbal paraphasia" was calculated. It was found to be different in the different aphasia subtypes. In Broca's aphasia, literal paraphasias are about 5 times more frequent than verbal paraphasias. In conduction aphasia, this relation is 10:1. In Wernicke's aphasia the ratio "phonemic paraphasia/verbal paraphasia" is close to 1. This means that the amount of phonemic and verbal paraphasias is roughly the same. In extrasylvian motor aphasia literal paraphasias are virtually absent, and only sporadically verbal paraphasias are recorded. In anomia, literal paraphasias are practically non existing and the ratio "phonemic paraphasia/verbal paraphasia" is close to zero. As a matter of fact, the definition of anomia supposes the presence of verbal but not literal paraphasias.

In summary, even though some deviations tend to predominate in certain aphasia subtypes, the relationship between aphasia type and paraphasia type is not simple. Furthermore, the frequency of paraphasias analyzed above corresponds to Spanish. Nonetheless, it can be conjectured that Broca's aphasics in any language will present a significant number of phonemic paraphasias particularly as a result of phoneme omissions. By the same token, it can be anticipated that conduction aphasia patients will present a very high frequency of literal paraphasias, specially observed in repetition tasks, associated with self-corrections and approximations. In any language, it can be expected that Wernicke's aphasics will present a significant amount of both, phonemic and verbal paraphasias. In extrasylvian motor aphasia, only verbal changes are expected. In anomia, language deviation must correspond to semantic substitutions; this type of change is usually included in the definition of anomia.

Morphosyntax

To the best knowledge of the author of this paper, only three research studies dealing with agrammatism in Spanish-speaking aphasics have been published in the international literature (Reznik, Dubrovsky & Maldonado, 1995; Benedet, Christiansen & Goodglass, 1998; Ostrosky-Solis, Marcos-Ortega, Ardila, Rosselli & Palacios, 1999). Obviously, agrammatism in Spanish, as in any other language, has certain specific characteristics. There are grammatical aspects shared by every language, but also specific grammatical idiosyncrasies in every language. Intuitive clinical observations suggest the following comments:

1. In Spanish-speaking aphasics, article omissions represent the most evident sign of agrammatism. It is very easy to observe in spontaneous language, or even in naming tasks (Spanish speakers usually name using the article plus the name). It is interesting to note that patients with Wernicke's aphasia, even though unable to find nouns, may correctly select the article (in Spanish there are masculine and feminine nouns and corresponding articles) (e.g., they fail in naming la mesa -the table; but they know it is la -feminine, not el -masculine)

2. Spanish has flexible word order. However, in cases of agrammatism, flexibility in word order can be impaired. Patients with Broca's aphasia can produce and understand sentences with a canonical word order, but they fail with other non-canonical word orders.

Reznik, Dubrovsky, and Maldonado (1995) reported the case of a 55-year-old right-handed woman with a large right parietal-temporal, cortical-subcortical lesion extending to the occipital and frontal lobes. Initially a severe aphasia and anarthria were found. It was assumed that the patient presented with a crossed aphasia. Three months later, a significant improvement was found. A diagnostic of Broca's aphasia was proposed. A 535-word oral language sample was analyzed. In this language sample, 51.03% of the words corresponded to open class (lexical items) and 48.97% to closed class words (grammatical elements). This distribution was similar to the distribution found in normal language. Two different types of defect, however, were found: (1) frequent omission of clitic pronouns, and (2) difficulty in producing sentences with a canonical order.

This is an extremely unusual case that in no way can be considered typical of Spanish agrammatism. The patient suffered an extensive right hemisphere lesion and three months later her language was nearly normal.

As a matter of fact, the patient did not present any evidence of agrammatism, and maybe she did not even present any evident aphasia. Word order in sentence is extremely flexible in Spanish. In cases of agrammatism in Broca's aphasia the opposite situation is usually found: only canonical order is accessible to the patient. Frequent production of a non-canonical order cannot be interpreted as agrammatism. Only clitic pronoun omission could be accepted as indicative of agrammatism. Nonetheless, it would be an extraordinary selective form of agrammatism that cannot be interpreted as the usual agrammatism found in Broca's aphasia (Benson & Ardila, 1996). Even if the patient presented aphasia and agrammatism, crossed aphasia is not a good model to study agrammatism.

Benedet, Christiansen and Goodglass (1998) selected six Broca agrammatic aphasics. A Spanish version of the Morphosyntactic Battery developed by Goodglass, Christiansen and Gallagher (1993) was administered. It was found that the relative order of difficulty in production as well as in comprehension of grammatical morphemes, was similar to that reported in English. Nonetheless, two significant exceptions were found: (1) Spanish-speaking aphasics had a better subject-verb concordance; and (2) comprehension of active and passive sentences was worse in Spanish than in English. In Spanish, a verbal form is more dependent on the pronoun than in English (e.g.., yo tengo, tú tienes, él tiene, etc; I have, you have, he has, etc.). It seems understandable that the relationship between subject and verb can be stronger and more resistant in Spanish than in English. By the same token, passive constructions are more frequent in English than in Spanish. In consequence, it seems understandable that they are stronger and more resistant in English than in Spanish. Ostrosky et al. (1999) analyzed the syntactic and nonsyntactic strategies used for understanding sentences by Spanish-speaking Broca's aphasic patients. A linguistic instrument was applied to 10 patients with Broca's aphasia. A forced choice task was used in which the patient listened to 190 different reversible sentences and was asked to select one of four options presented on a plate; each option contained a pair of animals performing a specific act and only one option was correct. The results showed significant differences in the use of syntactic and nonsyntactic strategies. Broca's aphasic patients used only morpho-syntactic marks with high cue validity. No significant effects of word order were found. Different strategies were observed in understanding sentences. The first depends on grammatical knowledge of the function of the preposition "*a*" (to) as a sign of the direct object. Another strategy depends, it would seem, on intuitions concerning the canonical grammatical structure, and is observed in a tendency to interpret as a subject (agent) the nominal phrase that precedes the transitive verb, and as the object (patient), the one that appears immediately after the verb. However, when the word order is changed from SVO to VSO, the role of patient is assigned to the noun that follows the verb.

Spanish speaking patients with Broca's aphasia, unlike normal subjects, did not use structural strategies in active sentences, such as the canonical word order of the sentence. They used free functors such as articles. Nor could they process passive sentences. Neither syntax complexity nor canonical word order affected their performance. As long as the preposition "a" was present, the subjects performed at the same level on sentences in which the order was canonical (TV-Pat) or not (Pat-TV). Likewise, both in simple sentences such as active, and in pseudocleft sentences, the only significant factor was the uncontracted preposition, and there were no significant differences of order or definiteness. The absence of use of these other strategies produced comprehension alterations. However, even in active sentences containing a preposition, the performance of the aphasic patients was less efficient than that of normal subjects (70% accuracy vs. 98% in normals). This means that in Broca's aphasics, free functor morphemes are available for processing. However the patients do not process all the morphology because in passive sentences that contain two signs "*por*" and the verbal ending "*-ado*", the results obtain by chance. Nor was a significant effect found in the processing of sentences with the contracted preposition "*al*", which suggests that the coalescence a+el could be affecting performance. Apparently the preposition "*a*" is resilient to brain damage because it is a crucial source of information for thematic assigment in Spanish.

In contrast to studies conducted in other languages with Broca's aphasics, Spanish-speaking patients use no principle of word order or surface markers such as the determiner. The fact that comprehension strategies are different seems to follow from this.

Conclusions

This paper has attempted to summarize the main studies dealing with aphasia in Spanish-speakers. As in any language, certain phonological, lexical and morphosyntactic idiosyncrasies are found in Spanish. Some tentative conclusions can be drawn:

1. Phonological errors in aphasia more frequently involve vowels than consonants. This is particularly true in motor types of aphasia. Reading and writing errors in normal subjects and disabled children are more unfrequently found in consonants than in vowels. This is related with the salience of vowels observed in Spanish. Syllables are assembled around the vowels.

2. Phonological paraphasias are about 10 times more frequent than verbal paraphasias in conduction aphasia. In Broca's aphasia, they are only five times more frequent, whereas in Wernicke's aphasia the number of phonemic and verbal paraphasias is roughly the same. In anomic patients, a significant number of verbal, especially semantic paraphasias are observed, whereas phonological paraphasias are virtually absent. It is difficult to know how well this distribution fits in other languages, due to the absence of cross-linguistic comparisons.

3. Agrammatism in Spanish has certain distinguishing characteristics, particularly due to the significant flexibility of the word order in the sentence and the use of some preposition to distinguish the object from the subject. Relatively significant morphological complexity may play a certain role in Spanish agrammatism. Certain aspects of Spanish grammar are relatively resistant in cases of brain pathology, such as the subject-

verb concordance. Some relatively unusual types of sentences, such as passive sentences, are significantly impaired in cases of agrammatism. Obviously, those grammatical aspects that are stronger (i.e., more crucial to distinguish the agent and the patient, such as the use of the preposition "*a*") are also better preserved in cases of Broca's aphasia associated with agrammatism.

Address correpondence to: Alfredo Ardila, Ph.D., 12230 NW 8 Street, Miami, Florida 33182, USA. E-mail: AArdila@compuserve.com

References

Ardila, A., Monta-Fles, P., Caro, C., Delgado, F., & Buckingham, H.W. (1989). Phonological transformations in Spanish-speaking aphasics. *Journal of Psycholinguistic Research, 18,* 163-180.

Ardila, A., & Rosselli, M. (1992). Repetition in aphasia. *Journal of Neurolinguistics, 7,* 1-11.

Ardila, A., & Rosselli, M. (1993). Language deviations in aphasia: A frequency analysis. *Brain and Language, 44,* 165- 180.

Benedet, M.J., Christiansen, J.A. & Goodglass, H. (1998). A cross-linguistic study of grammatical morphology in Spanish and English-speaking agrammatic patients. *Cortex, 34,* 309-336.

Benson, D.F. & Ardila, A. (1996). *Aphasia: A clinical perspective*. New York: Oxford University Press.

Blumstein, S. (1973). *A phonological investigation of aphasic speech*. The Hague: Mouton.

Bravo-Valdivieso, L. (1982). Dislexia, maduracio'n e integración de funciones cerebrales. *Avances en Psicologia Clínica Latinoamericana, 1,* 111-127.

Bravo-Valdivieso, L. (1988). Las dislexias: investigacio'n en Latinoamerica. In A. Ardila & F. Ostrsoky-Solís (Eds.), *Lenguaje oral y escrito* (pp. 172-193). Mexico: Trillas.

Buckingham, H.W. (1989). Mechanisms underlying aphasic transformations. In A. Ardila & F. Ostrosky (Eds.), *Brain organization of language and cognitive processes* (pp. 123-145). New York: Plenum.

Goodglass, H., Christiansen, J.A. & Gallagher, R. (1993). Comparison of morphology and syntax in free narrative and structured tests: Fluent versus nonfluent aphasics. *Cortex, 29,* 377-407.

Goodglass, H., & Kaplan, E. (1979). *Evaluación de las afasias y de transtornos similares*. Buenos Aires: Editorial Me'dica Panamericana..

Jakobson, R. (1964). Towards a linguistic typology of aphasic impair-ments. In A. De Reuck & M. O'Connor (Eds.), *Disorders of language*. London: Churchill.

Lecours, A.R. (1975). Methods for the description of aphasic transforma-tion of language. In E.H. Lenneberg & E. Lenneberg (Eds.), *Foundations of language development*, vol. 2 (pp. 75-94). New York: Academic Press.

Lecours, A.R., & Caplan, D. (1975). A review of 'A phonological investigation of aphasic speech' by S.E. Blumstein (1973). *Brain and Language, 2,* 237-254.

Lecours, A.R., & Lhermitte, F. (1969). Phonemic paraphasias: Linguistic structures and tentative hypotheses. *Cortex, 5,* 193-228.

Luria, A.R. (1976). *Basic problems of neurolinguistics*. The Hague: Mouton.

Marcos, J. & Ostrosky, F. (1995). Estrategias para la asignación de papeles temáticos en la interpretacio'n de enunciados en español. In D. Pool (Ed.), *Estudios en linguística formal*. Mexico, D.F.: El Colegio de Mexico.

Ostrosky-Solis, F., Marcos-Ortega, J., Ardila, A., Rosselli, M., & Palacios, S. Syntactic comprehension in Broca's Spanish-speaking aphasics: Null effect of word-order. *Aphasiology, 13,* 553-571.

Reznik, M., Dubrovsky, S., & Maldonado, S. (1995). Agrammatism in Spanish: A case study. *Brain and Language, 51,* 355-358.

Ryalls, J., Valdois, S., & Lecours, A.R. 1988. Paraphasia and jargon. In F. Boller, J. Grafman, G.Rizzolati, & H. Goodglass (Eds.), *Handbook of neuropsychology*, vol 1 (pp. 367-373). Amsterdam: Elsevier Sciences

Agrammatic verb errors in Spanish speakers and their normal discourse correlates[1]

José G. Centeno[*], Loraine K. Obler[°]

[*]*St. John's University, Jamaica, NY;* [°]*City University of New York Graduate Center, New York, NY*

Abstract—Agrammatic verb errors are characterized by a reliance on simple verb forms without elaborated inflectional markings. Yet agrammatism studies on verbs have not addressed the possible correlations that might exist between pre-morbid verb use patterns and agrammatic verb production, especially frequency in oral discourse. Spanish, a language with a highly inflected verb system, is a useful context to explore this interaction. This study investigated agrammatic and normal verb use for those Spanish verb tenses found in daily conversation (Silva-Corvalán, 1983; Bentivoglio and Sedano, 1992). We analyzed agrammatic verb performance in spoken discourse and a sentence repetition task, and compared it with verb use in normal spoken and printed narratives.

Findings suggested that the present was the most frequently used tense by both agrammatics and normals. The preterit, the second most frequent tense in normals, was similarly employed correctly by agrammatic subjects in the repetition task but was not present in their discourse. All other verb tenses, minimally found in normal texts, were similarly never produced in agrammatic discourse or minimally produced correctly in agrammatic sentence repetition. These results suggest that daily verb use patterns have a facilitating effect on verb use by Spanish-speaking agrammatic subjects. They agree with earlier arguments supporting the resistance of high-frequency words to errors in normal and aphasic speakers (Hall, 1954; Howes, 1964; Rochford & Williams, 1984), possibly a reflection of an automatic, routinized, and overlearned nature due to their early acquisition (Schnitzer, 1989), and a significant degree of lexical strength (Bybee, 1985; 1995; Stemberger & MacWhinney, 1986).

Agrammatism, a language disorder secondary to acquired brain damage, has been described as a simplification of sentence structure due to "a limited output use of the syntactic and morphological resources of the language" (Menn & Obler, 1990, p.3). Specifically, oral expression in agrammatic speakers is limited by the presence of one or several morphosyntactic deficits such as the omission of free morphemes or functors (e.g., prepositions, conjunctions, and articles), bound morphemes (e.g., verb inflections), and modifying terms (e.g., adjectives and adverbs).

In terms of verb use, agrammatic English speakers have been observed to rely on simple verb forms, such as the uninflected infinitive and the *-ing* forms (i.e., *go*, *going*), at the expense of complex verb inflectional markings and use of the auxiliary (Goodglass, 1976). Similarly, in languages with a highly inflected verb system, agrammatic individuals display a reduction in the complexity of their spoken verb forms with a prominent use of infinitives, as reported in French speakers (Tissot, Mounin, & Lhermitte, 1973; Nespoulous, Dordain, Perron, Jarema, & Chazal, 1989); and number, gender, person, and tense errors as reported in both French and Italian speakers (Jarema & Kehayia, 1992; De Bleser & Luzzatti, 1994).

Indeed, Spanish, with a highly inflected verb system similar to that of other Romance languages, such as French and Italian, has been shown to have a similar agrammatic profile for verbs. For example, in a preliminary study by the first author summarized in Centeno (1996), a severely agrammatic Spanish Venezuelan speaker, AC, generated the following narrative after being asked what her work activities were before her CVA:

Cosía ... casa ... a trabajo ... algo ... a cocinar ... a fregar ... este ...
[he/she] was sewing... house... at work... something... to cook... to wash [dishes]... this ...
a cocinar ... yo cocino la casa ... cocinar bien.
to cook ... I cook the house... to cook well.

As in French and Italian agrammatism, verb use by the above agrammatic Spanish speaker was characterized by the reliance on simple verb forms without elaborated inflectional markings to indicate the time or person associated with the actions expressed by the verb. Verb forms in her narrative included the infinitive (fregar/to wash [dishes], cocinar/to cook), the present (cocino/I cook), and the imperfect (cosía/[he/she] was sewing).

Several explanations have been advanced to explain agrammatic verb errors in French and Italian. In French, Jarema and Kehayia (1992) argue that the mental organization of verbs might involve an uninflected stem to which those inflectional possibilities allowed for each stem of the verb can be appended. Their assertion is based on the errors for tense and aspect markers that agrammatic French-speaking subjects produced in repetition and sentence-production tasks involving one- or two-root French verbs. Error patterns led these authors to claim that "lexical storage reflects the internal morphological structure and idiosyncrasies of verbal lexical items" (p. 559). In this manner, one-root verbs (e.g., *manger* [to eat]: *mang-*) and their inflectional options would be stored in one common storage unit whereas two-root verbs (e.g., *partir* [to leave]: *par-* or *part-*) would have two separate, yet linked, storage units for each root and its respective inflectional options.

Jarema and Kehayia's investigation provided additional important evidence for the study of agrammatism. The variability in the types of substitutions generated by the subjects for the target inflections, for instance, the present and imperfect tenses for the past and future tenses for one-root verbs, and the infinitive for two-root verbs, demonstrated that the infinitive or the gerund are not the only verb forms to which agrammatic speakers might resort in their oral expression. Other inflections permitted by the wide range of inflectional possibilities in the paradigm of a particular verb can be erroneously accessed. Consistent with Jarema and Nespoulous (1984), who reported that the infinitive is not the only substituting form used by French-speaking agrammatics, Jarema and Kehayia's findings markedly contrast with the agrammatic reduction of verb use in English, a less inflected language than French, to two characteristic verb forms; the infinitive and *-ing* forms.

The inflected Italian verb system has also served as research tool to address the question of verb inflections in agrammatism. In an investigation of the required gender and number markings of the past participle in Italian verbs, De Bleser and Luzzatti (1994) observed that the rate of success exhibited by agrammatic Italian-speaking subjects depended on the syntactic complexity of a sentence. Agrammatic subjects performed better with simple sentences than in complex sentences in cloze tasks requiring the production of the appropriate participial inflection. In Italian, gender and number inflectional assignment for the past participle requires the interpretation of the grammatical features of an appropriate antecedent, such as a noun or a pronoun.

Based on the deficient inflectional marking of the past participle in complex sentences, De Bleser and Luzzatti claim that agrammatic speakers might not be able to access the full syntactic representation of the argument structure of verbs in complex sentences since the two subjects participating in the study used a minimal-distance solution or random selection to assign gender and number inflections to the past participle used in the sentence context. They place the possible locus of the impairment at the positional level in Garrett's (1980) sentence production model in which grammatical suffixes are mapped onto functional representations.

Only a very small number of studies has particularly addressed the production of verb inflections by agrammatic Spanish speakers. In fact, there is a considerable paucity in the aphasia literature on aphasic symptoms in Spanish speakers (see Ardila, 2001). Regarding verbs, Schnitzer (1989) attempted to provide some insight into the use of verbal inflectional markings by Spanish-speaking aphasics. In his study of an undifferentiated aphasic group of monolingual Spanish and bilingual Spanish-English Puerto Rican individuals, Schnitzer reported inflectional errors in the spoken modality for most of the grammatical and semantic features in the Spanish verb structure, which will be discussed later in this chapter. These findings, which included errors of tense-aspect, person, and number markings, led Schnitzer to support a regression to a Givonian "pragmatic" [2], "conversational interpretation" of language (p.140) to explain aphasic verb use.

Because Schnitzer's investigation employed an unselected subject population, we cannot delimit specific information concerning verb use by Spanish-speaking agrammatic individuals. Yet, his investigation provided an important observation in that it suggested that poor performance in some of the investigated tense-aspect forms, such as the future, conditional, and present perfect, might have resulted from their limited frequency in ordinary communication and the use of alternative verb forms to convey their meaning. For instance, he reports that the inflected future tense (e.g., comeré[he/she/it will eat]) is rarely used conversationally in Puerto Rican Spanish. Rather, the construction *"ir a"* (to be going + infinitive) is generally used instead. This finding is consistent with observations of informal, spoken Spanish in Venezuela (Sedano, 1994).

Other studies have specifically addressed morphosyntactic agrammatic errors in Spanish. Reznik, Dubrovsky, and Maldonado (1995) analyzed the spontaneous narrative sample generated by an agrammatic Argentinean speaker. In particular, this speaker exhibited no morphological errors but difficulty with word order (e.g., " *encontré no a una hermana mí" [no encontré a mi hermana]/found no to a sister my [I didn't find my sister], p. 364) and clitic pronouns (" *hermano mío"[mi hermano]/brother mine [my brother], p. 363). Reznik et al. do not provide a theoretical explanation to account for the word order deficits in this agrammatic speaker but argue that, for clitic pronoun restrictions, Chomsky's Government Binding principles can have an explanatory value. In particular, clitic pronoun deficits seem to emerge when the speaker has to process null elements (*e*) as in the expression "Pedro la entregó" (Pedro gave it). In syntactic terms, this expression can be represented as "Pedro la_i entregó e_i" in which there is a relationship between the clitic *la* and the null element *e*.

Other research on agrammatic Spanish verb errors invokes the role of morphological structure as a relevant factor. Based on results from a sentence repetition task (which were analyzed in a different fashion for this chapter), Obler, Harris, Meth, Centeno, and Matthews (1999) argue that agrammatic verb errors may stem from production difficulties involving the structural length of the verb inflection. Results showed that agrammatic Spanish speakers experienced more difficulty as the syllabic length of the inflectional affixes increased.

In this chapter, we demonstrate the role of discourse frequency as a facilitating factor in agrammatic Spanish verb use. We present evidence suggesting that agrammatic verb errors can reflect premorbid uses of verb forms when we compare agrammatic and normal verb use for those verb tenses occurring in daily conversation. We will begin with a description of the discourse characteristics of Spanish verbs. Then, we will present findings from the aphasia and Spanish language development literature suggesting the possible facilitating role of lexical frequency of occurrence in aphasic language use. Finally, we will discuss our study, its findings, and its possible implications for the understanding of verb use in agrammatism in Spanish speakers.

Discourse Features of Spanish Verbs

The Spanish verb system, like that of French and Italian, is highly inflected. Spanish verbs encode several morphosemantic notions: tense, mood, aspect, person, and number. In addition, each Spanish verb involves a "thematic vowel", *a*, *e*, and *i,* easily recognized in the infinitive (e.g., *tomar*/to drink, *comer*/to eat, *subir*/ to move up, to go up). According to their thematic vowel, Spanish verbs can be classified into first, second, and third conjugation classes depending on whether their inflectional endings follow the *-ar*, *-er*, or *-ir* inflectional patterns, respectively. Also, Spanish verbs are subject to the stress-assignment rules of the language, generally carrying a strong-weak syllable pattern. For an in-depth discussion of these features, the reader is advised to refer to Centeno (1996), Qüilis and Hernández-Alonso (1990), and Stockwell, Bowen, and Martin (1965). Here, we focus on an additional factor having an impact on the use of Spanish verbs, namely, frequency patterns in daily discourse.

Some Spanish verb forms are employed more frequently than others in informal conversation, as shown by sociolinguistic research. Silva-Corvalán (1983) reported the prominent use of certain verb tenses in the narratives produced by Chilean and Mexican speakers. She observed that despite the frequent alternated use of the present [*presente*[3]], the preterite [*pretérito perfecto simple*], and the imperfect [*pretérito imperfecto*] tense-aspect forms in spoken discourse, the preterite-present alternation emerged as the most prominent shift. Silva-Corvalán argued that, by bringing past events into the present time, it helped the speaker describe past events in a "more vivid and dramatic" (p. 775) manner, as if they were occurring in the present time in front of the narrator. Inspection of the language samples provided by Silva-Corvalán revealed that other tense-aspect forms, including the *condicional* and *pretérito pluscuamperfecto*, were produced by the speakers in conversation less frequently than the present, preterite, and imperfect.

Bentivoglio (1987) and Bentivoglio and Sedano (1992) provide similar evidence confirming the use of the above tense-aspect forms (i.e., *presente, pretérito perfecto simple, pretérito imperfecto, condicional*, and *pretérito pluscuamperfecto*) and, in the case of Bentivoglio and Sedano (1992), utterances indicate the presence of an additional form, the *pretérito perfecto compuesto*, in the informal spoken language samples of Venezuelan speakers. These tense-aspect forms used in informal conversation by Spanish speakers are summarized in Appendix A.

Lexical Frequency of Occurrence and Aphasic Language Use

Studies on agrammatic verb errors have not addressed the possible correlations that might exist between agrammatic verb use and pre-morbid verb use patterns, especially frequency in spoken discourse. There is evidence supporting the importance of frequency of occurrence for lexical items in normal language processing and aphasia. Specifically, high-frequency forms seem to be resistant to errors in normal language processing. For instance, Hall (1954) reported that high-frequency words are much easier to recall than low-frequency words in a free-recall task. In terms of aphasic language, Howes (1964) showed that aphasics favored the use of high-frequency vocabulary instead of low-frequency lexical items in their free speech. Rochford and Williams (1965) found that the effect of frequency of usage favoring high-frequency words held for both verbs and nouns in a pictured naming task given to aphasics. Goodglass (1976) and Stemberger (1984) suggest the possibility that the hierarchy of loss errors in agrammatism might be sensitive to usage frequency patterns. In particular, the plural suffix *-s*, the 3sg. pres. suffix *-s*, and the possessive clitic *-s* are differentially affected in this order. The plural, the most frequent, is the least affected; the present, with an intermediate frequency, is moderately affected; and the possessive, the least frequent, is the most commonly affected. Finally, Miceli and Caramazza (1988) found that an Italian agrammatic speaker's word repetition was better for frequent units than for infrequent units.

Some pyscholinguistic principles have been proposed to account for the resistance of high-frequency vocabulary to errors. Stemberger and MacWhinney's (1986) analyses of spontaneous speech errors showed that high-frequency inflected forms are less susceptible to at least one type of inflectional error - the no-marking error (e.g., "need" for "needed"). These findings led the investigator to argue that frequency is encoded in terms of "strength" (p. 24) or degree of semantic or pragmatic activation which protects the item from error. Hence, high-frequency items, involving higher activation levels than low-frequency items, would be less vulnerable to phonological and inflectional errors than those forms with a low frequency.

In line with Stemberger's argument, Bybee (1985, 1995) similarly advances the notion of "strength" in morphological processing in the lexicon. To Bybee, an item that occurs frequently in actual language usage would have a high lexical strength, would be easy to access, have more morphological fusion, and exhibit an autonomy that makes it resistant to change and prone to semantic independence.

In sum, frequency of occurrence, not investigated in earlier studies of agrammatic verb errors, might seem to be an important factor. The above discussion illustrated that high- and low-frequency lexical items, involving different degrees of morphological fusion, have a different "strength" to resist impairment and, in turn, could result in different production patterns in agrammatic expression.

Frequency Patterns in Spanish Acquisition and Discourse

The relationship between verb acquisition and discourse patterns can also be incorporated in the study of agrammatic verb impairment. In particular, the frequency patterns observed during the development of verb inflections in Spanish-speaking children and their usage patterns later observed in the discourse of Spanish-speaking adults deserve our attention. It is possible that the frequency parallels observed in early acquisition and maintained in adult language usage might have an important role in facilitating the production of certain verb forms. In this regard, grounded in Givón's (1979) proposal on a language performance, Schnitzer (1989) advances the notion that early acquisition and frequency of use might interact. Early emerging forms prominently occurring in daily conversation might be associated with an "overlearned", "automatic", and "routinized" processing (p. 6, 136) thus being able to withstand linguistic dissolution in aphasia.

Descriptive studies looking at the sequential acquisition of grammatical morphemes in Spanish appear to be in agreement that the first tense and inflection used by Spanish-speaking children is the present tense and the third person singular as suggested by the use of forms such as "*Habla*"[he/she speaks], "*Va*"[he/she goes, and "*Tiene*"[s/he has] (Gonzalez, 1980; Kvaal, Shipstead-Cox, Nevitt, Hodson, & Launer, 1988; Maéz, 1981).

Findings on narrative production in normal Spanish-speaking children and adults are consistent with the above observations. Based on spoken narrative texts in children and adults, Sebastián and Slobin (1994) reported findings supporting Silva-Corvalán's (1983) observations on oral narratives in Spanish-speaking adults. These authors showed that, despite an oscillation between the present and the past in choice of dominant tense until age 5, the present stabilized as the most frequently used tense in the narrative of the 9-year-old children, the oldest group of children in the study, as it was in adult discourse. Similarly, Bybee's (1985) survey of Spanish adult narratives suggests that the four most frequent verb forms in Spanish correspond to singular inflections for the present and past tenses in the indicative mood (*presente* and *pretérito perfecto simple* in this study).

In sum, early acquisition patterns in Spanish verb tenses seem to be reflected in the frequency of adult spoken verb usage. Consistent with the argument suggesting a resiliency of early-acquired, frequently-used language forms to impairment (Schnitzer, 1989), studies on agrammatic verb deficits should also consider the implications that these observations might have on the facilitation of the production of certain verb inflections. In particular, for this study, we predicted that those verb tenses most frequently employed in daily discourse, namely, *presente* and *pretérito* (Silva-Corvalán,

1983), with an early acquisition history, would similarly occur in agrammatic utterances for their resilient nature to aphasic breakdown.

Investigation of Verb Errors
Method
Normal Speakers

Samples: In order to determine frequency of verb tenses in daily use, two types of samples, were employed, namely, newspaper texts and soap opera dialogues. These samples were selected for their average level of linguistic complexity. Specifically, fifty randomly-selected paragraphs from different Venezuelan newspaper articles and 45 minutes of spoken dialogue from three different popular Venezuelan soap operas were analyzed for the verb forms employed in their written and spoken discourse, respectively.

Procedures and Data Analysis: Each time a verb tense was used in each text for newspaper articles and soap operas was counted to calculate an overall total and percentage of occurrence for each verb tense (Table 1).

Agrammatic Speakers

All subjects participating in the tasks below were monolingual Spanish speakers with an average level of education. They were clinically categorized as agrammatic using the guidelines provided by the Boston Diagnostic Aphasia Examination (Goodglass & Kaplan, 1974) and the Cross-Language Agrammatism Study (Menn & Obler, 1990). Their speech was halting but intelligible. Their comprehension was adequate for conversation and the tasks presented. All subjects had a single, unilateral, left-sided, cortical lesion. They had no history of alcohol or substance abuse, psychiatric illness, or learning disabilities. In addition, their hearing was assessed to be within normal limits. Finally, subjects were alert, attentive, and cognitively intact.

(A) *Spoken Discourse Samples*

Subjects: Six subjects, three normal and three agrammatic speakers, participated in this task. All subjects were matched for age and Spanish dialect (i.e., Mexican, Puerto Rican, and Venezuelan).

Procedures: Following a format similar to the one used by the Cross-Language Agrammatism Group (Menn & Obler, 1990), subjects were asked to describe the Cookie Theft picture of the BDAE, provide a rendition of a popular folktale ("Little Red Riding Hood"), and participate in conversation regarding their routine activities before their CVA.

Data Analysis: All subjects' utterances were audiotaped and transcribed, and the verbs were transcribed by speech/language professionals, all native speakers of the subjects' Spanish dialect. All intelligible verb utterances were included in the analysis. When literal paraphasias were produced (e.g, "sememos" for "comemos"), the analysis focused on the integrity of their inflections. All verb forms were tallied for each verb tense generated by the subjects. Percentages were calculated with the numerator representing the total number of times the verb form was employed by all agrammatic speakers and the denominator representing the total number of verb forms employed in their narratives (Table 1).

(B) *Sentence Repetition Task*[7]

Subjects: Twelve Venezuelan subjects, six normal and six agrammatic speakers, participated in this task. Both subject groups were matched for age and Venezuelan Spanish dialect.

Procedures: Each subject was asked to repeat 216 audiotaped sentences divided into three 72-sentence blocks to prevent their fatigue. The sentences consisted of 36 for each of the 6 verb tenses found in daily discourse (i.e., 36 sentences x 6 verb tenses = 216 sentences). These sentences were constructed to have an equal number of verbs for each thematic vowel (see "Discourse Features of Spanish Verbs"), have a short SVO structure, and contain the verb tenses found in daily discourse: presente (P[4]), pretérito perfecto simple (PR), pretérito imperfecto (PRI), condicional (C), pretérito perfecto compuesto (PRP), and pretérito pluscuamperfecto (PRC) (Bentivoglio, 1983; Bentivoglio & Sedano, 1992; Silva-Corvalán, 1983). All verbs were high frequency (Márquez-Villegas, 1975), concrete, regular, transitive, and short in structure (i.e., 2-syllable infinitive).

Data Analysis: a format similar to the one described for spoken agrammatic samples above was employed. In this case, all verb forms were tallied for each verb tense repeated correctly by the subjects. Percentages were calculated with the numerator representing the total number of times the target verb form was repeated correctly by all agrammatic subjects and the denominator representing the total number of stimuli for each verb tense presented to the six subjects for repetitions (i.e., 36 sentences for each verb tense x 6 subjects = 216 sentences) (Table 1).

Table 1: Production of Verb Tenses by Normal and Agrammatic Spanish Speakers

	NORMAL	AGRAMMATIC	
Verb Tense	Newspapers + Soap Operas (%)	Spoken Discourse (%)	Sentence Repetition (%)
PRESENTE (P)	53.5 (265/495)	92.8 (26/28)	59.2 (128/216)
PRETÉRITO PERFECTO SIMPLE (PR)	25.4 (126/495)	0	50 (108/216)
PRETÉRITO IMPERFECTO (PRI)	4.8 (24/495)	7.1 (02/28)	20.8 (45/216)
FUTURO (F)	1.2 (06/495)	0	*
CONDICIONAL (C)	3.2 (16/495)	0	19.9 (43/216)
PRETÉRITO PERFECTO COMPUESTO (PRP)	4.4 (22/495)	0	9.7 (21/216)
PRETÉRITO PLUSCUAMPERFECTO (PRC)	1.6 (08/495)	0	2.3 (05/216)
CONDICIONAL PERFECTO (CP)	0.4 (02/495)	0	*

The percentages shown indicate the number of times that a verb form was produced by the speaker. Verb tenses that were not produced (0) or not employed in this investigation (*), since they did not occur in normal daily discourse (Bentivoglio, 1983; Bentivoglio & Sedano, 1992; Silva-Corvalán, 1983), are also shown.

Results and Discussion

Regarding normal discourse in the current study, the present tense, *presente* (e.g. yo como [I eat]), was the most frequently employed verb form followed by the preterite, *pretérito perfecto simple* (e.g. yo comí [I eat]). All other verb tenses occurred minimally in the samples (Table 1).

In terms of the agrammatic speakers, we had predicted that those verb tenses most prominently used in normal conversation in Spanish, that is, the present and the preterite (Silva-Corvalán, 1983), would be more likely to be employed by agrammatic speakers in their verb attempts. Indeed, as in normal speakers, the *presente* consistently was the most frequently used tense by the agrammatic subjects. The *pretérito perfecto simple,* the second most frequent tense in normal speakers, was similarly employed correctly by agrammatic subjects in the repetition task but was not present in their discourse despite the fact that it could have been used for the stimuli given. All other verb tenses, minimally found in normal texts, were similarly never produced in agrammatic discourse or minimally produced correctly in agrammatic sentence repetition.

These results suggest that daily verb use patterns have a facilitating effect on verb use by agrammatic speakers. They also agree with earlier arguments supporting the resistance of high-frequency words to errors in normal and aphasic speakers (Goodglass, 1976; Hall 1954; Howes, 1964; Miceli & Caramazza, 1988; Rochford & Williams, 1965; Stemberger, 1984), possibly a reflection of an automatic, routinized, and overlearned nature due to their early acquisition (Schnitzer, 1989) and a significant degree of lexical strength (Bybee, 1985; 1995; Stemberger & MacWhinney, 1986).

In sum, agrammatic verb profiles for Spanish speakers are similar to those reported for speakers of other Romance languages, such as French and Italian, with a similar degree of inflectional complexity in their verb systems (De Bleser & Luzzatti; 1994; Jarema & Kehayia, 1992; Nespoulous et al., 1989; Tissot et al., 1973). As in French and Italian agrammatism, verb use by agrammatic Spanish speakers can be characterized by a reliance on a limited repertory of simple verb forms, such as the infinitive and the imperfect, at the expense of other verb forms requiring more complex inflectional markings to encode the different morphosyntactic and semantic features of Spanish verbs (Centeno, 1996). Yet, the complex inflectional paradigm of Spanish verbs allowed us to investigate the possible correlations between pre-morbid verb use in spoken discourse and agrammatic verb production, an interaction not studied in earlier investigations on agrammatism. Our findings, supporting a possible facilitating role of frequency of verb use in daily oral discourse in verb production by agrammatic Spanish speakers, provide a plausible account that might likely hold for agrammatic verb production in other languages, and probably beyond the verb system, as well.

Footnotes

[1]A version of this paper was presented at the 5to Congreso Latinoamericano de Neuropsicología, Guadalajara, Mexico, October, 1997; and will be published in Matute, E., & Leal, F. (In preparation). *Introducción al Estudio del Español desde una Perspectiva Multidisciplinaria.* México: Fondo de Cultura Económica y Universidad de Guadalajara.

[2] In general terms, Givón (1979), looking at language from a phylogenetic and ontogenetic point of view, describes a communicative continuum consisting of three levels; a monopropositional level, restricted to time and space and associated with concrete concepts; a pragmatic level, involving conversational interpretation of sentences, and a syntactic level, responsible for morphosyntactic language descriptions.

[3]Tenses have been labeled using the terminology of the Real Academia Española (1985), RAE.

[4]Abbreviations (P, PR, PRI, etc.; see Appendix A) are only given for those verb forms that are used in the experimental stimuli of this study.

[5] The inflected form of the future (e.g., comeré [will eat]), rather than its periphrastic form (e.g., ir a comer [going to eat]), is shown on this table since the inflected form is the one receiving morphological markings.

[6]The verb conjugations provided are only for those tenses included in this investigation.

[7]The data presented here were analyzed differently in an earlier and larger investigation of verb use by Spanish-speaking agrammatic subjects (Centeno, 1996).

Address correspondence to: José G. Centeno, Ph.D., New York Speech Pathology Clinic, 145 East 15th St., New York, NY 10003, U.S.A. E-mail: frontier2@mindspring.com

References

Ardila, A. (2001). The manifestation of aphasic symptoms in Spanish. In M. Paradis (Ed.), *Manifestations of aphasic symptoms in different languages*. Oxford: Pergamon Press.

Bentivoglio, P. (1987). *Los sujetos pronominales de primera persona en el habla de Caracas.* Caracas: Universidad Central de Venezuela.

Bentivoglio, P., & Sedano, M. (1992). Morfosintaxis. In A. Alvarez, P. Bentivolgio, E. Obediente, & M. Sedano, M.J. Tejera (Eds.), *El idioma Español de la Venezuela actual.* Caracas: Lagoven.

Bybee, J. (1985). *Morphology: A study of the relation between meaning and form.* Amsterdam: John Benjamins.

Bybee, J. (1995). Regular morphology and the lexicon. *Language and Cognitive Processes, 10,* 425-455.

Centeno, J. (1996). Use of verb inflections in the oral expression of agrammatic Spanish-speaking aphasics. Unpublished doctoral dissertation, City University of New York

De Bleser, R., & Luzzatti, C. (1994). Morphological processing in Italian agrammatic speakers' syntactic implementation of inflectional morphology. *Brain and Language, 46,* 21-40.

Garrett, M.F. (1980). Levels of processing in sentence production. In B. Butterworth (Ed.), *Language Production,* vol. 1. London: Academic Press.

Garrett, M.F. (1975). The analysis of sentence production. In G. Bower (Ed.), *Psychology of Learning and Motivation,* vol. 9. New York: Academic Press.
Givón, T. (1979). *On understanding grammar*. New York: Academic Press.
Gonzalez, G. (1980). The acquisition of verb tenses and temporal expressions in Spanish children age 2.0 to 4.6. *Bilingual Education Paper Series*, *4*(2).
Goodglass, H.(1973). Studies on the grammar of aphasics. In H. Goodglass & S. Blumstein (Eds.), *Psycholinguistics and aphasia*. Baltimore: John Hopkins University Press.
Goodglass, H. (1976). Agrammatism. In H. Whitaker & H. A. Whitaker (Eds.), *Studies i n Neurolingistics*, vol. 1. New York: Academic Press.
Goodglass, H., & Kaplan, E. (1974). *Evaluación de la afasia y de trastornos similares.* (Translated by Sylvia Cuschnir de Fairman). Buenos Aires: Editorial Médica Panamericana.
Grodzinsky, Y. (1990). *Theoretical perspectives on language deficits*. Cambridge, MA: MIT Press.
Hall, J.F. (1954). Learning as a function of word frequency. *American Journal of Psychology, 67,* 138-140.
Howes, D. (1964). Application of the word frequency concept to aphasia. In A.V.S. DeReuck & M. O'Connor (Eds.), *Disorders of language*. London: Churchill
Jarema, G., & Kehayia, E. (1992). Impairment of inflectional morphology and lexical storage. *Brain and Language, 43,* 541-564.
Jarema, G., & Nespoulous, J.-L. (1984). Infinitif et flexions verbales chez l'aphasique agrammatique. *La Linguistique, 20* (Fasc. 2), 99-113.
Kvaal, J.T., Shipstead-Cox, N., Nevitt, S.G., Hodson, B.W., & Launer, P.B. (1988). The acquisition of 10 Spanish morphemes by Spanish-speaking children. *Language, Speech, and Hearing Services in Schools, 19,* 384-394.
Maéz, L.F. (1981). Spanish as a first language: The early stages. Unpublished doctoral dissertation, University of California, Santa Barbara, CA.
Marcos-Marín, F. (1975). *Aproximación a la gramática Española*. Madrid: Cincel.
Marquéz-Villegas, L. (1975). *Vocabulario del Español Hablado*. Madrid: Sociedad General Española de Librería.
Menn, L., & Obler, L.K.(1990). *Agrammatic aphasia,* vol. 1-3. Amsterdam: John Benjamins.
Miceli, G., & Caramazza, A. (1988). Dissociation of inflectional and derivational morphology. *Brain and Language, 35*, 24-65.
Miceli, G., & Mazzucchi. (1989). Agrammatism in Italian: Two case studies. In L. Menn & L.K. Obler (Eds.), *Agrammatic aphasia,* vol. 1. Amsterdam: John Benjamins.
Nespoulous, J-L., Dordain, M., Perron, C., Jarema, G., & Chazal, M. (1989). Agrammatism in French: two case studies. In L. Menn & L.K. Obler (Eds.), *Agrammatic aphasia,* vol. 1. Amsterdam: John Benjamins.
Obler, L. K., Harris, K., Meth, M., Centeno, J., & Matthews, P. (1999). The phonology-morphosyntax interface: Affixed words in agrammatism. *Brain and Language, 68*, 233-240.
Qüilis, A., & Hernández-Alonso, C. (1990). *Lingüística Española aplicada a la terapia del lenguaje*. Madrid: Gredos.
Real Academia Española. (1985). *Esbozo de una gramática de la Lengua Española*. Madrid: Espasa-Calpe.
Reznik, M., Dubrovsky, S., & Maldonado, S. (1995). Agrammatism in Spanish: A case study. *Brain and Language, 51*, 355-368.
Rochford, G., & Williams, M. (1965). Studies in the development and breakdown of the use of names. IV: The effect of word frequency. *Journal of Neurology, Neurosurgery, and Psychiatry, 28,* 407-413.
Schnitzer. M.L. (1989). *The pragmatic basis of aphasia*. Hillsdale, NJ: Lawrence Erlbaum.
Sebastián, E., & Slobin, D. (1994). Development of linguistic forms: Spanish. In R. A. Berman & D. I. Slobin (Eds.), *Relating events in narrative: A crosslinguistic developmental study.*

Hillsdale, NJ: Lawrence Erlbaum.
Sedano, M. (In press). El futuro morfológico y la expresión *ir a + infinitivo* en el Español hablado de Venezuela. *Verba.*
Silva-Corvalán, C. (1983). Tense and aspect in oral Spanish narrative. *Language*, 59, 760-780.
Stemberger, J.P. (1984). Structural errors in normal and agrammatic speech. *Brain and Language, 1,* 281-313.
Stemberger, J.P., & MacWhinney, B. (1986). Frequency and the lexical storage of regularly inflected forms. *Memory and Cognition, 14,* 17-26.
Stockwell, R.P., Bowen, J.D., & Martin, J.W. (1965). *The grammatical structures of English and Spanish.* Chicago: University of Chicago.
Tissot, R.J., Mounin, G., & Lhermitte, F. (1973). L'agrammatisme. Brussels: Dessart.

Appendix A: Examples of Verb Conjugations[6]

Indicative Mood

Simple Tenses

		-AR (Tomar/ to drink)		-ER (Comer/ to eat)		-IR (Subir/ to move up)	
PRESENTE[1] (P)	Yo/I	TOM	o	COM	o	SUB	o
	Tú/You		as		es		es
	El/He Ella/She		a		e		e
	Nosotros/We		amos		emos		imos
	Ustedes/You		an		en		en
	Ellos/They		an		en		en
Example:	Yo tomo agua todos los dias I drink water everyday						
PRETÉRITO PERFECTO SIMPLE (PR)	Yo/I	TOM	é	COM	í	SUB	í
	Tú/You		aste		iste		iste
	El/He Ella/She		ó		ió		ió
	Nos./We		amos		imos		imos
	Ustedes/You		aron		ieron		ieron
	Ellos/They		aron		ieron		ieron
Example:	Yo tomé mucha agua ayer I drank a lot of water yesterday						

Appendix A: Examples of Verb Conjugations (Continuation)

PRETÉRITO IMPERFECTO (PRI)	Yo/I	TOM	aba	COM	ía	SUB	ía
	Tú/You		abas		ías		ías
	El/He Ella/She		aba		ía		ía
	Nos./We		ábamos		íamos		íamos
	Ustedes/You		aban		ían		ían
	Ellos/They		aban		ían		ían
Example:	Yo tomaba agua cuando ella llegó I was drinking water when she arrived						
CONDICIONAL (C)	Yo/I	TOM	aría	COM	ería	SUB	iría
	Tú/You		arías		erías		irías
	El/He Ella/She		aría		ería		iría
	Nos./We		aríamos		eríamos		iríamos
	Ustedes/You		arían		erían		irían
	Ellos/They		arían		erían		irían
Example:	Yo tomaría agua si estuviera fría I would drink water if it were cold						

Appendix A: Examples of Verb Conjugations (Continuation)
Compound Tenses

			-AR (Tomar/ To drink)	-ER (Comer/ To eat)	-IR (Subir/ To move up)
PRETÉRITO PERFECTO COMPUESTO (PRP)	Yo/I	he	tomado	comido	subido
	Tú/You	has	"	"	"
	El/He Ella/She	ha	"	"	"
	Nos./We	hemos	"	"	"
	Ustedes/You	han	"	"	"
	Ellos/They	han	"	"	"
Example:	Yo he tomado mucha agua hoy I have drunk a lot of water today				
PRETÉRITO PLUSCUAMPERFECTO (PRC)	Yo/I	había	tomado	comido	subido
	Tú/You	habías	"	"	"
	El/He Ella/She	había	"	"	"
	Nos./We	habíamos	"	"	"
	Ustedes/You	habían	"	"	"
	Ellos/They	habían	"	"	"
Example:	Yo había tomado agua antes que ella llegara I had drunk water before she arrived				

Grammatical features of aphasia in Swedish

Ann-Christin Månsson and Elisabeth Ahlsén

Department of Linguistics, Göteborg University

Abstract—Grammatical features in four Swedish aphasic patients with agrammatism were analyzed in conversations and elicited narratives. The most salient features of agrammatism in Swedish are problems with the V + S (i.e., reversed) word order, which is sometimes obligatory; omissions and substitutions affecting auxiliaries and "to have" and "to be", subjects, prepositions and pronouns; and substitutions affecting main verbs. These features were found in all four subjects. Non-use of the obligatory reversed word order (Adv + V + S replaced by Adv + S + V), omission of main verbs, changing inflected forms to root morphemes, omission of the object, and omission and substitution of the indefinite article were also salient features in the production of some of the agrammatic subjects.

Keywords: Aphasia, Agrammatism, Swedish, Omission, Substitution

1. Summary of Relevant Features of Swedish Grammar

Swedish is a Germanic language with a basic SVO word order for main and subordinate clauses. There is a verb-second constraint in main clauses, i.e., a clause starting with an adverbial expression requires VS order. Subjects must be expressed. Adjectives precede the noun. Prepositions are used. Negation is placed after the main verb (or first auxiliary).

Verb morphology: The verb stem + *r* makes up the present indicative active, while the verb stem + *a* (or the verb stem alone) forms the infinitive. The verb is not marked for person or number. There are two kinds of verbs: weak (regular) verbs form past tense by combining the stem with past tense suffixes (*-de*, *-te* or *-dde)*. Strong (irregular) verbs form past tense by changing the stem vowel.

The compound tenses are perfect tense, formed by *ha* (have) + participle; pure future tense, formed by *kommer att* (come to) + infinitive; future of intention or determination, formed by *skall* (shall) + infinitive; and personal passive, formed by *bli* (become) + participle. Other auxiliaries, mainly the modals *vill* (want to), *kan* (can, be able), and *måste* (must), are followed by the infinitive of the main verb.

Noun morphology: Swedish has two genders: common (utrum) and neutral (neutrum), which are marked only in the singular. They are grammatically (rather than naturally or semantically) defined, and must be learned and memorized for each noun. The plural is formed by the stem + *-r, -or, -ar, -er, -r, -n*, a stem change, or no marking. The genitive suffix is *-s*; on plurals it is added after the plural marker.

Adjective morphology: Adjectives are inflected for gender and number to agree with the noun. The suffixes are *-a* for definite and for plural, and *–t* for neuter singular.

Articles: In Swedish, a noun is usually accompanied by an article. The indefinite article *en* (a)/*ett* (an) is a free morpheme and the definite article *-en*/*-et* is a bound suffix. The articles have different forms depending on the grammatical gender of the noun. If the indefinite article is *ett*, the definite article has a form with *-et* or *-t* (utrum), instead of a form with *-en* or *-n* (neutrum). Example (1) shows the use of the indefinite article and example (2) of the definite article.

(1) Target: Jag köper ett äpple och en banan
Gloss: I (pro) buy (V pres) an apple (indef art N) and (conj) a banana (indef art N)
Target English equivalent: I buy an applc and a banana

(2) Target: Jag äter äpplet men inte bananen
Gloss: I (pro) eat (V pres) apple-the (N def art) but (conj) not (neg) banana-the (N def art)
Target English equivalent: I eat the apple but not the banana

Possessive adjectives: These forms are used for the possessive of the first and second persons and reflexive pronouns. Their endings agree with gender of the object possessed.

Pronouns: Masculine pronouns (forms of *han* (he)) and feminine pronouns (forms of *hon* (she)) are used for natural gender human nouns. *Den* is used for common-gender non-human nouns, and *det* for neuter-gender human nouns (see "Noun morphology" above). The plural pronoun is *de* (they).

2. Earlier Descriptions of Grammar in Swedish Aphasics

2.1 The Cross Language Aphasia Study

The first study of agrammatism in Swedish was provided by Ahlsén and Dravins (1990) as part of the Cross Language Aphasia Study (CLAS) (Menn & Obler, 1990). The Swedish findings were in accordance with the main general cross-linguistic findings. Agrammatic speech was found to be characterized by short phrase length and slow speech rate. Free grammatical morphemes were sometimes omitted and occasionally substituted. Bound grammatical morphemes were occasionally omitted and infinitive verb forms were used. Bound grammatical morphemes were more likely to be substituted than omitted. Certain free grammatical morphemes, e.g., conjunctions and adverbs, were used heavily. Lexical and syntactic factors interacted, e.g., main verbs differed from copulas, etc. More than 10% of main verbs were omitted. The subjects relied heavily on the simplest structures of the language (VO and SV).

Features of agrammatism in Swedish, for the subjects (MG and MB) in that study were as follows:

• Syntactic simplification, with short phrases, very simple NPs and underuse of prepositional phrases, relative phrases and subordinate clauses.
• Attempts to use adverbial clauses with word-order reversal (Adv + V + S order), but considerable problems in this context. The problems included broken-off clauses with restarts avoiding the initial adverb, a high percentage of morphological errors and, in one of the subjects (MG), word order problems, i.e., incorrect use of Adv + S + V order (cf. Ahlsén & Dravins, 1990; Comrie, 1990).
• Tense errors (incorrect mixture of tenses, i.e., sudden and unmotivated tense changes).
• Underuse of nouns, which are replaced by pronouns (compared to controls).
• Omission and substitution of pronouns.
• Omission of the preposed indefinite article *en* or *ett,* which is always a free-standing morpheme (e.g., *en bil* (a car)), more frequently than of the postposed definite article *-en* or *-et,* which is always a bound morpheme (e.g., *bilen* (the car)).
• Grammatical errors in writing and reading aloud.
• Over-employment of direct discourse (by MB only).

Example 3 below illustrates MG's word order problems in adverbial clauses.

(3) sen vakna jag → *sen jag vakna
(then woke up I) (then I woke up)

These features of agrammatism in Swedish suggested a basic difficulty in dealing with long units and complex constructions, which could most likely be caused by a general impairment related to cognitive and/or grammatical load and affecting processing on several levels. It was also clear that the subjects employed strategies to avoid problem areas, e.g., producing an initial noun and then restarting with pronoun + verb, restarting adverbial clauses in order to avoid the VS word order, or using direct discourse.

2.2 Cognitive Morphology in Swedish

A study on cognitive morphology in Swedish (Ahlsén, 1994) included an analysis of the agrammatic speech production data from the Cross Language Aphasia Study and agrammatic reading by a bilingual Swedish-Finnish subject. These findings were used in combination with two other sources of data: slips of the tongue by normal and aphasic speakers and results on three lexical-decision experiments with normal subjects. The study addressed the question of whole word processing and morphological processing of words in Swedish, as part of a project comparing Finnish and Swedish.

In the agrammatic production data (1,534 words), there were omissions and substitutions of grammatical morphemes (both affixes and function words). One subject (MG) changed inflected forms to base forms (see example 4), and also produced some non-words out of real morphemes.

(4) sover → sova
sleep (PRES) sleep (INF)

These changes may point to difficulties with ongoing morphological processing, rather than whole word processing. There were also examples of inflected forms being changed to root forms, as in example 5.

(5)	svimmade	→	*svim
	fainted		faint (root, but not a word)

This might also point to problems with morphological processing (cf. Badecker & Caramazza, 1991).

Finally, real morphemes were combined into non-words, which clearly points to difficulties with morphological processing, as in example 6.

(6)	hund-en	→	*hund-er
	dog+DEF		dog+PLUR (wrong declension)

In JS's agrammatic reading (cf. also Laine et al., 1994), regular morphological operations sometimes resulted in illegal morpheme combinations.

In the agrammatic data, then, the processes of morphological decomposition and composition did seem to be used by at least some subjects, possibly in combination with whole word production. In the database of 300 slips of the tongue, 10% were morphological, and there were some non-words consisting of real morphemes. This also points to possible morphological decomposition in speech production by non-aphasic speakers. The three lexical decision experiments yielded no evidence of morphological decomposition in the recognition of relatively simple Swedish words. (Jarvella & Wennstedt (1993) did, however, find morpheme effects in non-word lexical decision-making.) Lexical decision data for Swedish, thus, supports models such as the AAM (Augmented Addressed Morphology) (Caramazza et al., 1988), where morphological processing takes place only in extreme conditions, or the MRM (Morphological Race Model) (Stemberger, 1985), where there are two competing routes to processing. Processing seems to vary along a continuum, from whole word processing, which is automatized and used in relatively simple tasks, to morpheme-based processing, which is used less often and in less automatized contexts, e.g., agrammatic speech.

2.3 On Agrammatism and Telegram Style

In a study within the European Telegram Project (e.g., Tesak & Dittman, 1991; Tesak & Ahlsén, 1994), agrammatism in Swedish was compared to a corpus of simulated telegrams (Ahlsén, 1993). The similarities between the two types of language were the short phrase length and the occurrence of noun enumeration (which was, however, not dominant).

Substantial differences were also found. The highly regular use of short grammatical structures (mainly free-standing VPs and APs) in telegrams was not found in the agrammatic speech. The substitutions and changes in word order in agrammatic speech did not occur in telegrams. Thus, the Swedish data provided no support for the strong adaptation claim put forward by Isserlin (1922). In a weaker, more metaphoric sense, adaptation theory may be applicable, since there were some similarities. The study emphasized the importance of taking activity-based differences into consideration when comparing data from agrammatic speech with simulated telegrams. The channel (speech or writing) and the purpose and other circumstances of the activity are important differences that are likely to influence the linguistic output. The simulated telegrams can clearly be described as a conventionalized register. If agrammatic speech could be described simply as the same chosen register, more similarities should be expected and there should be no substitutions in agrammatic speech. These conclusions were in accordance with those of Tissot et al. (1973). Since activity differences in types of linguistic structures were found within corpora, e.g., for different telegram scenarios, one would expect even more differences between corpora of simulated telegrams vs. agrammatic speech.

2.4 Noun Phrases in Agrammatic Subjects—Swedish in a Cross-Linguistic Study

In a cross-linguistic experimental study within the CLAS (Ahlsén et al., 1996) that compared Swedish, French, German, Polish and English data, noun phrases of increasing complexity were elicited from agrammatic subjects. Two Swedish agrammatic subjects took part in this study. The increasingly complex NPs were elicited using contrastive naming. The most complex NP structure elicited in Swedish was Article + Adj + Adj + Noun.

The Swedish agrammatics make many more errors on the second adjective than on the first. Swedish prenominal adjectives tend to attract errors, including placement errors, where they are moved to a postnominal position, which is ungrammatical in Swedish (see example 7 below). (Interestingly enough, French agrammatics make many more grammatical errors on the first (prenominal) adjective than on the second (postnominal) one. Movement of prenominal adjectives to a postnominal position also occurs. If we look at French adjectives in postnominal position, however, very few substitution and omission errors occur. The "most vulnerable" adjective position in both languages is thus prenominal.) Prenominal adjectives might be more affected because they precede the head of the noun phrase (the noun), which determines their inflectional features. The production of postnominal adjectives, however, involves a lighter processing load.

(7)	en liten svart get	→	get svart liten
	(a small black goat)		(goat black small)

The Swedish agrammatic subjects produced a number of noun phrases with the noun in the initial position, not only omitting articles, but also placing the noun in front of the adjective(s), as in example 7. (This finding was also true of German, French and Polish.) In NP types where a plural noun was the target, surprisingly many singular nouns were produced, either as the first response, followed by a self-correction to plural, or as the only response.

A noteworthy finding was that the subjects did produce complex NP structures, sometimes completely correct, although at other times deviant. This signifies that not only syntactic categories but also more complex structures can be accessed, at least in this type of task, i.e., there is access to a certain hierarchical structure (cf. Caplan, 1983). A number of noun phrases containing two adjectives were correctly produced, i.e., all words were included and correctly inflected and word order was preserved. This shows that we are not just dealing with production of the citation form of the most salient item, followed by more or less random attribution of descriptive terms, but that more complex computation is also going on.

Substitutions of grammatical markers were numerous and, in combination with complex NP structures, they gave rise to partially correct noun phrases where grammatical forms and markers did not agree.

One of our hypotheses was that agrammatic patients would have problems even in producing isolated noun phrases accurately and this was true for the Swedish subjects (and for all the others).

Another hypothesis was that the number of errors produced by agrammatic patients would increase with increasing structural (syntagmatic and paradigmatic) complexity (here interpreted as increased processing load). The problems that our agrammatic aphasics had did increase with increasing complexity and length of the NPs. Since complexity and length are interdependent in this material, the possible role of memory problems should be further investigated (cf., however, Nespoulous & Dordain, 1992). There were quite stable cross-linguistic patterns in the production of noun phrases. Such patterns include word order and number deviations, i.e., preference for "noun first", "adjectives in postnominal position" and "singular first", the problems with the production of complex noun phrases, and the substitution of grammatical markers resulting in agreement errors.

Agrammatic subjects showed a tendency to start their speech production with something simple and salient (cf. Goodglass, 1968). This tendency seemed so strong that it overrode other input including features of the picture stimuli, e.g., a singular noun was first produced instead of a plural. The noun is most salient and tends to be produced first, while the adjectives are "pasted on" after the noun has been produced. Is this topic-comment-like structure simpler and more easily accessible than the ordinary language-specific NP structure? And is it the result of a structural change strategy affecting the NP as a whole; a fragmentation strategy dividing the production task into smaller pieces which are easier to handle sequentially, i.e., "procedural fragmentation" (cf. Nespoulous, 1994); or a combination of the two strategies? In many cases, agrammatic subjects pause between, for example, an initial noun and a following adjective. This could very well be the result of a fragmenting of the task into separate subtasks, e.g.: (1) produce the noun in singular form; (2) change the noun to plural form if necessary; (3) add adjectives if necessary. There were, however, also attempts at more advanced phrase construction, which were sometimes successful, but which more often caused a range of grammatical deviations, especially in moderate to mild agrammatic subjects, such as the Swedish sample. This could imply that "fragmentation" and more advanced phrase construction involving morphological and syntactic errors are strategies representing different degrees of severity of agrammatism.

3. Agrammatic Features in Swedish—Four Cases

3.1 Method

3.1.1 Subjects

The subjects in this study are two male and two female patients with aphasia, who were clinically classified as Broca's aphasics (in one case, mixed nonfluent) with agrammatism. Subjects 1 and 2 were also part of the CLAS Study (Ahlsén & Dravins, 1990), while subjects 3 and 4 were agrammatic subjects added for this study. All subjects were right-handed and monolingual. Two of the subjects were young (subjects 1 and 3) and two middle-aged (subjects 2 and 4). Two Swedish-speaking adults without any history of CVA were chosen as controls, one female, age 18, and one male, age 58.

Subject 1
Age: 21
Sex: Female
Time post onset: 18 months
Etiology: Vascular spasm after removal of aneurysm just under the carotid siphon
Aphasia type: Mild Broca with oral apraxia
Neurological data:
Pareses: Right hemiparesis
No sensory deficit
No visual deficit

Subject 2
Age: 45
Sex: Male
Time post onset: 1.5 months
Etiology: Occlusion of the left middle cerebral artery 1 cm from its departure from the carotid artery
Aphasia type: Mild Broca with anomic component
Neurological data:
Pareses: Right hemiparesis
No sensory deficit
No visual deficit

Subject 3
Age: 28
Sex: Male
Time post onset: 9 years and 9 months
Etiology: Skull fracture, subdural haematoma, fracture of frontal and parietal lobe and subcortical areas
Aphasia type: Mixed nonfluent, poor auditory comprehension, agrammatic
Neurological data:
Pareses: Severe right hemiparesis
Sensitivity: Mild right hemihypaesthesia
Vision: No visual field disturbance
Spatial problems
Mild dysarthria

Subject 4
Age: 58
Sex: Female
Time post onset: 4 months
Etiology: Large left hemisphere cerebral infarction
Localization of brain damage: Frontal arcuate fasciculus, frontal insula, anterior corona radiata
Aphasia type: Efferent motor aphasia (Broca's aphasia) with articulatory disorder, anomia
Neurological data:
Pareses: Moderate right hemiparesis of leg and foot, paralysis of right arm and hand
Sensitivity: Tactile gnosis missing in right hand

3.1.2 Data collection and transcription

The subjects with aphasia were video-recorded in a ten-minute conversation with their therapists, with separate sound recordings. The topics of the conversations were the history of the illness, a typical day, and the subject's occupation and hobbies. The narrative eliciting tasks were to tell the story of a picture sequence ("Man and leaves"), to describe what happens in a thematic picture ("Thieves"), and to tell "Little Red Riding Hood" by heart (if this was not possible, picture stimuli were used (Ahlsén, 1985)). The tapes were transcribed and the transcriptions were grammatically tagged by hand.

3.2 Result

3.2.1 Word order problems

Subjects 1 and 2 showed syntactic simplification, with short phrases, very simple noun phrases, and an underuse of prepositional phrases, relative clauses and subordinate clauses. In this study, subject 4 also showed the same pattern. All three subjects tried to use adverbial clauses, which are complex in Swedish since a word order reversal is required, but still a commonly used narrative strategy in normal-speaking subjects. An example from one of the controls in the CLAS study is example 8:

(8) Target: så bytte han
Gloss: then (adv) changed (V) he (pro)
Target English equivalent: then he changed

Agrammatic production is exemplified below (examples 9 and 10):

(9) Target: sen pratade jag
Gloss: then (adv) talked (V past) I (pro)
Target English equivalent: Then I talked

Subject 1: sen jag prata
Gloss: then (adv) I (pro) talk/talked (V inf/part)
* Word order reversed from aux pro Adv + N + V

10) Target: men nu ska jag ha
Gloss: but (conj) now (adv) shall (aux) I (pro) have (V inf)
Target English equivalent: but now I shall have

Subject 4: men nu jag ska ha
Gloss: but (conj) now (adv) I (pro) shall (aux) have (V)
* Word order reversed

Subjects 1 and 4 had word order problems in adverbial clauses. Subject 2 had preserved word order in adverbial clauses, but often interrupted himself and made new starts without adverbs, trying to avoid the problem in this manner. Subject 3 did not avoid adverbial clauses but omitted the verb in such structures. Thus, adverbial clauses, which require a word order reversal, caused problems for all the agrammatic subjects. Coordinate clauses starting with an adverb or conjunction were often followed by an omitted verb, an uninflected verb, or present instead of past tense in auxiliary and main verbs; sometimes the subject was omitted (see examples 11 to 13).

(11) Target: men jag kunde inte prata
Gloss: but (conj) I (pro) could (aux past) not (neg) talk (V inf)
Target English equivalent: but I could not talk

Subject 1: men kan inte prata
Gloss: but (conj) can (aux pres) not (neg) talk (V inf)
* Subject omitted
* Auxiliary verb in present instead of past tense

(12) Target: sen så gick jag under den här
Gloss: then (adv) so (filler) went (V past) I (pro) under (prep) this (pro)
Target English equivalent: then, so I went under this

Subject 2: sen så gå under den här
Gloss: then (adv) so (filler) go (V inf) under (prep) this
* Subject omitted
* Verb uninflected

(13) Target: å sen pratar jag å lägger bokstäver
Gloss: and (conj) then (adv) talk (V pres) I (pro) and (conj) lay down (V pres) letters (Noun)
Target English equivalent: and then I talk and lay down letters

Subject 3: å sen pratar jag å bokstäver
Gloss: and then talk I and [V missing] letters

Subject 2 also reversed word order in clauses beginning with a question word (example 14).

(14) Target: o vad är det fatt
Gloss: oh what (Q) is (to-be-verb) it (pro) matter (adj)
Target English equivalent: oh, what is the matter?

Subject 2: o vad det är fatt
Gloss: oh what it is matter

If we look at the argument structures used in clauses, all four participants in this study omitted the subject and subjects 1 and 3 also omitted the verb. Omissions will be covered in more detail below.

3.2.2 Substitution of "to have"/"to be"

"To be" was omitted in the present tense (example 15) as well as the past tense (example 16).

(15) Target: ja hon sa fan hon är knäpp
Gloss: yes she (pro) said (V past) devil (filler) she (pro) is (to-be verb) nuts (adj)
Target English equivalent: yes, she said, devil, she is nuts

Subject 1: ja hon sa fan hon knäpp
Gloss: yes she said devil she nuts
* *Är* ("to be" in the present tense) omitted

(16) Target: å sen var de en
Gloss: and (conj) then (adv) was (to-be verb past) it (pro) one (num)
Target English equivalent: and then there was one

Subject 3: å sen de en
Gloss: and then there one
* *Var* (to be in the past tense) omitted

"To have" and "to be" were omitted by all four subjects after the subject in the clause, but there were no examples of substitutions.

3.2.3 Omission and substitution of main verbs
All subjects substituted main verb forms: either the verb was changed to an infinitive instead of the present or past tense (see example 12 above), or to the present instead of the past. Main verbs were also omitted by subjects 1 and 3 (example 17).

(17) Target: va fan jag ska hem
Gloss: what (Q) devil (filler) I (pro) shall (V) home (adv)
Target English equivalent: what the devil, I shall go home

Subject 1: va fan jag hem
Gloss: what devil I [V omitted] home

All subjects, thus, had problems affecting main verbs.

3.2.4 Substitution of auxiliary verbs
There are a number of auxiliary verbs in Swedish. An auxiliary verb always precedes a main verb . Some of the most important Swedish auxiliary verbs are the following (where the infinitive form is followed by the present and past tenses in brackets): *kunna (kan, kunde)* "be able (can, could)", *vilja (vill, ville)* "want to (want to, wanted to)", *skola (ska, skulle)* "have to (shall, should)". All subjects omitted or substituted auxiliary verbs (examples are given in 18 and 19).

(18) Target: jag kunde inte gå
Gloss: I (pro) could (aux past) not (neg) walk (V inf)
Target English equivalent: I could not walk

Subject 1: jag kan inte gå
Gloss: I can (aux present) not walk
* Wrong tense, should be past tense; the sentence would be correct if she was speaking in the present

(19) Target: ja men jag kunde förstå nåt
Gloss: yes (filler) but (conj) I (pro) could (aux V past) understand (V inf) something (pro)
Target English equivalent: yes, but I could understand something

Subject 2: ja men jag kan förstå nåt
Gloss: yes but I can (aux V pres) understand something

3.2.5 Changes from inflected form to base form

All subjects changed inflected forms into the base form, i.e., the infinitive of the verb. See example 12 above and examples 20 to 22 below.

(20) Target: jag gick ut till
Gloss: I (pro) went (V past) out (adv) to (prep)
Target English equivalent: I went out to

Subject 2: Jag gå ut till
Gloss: I go (V inf) out to

(21) Target: hon gav blommor
Gloss: she (pro) gave (V past) flowers (N)
Target English equivalent: she gave flowers

Subject 3: hon ge blommor
Gloss: she give (V inf) flowers
* Infinitive instead of past tense

(22) Target: ja det går jättefint
Gloss: yes (filler) it (pro) goes (V pres) super fine (adj)
Target English equivalent: yes, it goes super well

Subject 4: ja gå jättefint går det
Gloss: yes go (V inf) super fine goes (V pres) it
* Infinitive instead of present tense
* It (formal subject) missing in the beginning

3.2.6 Change of inflected form to root morpheme

Only subject 2 produces a root morpheme instead of an inflected verb form (example 23).

(23) Target: Jag svimmade
Gloss: I (pro) fainted (V past)
Target English equivalent: I fainted

Subject 2: Jag svim
Gloss: I faint (V root form)
* Root but not a word, in fact a non-word

3.2.7 Omission and substitution of prepositions
All four subjects omitted (example 24) or substituted (example 25) prepositions.

(24) Target: jag bor på Källbergsgatan
Gloss: I (pro) live (V) on (prep) Källbergsgatan (N)
Target English equivalent: I live on Källbergs Road

Subject 3: jag bor Källbergsgatan
Gloss: I live [omitted prep] Källbergsgatan

(25) Target: sen ramla han av stolen
Gloss: then (adv) fell (V past) he (pro) off (prep) the chair (N)
Target English equivalent: then he fell off the chair

Subject 1: sen han ramla på stolen
Gloss: then he fell on [substituted prep] the chair

3.2.8 Omission and substitution of pronouns
Pronouns were omitted by all four subjects (see examples 11 and 12).

Pronouns were also substituted by all four subjects (see example 26, where subject 2 is telling the story of Little Red Riding Hood).

(26) Target: ja så går hon iväg
Gloss: yes (interj) so (adv) walks (V pres) she (pro) away (adv)
Target English equivalent: yes, so she walks away

Subject 2: ja så går han iväg
Gloss: yes so walks he [substituted pro] away

3.2.9 Indefinite and definite articles
The subjects in this study omitted only the indefinite articles, i.e., the preposed free-standing articles (see example 27). The definite article is better preserved for all four subjects. Subjects 1, 2 and 4 omitted, and subject 3 substituted, the indefinite article. Only subject 3 once substituted an indefinite article for a definite article (see example 28).

(27) Target: det är en sån blomma
Gloss: it (pro) is (to-be verb) a (art) such (pro) flower (N)
Target English equivalent: it is such a flower

Subject 2: det sån blomma
Gloss: it such flower

(28) Target: löven
Gloss: leaves-the (N plur def art)
Target English equivalent: the leaves

Subject 3: ett löv
Gloss: a leaf (indef art N)
* Singular noun instead of plural

The definite article, which is a bound morpheme (a suffix), was never omitted.

3.3 Summary

All four subjects had problems with clauses requiring reversed word order. All four also substituted main verbs and changed inflected forms into base forms. They omitted and substituted auxiliaries, mainly modals, and they also omitted "to have"/"to be" verbs. They all omitted subjects and omitted and substituted pronouns. All four had problems (substitutions and/or omissions) affecting the indefinite, free-standing article, but no problems with the definite, bound article.

Features that were found in some, but not all, of our four agrammatic subjects were: change of inflected form to root morpheme (subject 2), omission of main verbs (subjects 1 and 3), omission of the object (subject 4), omission of the indefinite article (subjects 1, 2 and 4), and substitution of the indefinite article (subject 3).

4. Conclusions

All four subjects produced pauses longer than three seconds or self-interruptions when there was something problematic in the clause they were attempting to produce. Verbs in the same clause were either omitted or substituted. Uninflected infinitives replaced the present or past tense and present tense forms replaced the past. Auxiliary verbs, mainly modals in the past tense, were omitted or substituted by all subjects. "To have" and "to be" after the subject were omitted by all four. The verbs that our subjects used were very frequent and simple; in fact, they were the same verbs that are used by children acquiring Swedish as their first language. Changes from inflected forms to the base form were made by all subjects. The argument structure of the clause was affected by the omission of the subject. The verb seems to be the most powerful element in the argument structure; the subject was omitted more often than the verb. This may be an attempt at economy of effort, because sometimes only the verb was used in a clause. Argument structure may be the principle by which the lexicon is organized. All four aphasic subjects omitted or substituted prepositions and pronouns. One subject changed an inflected form into a root morpheme, which was a non-word in Swedish. Subjects 1 and 3 omitted main verbs. The indefinite article was omitted by subjects 1, 2 and 4 and substituted by subject 3. The definite article was well preserved for all subjects. This is in accordance with Ahlsén and Dravins's (1990) finding that omission of the preposed, free-standing indefinite article is more frequent than omission of the postposed, bound definite article. Nouns were replaced by pronouns. Noun morphology was well preserved, but again, very simple and frequent words were used.

Subject 3, for whom the longest time had elapsed post onset, made fewer grammatical errors than the other subjects in his spontaneous speech sample, but more grammatical errors when doing the picture description task. He had somehow developed a strategy to avoid grammar that he knew he would not be able to cope with in spontaneous speech. Irregular verbs were more difficult for him than regular verbs. Some grammatical forms that could be memorized were used correctly, but this was not a pattern or strategy that the other subjects used.

Bound grammatical morphemes were more often substituted than omitted, but omissions did occur.

All subjects used short phrases, with very simple NPs, and all underused prepositional phrases, relative clauses and subordinate clauses. All subjects tried to use adverbial clauses, which are complex in Swedish, since a word order reversal is required, and all encountered problems with these clauses. The word order Adverb + Subject + Verb is, according to several researchers, used by second language learners of Swedish (Hyltenstam, 1977; Bolander, 1988; Håkansson, 1997), including children learning Swedish as their second language (Håkansson, 1997). It is also used by children with SLI (Hansson & Nettelbladt, 1995; Håkansson, Nettelbladt & Hansson, 1991). In Swedish, SVO word order is rarely used (Håkansson, 1997), except in sentences out of context. In communicative situations, sentences are often linked by means of adverbs, which reverses the word order. Håkansson also mentions that children learning Swedish as their first language used 64% SVO and 36% reversed word order, which was similar to adults with Swedish as their native language. Second language users produced SVO order in 95% of all sentences.

5. Summary of Findings for Agrammatism in Swedish

In Swedish agrammatic speech, we find short and simple phrase structures; however, there is no highly regular use of only VPs and APs (as in telegrams). The SV structure is important.

The most salient features in the speech of agrammatic Swedish speakers are problems with the V + S (i.e., reversed) word order, which is sometimes obligatory; omissions and substitutions affecting auxiliaries and "to have" and "to be", subjects, prepositions and pronouns; and substitutions affecting main verbs. These features were found in all four subjects.

Non-use of the obligatory reverse word order (Adv + V + S replaced by Adv + S + V), omission of main verbs, changing inflected forms to root morphemes, omission of the object, and omission and substitution of the indefinite article were also salient features in the production of some of the agrammatic subjects. Swedish agrammatic subjects do omit some main verbs. There is some evidence in agrammatic speech of morphological decomposition and difficulties in morphological processing, e.g., the production of non-words consisting of real morphemes.

In complex phrases, there are substantial problems. Examples of this are as follows:

- The verbs used are mostly uninflected infinitive forms replacing present or past tense forms, or present tense replacing past tense forms.
- There is considerable difficulty with the V2 constraint, i.e., the Adv + V + S structure is problematic and leads to restarts without the adverb and/or changes to S + V word order, as well as to more morphological errors.
- In complex NPs (which generally occur only when they are elicited in experimental studies), preposed adjectives are vulnerable, especially the second adjective, which directly precedes the noun.
- NPs tend to be simplified by starting with something salient first, e.g., the noun or the singular form. This leads to word order problems.
- In free narration, we find overuse of direct discourse, which also leads to less complex syntax.

As we have seen, difficulty with an increasing cognitive and/or syntactic load, associated especially with complex structures, can lead to the simplification of several features. Many of these features, e.g., the simplification of noun phrases, can be interpreted as the result of adaptation (cf. Kolk & Heeschen, 1990). When complex structures are used, a number of problems, e.g., morphological substitutions and self-interruptions, are associated with them, pointing more directly to processing difficulties.

Address correspondence to: Dr. Elisabeth Ahlsén, Department of linguistics, University of Göteborg, Box 200, SE-405 30 Göteborg, Sweden. E-mail: Eliza@ling.gu.se

References

Ahlsén, E. (1985). Discourse patterns in aphasia. *Gothenburg Monographs in Linguistics 5*. Department of Linguistics, University of Göteborg, Sweden.

Ahlsén, E. (1993). On agrammatism and telegram style—An exemplifying discussion of Swedish data. *Nordic Journal of Linguistics*, *16*, pp. 137-152.

Ahlsén, E. 1994. Cognitive morphology in Swedish. *Nordic Journal of Linguistics*, *17*, 61-73.

Ahlsén, E., Nespoulous, J-L., Dordain, M., Stark, J., Jaréma, G., Kadzielawa, D., Obler, L., & Fitzpatrick, P. (1996). Noun phrase production by agrammatic patients: A cross linguistic approach. *Aphasiology, 10*, 543-559.

Ahlsén, E., & Dravins, C. (1990). Agrammatism in Swedish speaking aphasics. In L. Menn and L. Obler (Eds.), *Agrammatic aphasia: A cross language narrative sourcebook*. Amsterdam: John Benjamins.

Badecker, W., & Caramazza, A. (1991). Morphological composition in the lexical output system. *Cognitive Neuropsychology*, *8*, 335-367.

Bolander, M. (1988). Is there any word order in Swedish learner language? *Journal of Multilingual and Multicultural Development*, *9*, 97-113.

Caplan, D. (1983). Syntactic competence in agrammatism—A lexical hypothesis. In M. Studdert-Kennedy (Ed.), *Psychobiology of language*. Cambridge, MA: MIT Press.

Caramazza, A., Laudanna, A., & Romani, C. (1988). Lexical access and inflection morphology. *Cognition*, *28*, 297-332.

Comrie, B. 1990. Word order in the Germanic languages - subject-verb or verb-second?: evidence from aphasia in Scandinavian Languages. In L. Menn and L. Obler (Eds.), *Agrammatic aphasia: A cross language narrative sourcebook* (pp. 1357-1364). Amsterdam: John Benjamins.

Goodglass, H. (1968) Studies on the grammar of aphasics. In S. Rosenberg and J.H. Koplin (Eds.), *Developments in applied psycholinguistics research*. New York: MacMillan Co.

Hansson, K., & Nettelbladt, U. 1995. Grammatical characteristics of Swedish children with SLI. *Journal of Speech & Hearing Research*, *38*, 589-598.

Håkansson, G. 1997. Barnets väg till svensk syntax. In R. Söderbergh (Ed.), *Från joller till läsning och skrivning*. Malmö: Gleerups Förlag.

Håkansson, G., Nettelbladt, U., & Hansson, K. 1991. Variation and deviation in language acquisition. Some hypotheses and preliminary observations. *Working Papers*, *38*, 83-95. Department of Linguistics. Lund University.

Hyltenstam, K. 1977. Implicational patterns in interlanguage syntax variation. *Language Learning*, *27*, 383-411.

Isserlin, M. 1922. Über Agrammatismus. *Zeitschrift für die gesamte Neurologie und Psychiatrie*, *75*, 332-410.

Jarvella, R., & Wennstedt, O. 1993. Recognition of partial regularity in words and sentences. *Scandinavian Journal of Psychology*, *34*, 76-85.

Kolk, H.H.J. & Heeschen, C. 1990. Adaptation symptoms and impairment symptoms in Broca's aphasia. *Aphasiology*, *4*, 221-231.

Laine, M., Niemi, J., Koivuselkä-Sallinen, P., Ahlsén, E., & Hyönä, J. 1994. A neurolinguistic analysis of morphological deficits in a Finnish-Swedish bilingual aphasic. *Clinical Linguistics and Phonetics*, *8*, 177-200.

Menn, L. & Obler, L. 1990. Cross-language data and theories of agrammatism. In L. Menn and L. Obler (Eds.), *Agrammatic aphasia: A cross language narrative sourcebook* (pp. 1369-1380). Amsterdam: John Benjamins.

Nespoulous, J.-L. 1994. Procedural fragmentation and the production of complex NPs. Paper presented at the International Summer Session of Université de Montréal, Jouvence.

Nespoulous, J.-L., & Dordain, M. 1992. Le traitement de syntagmes nominaux par l'aphasique agrammatique: Une illustration des corrélations (directes?) existant entre "complexité structurale" et "complexité procédurale". *Revue de Neuropsychologie*, *2*, 395-417.

Stemberger, J. 1985. An interactive-activation model of language production. In A. Ellis (Ed.), *Progress in the psychology of language,* vol. 1. London: Erlbaum.

Tesak, J., & Ahlsén, E. 1994. Telegram style in telegrams, agrammatism and child speech. Evidence from Swedish, German and Dutch. In J. Allwood (Ed.), *Papers from the Fourteenth Scandinavian Conference of Linguistics*. Göteborg University, Department of Linguistics.

Tesak, J, & Dittman, J. 1991. Telegraphic style in normals and aphasics. *Linguistics*, *29*, 1111-1137.

Tissot, R., Mounin, G., & Lhermitte, F. 1973. *L'agrammatisme*. Brussels: Dessart.